TREATING THE HEADACHE PATIENT

TREATING THE HEADACHE PATIENT

EDITED BY

ROGER K. CADY
Shealy Institute for Comprehensive Health Care
Springfield, Missouri

ANTHONY W. FOX
Cypros Pharmaceutical Corporation
Carlsbad, California

Marcel Dekker, Inc.   New York • Basel • Hong Kong

Library of Congress Cataloging-in-Publication Data

Treating the headache patient / edited by Roger K. Cady, Anthony W. Fox.
    p.   cm.
    Includes bibliographical references and index.
    ISBN 0-8247-9109-6 (alk. paper)
    1. Headache.   I. Cady, Roger.   II. Fox, Anthony W.
    [DNLM: 1. Headache—therapy.   WL 342 T784 1994]
RC392.T72 1994
616.8'491—dc20
DNLM/DLC   94-25658
for Library of Congress   CIP

The publisher offers discounts on this book when ordered in bulk quantities. For more information, write to Special Sales/Professional Marketing at the address below.

This book is printed on acid-free paper.

Marcel Dekker, Inc.
270 Madison Avenue, New York, New York 10016

Current printing (last digit):
10 9 8 7 6 5 4 3 2 1

PRINTED IN THE UNITED STATES OF AMERICA

Preface

Headache is an ancient, universal human experience. Paradoxically, the validity of headache as a medical disease has been questioned until recent neuroscientific findings captured the medical community's attention. Patients, too, are learning more about the disease, placing new expectations for intervention upon the primary-care physician. In addition, patients are seeking recognized experts in headache. *Treating the Headache Patient* is a practical guide to headache management.

This book is a comprehensive guide for physicians managing headache patients in the context of a more general practice. We have tried to integrate the scientific and therapeutic advances in headache management with the practicalities of daily practice.

Headache is a valid neurobiological disorder. Advances in neurobiology and receptor chemistry have expanded the pathophysiological understanding of this disease and created rational treatment approaches for primary care. However, many biases and misconceptions remain among headache sufferers and physicians. *Treating the Headache Patient* dispels these, challenging physicians to take an active role in improving the lives of those with headache.

The chapters are arranged systematically to present the knowledge, experience, and choices available for effective treatment and problem-solving. The first of the book's four sections is directed to the question "What is migraine?" It begins with an in-depth review of clinical manifestations of the migraine syndrome and correlates these with available pathophysiological models. From this review of the acute migraine attack, the scope of migraine broadens. Studies of epidemiology, migraine comorbidity, and quality of life are used to create a graphic description of migraine's impact. This expanded view is described as the "migraine spectrum." Indeed, several chapters address how to distinguish migraine from kindred disorders. Factors involved in transforming migraine from an episodic to chronic disorder are reviewed, and special attention is directed to the role of medication in migraine transformation. This section concludes with a proposed classification system for chronic headache disorders. (Portions of the International Headache Society (IHS) definitive classification criteria for many head and facial pain disorders are included as an appendix at the end of the book.)

The second section of the book is devoted to clinical diagnosis and available treatment of migraine and cluster headache. A comprehensive management model for headache care is proposed. Acute and prophylactic pharmacological treatment of headache is discussed in detail in a presentation designed for easy use. Special attention is directed to serotonin and the role of serotonin agonists in migraine therapy.

The third section is devoted to chronic headache disorders, myofascial headache, and temporomandibular dysfunction. These syndromes, often considered in the domain of chronic pain, frequently present as diagnostic and therapeutic dilemmas to clinicians. By reviewing the role of peripheral and central factors, physicians gain practical advice for identification, management, and prevention of these conditions.

The fourth section develops the role of behavioral factors in the management of headache patients. These frequently add significant morbidity to the disease of headache. Early identification of psychological and lifestyle interventions are important issues in headache management. Biofeedback is reviewed in detail and realistic guidelines for its use are provided. Finally, the roles of consultation, referral, headache specialists, and integrated-care models are reviewed.

Clearly, the field of headache is only beginning to unfold. As an introduction to headache, this book leaves many unresolved questions and dilemmas to be addressed by future medical scientists. If *Treating the Headache Patient* generates interest and encourages optimal headache care, then all who have contributed to this endeavor have been successful.

Roger K. Cady
Anthony W. Fox

Contents

OTHER HEADACHE DISORDERS

BEHAVIORAL ASPECTS

CONSULTATION AND FUTURE DIRECTIONS

Contributors

Steven Baskin, Ph.D.   Co-Director, New England Institute for Behavioral Medicine, Stamford, Connecticut

Roger K. Cady, M.D.   Medical Director, Shealy Institute for Comprehensive Health Care, Springfield, Missouri

James R. Couch, Jr., M.D., Ph.D.   Professor and Chairman, Department of Neurology, University of Oklahoma Health Sciences Center, Oklahoma City, Oklahoma

Kenneth L. Everett, R.N., B.S.N.   Clinical Research Administrator, Shealy Institute for Comprehensive Health Care, Springfield, Missouri

Kathleen Farmer, Psy.D.   Head, Psychology Department, Shealy Institute for Comprehensive Health Care, Springfield, Missouri

Anthony W. Fox, M.D., Ph.D., M.F.P.M.   Vice-President, Drug Development, Cypros Pharmaceutical Corporation, Carlsbad, California

Michael L. Gelb, D.D.S., M.S.   Clinical Associate Professor, Department of Oral Medicine and Pathology, and Director, TMJ and Orofacial Pain Program, New York University College of Dentistry, New York, New York

Donna L. Gutterman, Pharm.D. Director, Cardiovascular and Migraine Medical Affairs Department, Glaxo Inc. Research Institute, Research Triangle Park, North Carolina

Gary W. Jay, M.D. Medical Director, Headache and Neurological Rehabilitation Institute of Colorado, Denver, Colorado

David Kudrow, M.D. Co-Director, California Medical Clinic for Headache, Encino, California

Lee Kudrow, M.D. Director, California Medical Clinic for Headache, Encino, California

Richard B. Lipton, M.D. Associate Professor of Neurology, Epidemiology, and Social Medicine, Albert Einstein College of Medicine, and Co-Director, Headache Unit, Montefiore Medical Center, Bronx, New York

Ninan T. Mathew, M.D., F.R.C.P.(C) Clinical Professor, Restorative Neurology and Human Neurobiology, Baylor College of Medicine, and Director, Houston Headache Clinic, Houston, Texas

Jane T. Osterhaus, Ph.D. Director, Pharmacoeconomics, Glaxo Inc. Research Institute, Research Triangle Park, North Carolina

Joseph D. Sargent, M.D. Director, Department of Internal Medicine and Neurology, Menninger Clinic, Topeka, Kansas

C. Norman Shealy, M.D., Ph.D. Director, Shealy Institute for Comprehensive Health Care, Springfield, Missouri

Robert Smith, M.D. Professor and Director Emeritus, Department of Family Medicine, and Director, Headache Center, University of Cincinnati College of Medicine, Cincinnati, Ohio

Seymour Solomon, M.D. Professor of Neurology, Albert Einstein College of Medicine, and Director, Headache Unit, Montefiore Medical Center, Bronx, New York

Egilius L. H. Spierings, M.D., Ph.D. Director, Headache Section, Division of Neurology, Brigham and Women's Hospital, and Department of Neurology, Harvard Medical School, Boston, Massachusetts

Paul Stang, Ph.D., PA-C Associate Director, Applied Healthcare Research, Glaxo Inc. Research Institute, Research Triangle Park, and Adjunct Assistant Professor, Department of Epidemiology, The

University of North Carolina at Chapel Hill School of Public Health, Chapel Hill, North Carolina

Walter F. Stewart, Ph.D., M.P.H. Assistant Professor, Department of Epidemiology, Johns Hopkins University School of Medicine, Baltimore, Maryland

Randall E. Weeks, Ph.D. Co-Director, New England Institute for Behavioral Medicine, Stamford, Connecticut

1

Introduction

Roger K. Cady and Kenneth L. Everett

Shealy Institute for Comprehensive Health Care
Springfield, Missouri

Headache is a universal part of the human condition. A plague as old as humankind, it is one of the most common ailments confronting the primary care physician. Headache may be insignificant or herald life-threatening illness. Its diagnosis may be straightforward or challenge the most experienced clinician.

The complexity of headache has been explored for centuries by many of the greatest minds in medicine, yet it continues to intrigue and bewilder modern science. The fact is, despite all efforts, headache remains a disabling and poorly understood medical condition afflicting the lives of millions of people.

Those with headache have often found medical therapy ineffective. Impediments to quality care deprive many of successful therapy. Biases and misconceptions about headache further confound communication between physician and patient. Despite the availability of many successful therapies, most migraineurs remain outside the medical system, suffering significant disability attributable to their disease (1).

1

The age-old mysteries of headache are beginning to unfold. Recent advances in pathophysiology and therapy are providing new insights and better treatment. Research into headache is validating the neurochemical nature of the disease process and offers understanding of many treatment mechanisms. Comprehending the global impact of headache on patients' lives supports a new medical paradigm: priority on quality of life rather than curing disease.

No disease has haunted human existence longer than headache, and no disease has remained as obscure in its etiology (Figure 1). Headache is often regarded as a fact of life—the consequences of uncontrolled headache pervade the lives of almost everyone. Work absenteeism, lost holidays, and family disruption are only part of the price. Headache has a major impact on our entire society. With understanding and proper medical care, clinicians can reduce the impact and suffering of headache. Ironically, no disease has more to teach us about caring for patients.

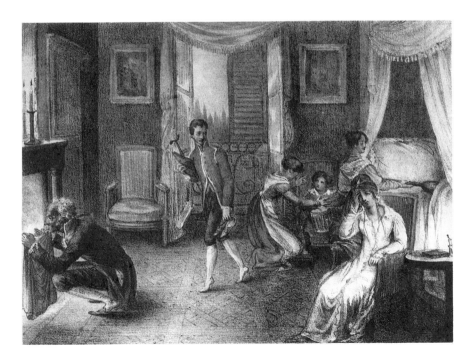

Figure 1 A 19th-century French illustration, "La Migraine," depicts a family's effort to comfort the suffering of migraine.

HISTORICAL OVERVIEW

Trepanation

In 1867, Ephraim George Squier, an American journalist and amateur archaeologist, unearthed from an ancient Peruvian graveyard a skull that had been surgically incised (2). Other archaeological expeditions have since discovered similar holes in prehistoric skulls, dating back as far as 7000 B.C., in Europe, Asia Minor, North Africa, and the Americas. Paul Broca (1824–1880), a French physician and anthropologist, demonstrated that many of these skulls showed evidence of healing, suggesting that this surgery, called trepanning, had been performed on living human beings (3). Using stone knives, he demonstrated that early surgeons could complete the trepanning procedure within 30 to 45 minutes, minimizing blood loss and helping to account for the observation that as many as 50% of trepanned subjects survived: an amazing feat, considering that the procedure was done without anesthesia or sterile surgical technique. If trepanning was the earliest treatment of headache, it was almost certainly based on the belief that headache could be cured by releasing demons trapped inside the head (2) (Figure 2).

Headache as a Curse

The belief that headache was a curse from the gods was common in many early cultures (Figure 3). A Sumerian record from about 4000 B.C. offers the following prescription (quoted in Ref. 4):

> Take the hair of a kid. Let a wise woman spin it on the right side and double it on the left, and tie it twice seven knots. Perform the incantation of Eridu. Bind therewith the head of the sick man . . . cast therewith the water of incantation over him, that the headache may ascend to heaven.

Similar therapies were prescribed by the Egyptians. Discovered in a tomb at Thebes, the Ebers Papyrus, which dates back to about 1200 B.C., describes migraine and cranial neuralgias. It advises the physician to "bind a crocodile made of clay, with an eye of faience, and straw in its mouth, to the head using a strap of fine linen upon which has been inscribed the names of the gods, and he shall pray" (5).

Offerings to the gods and magical symbols were also common in early Greek medicine. Remedies for headache offered by Pliny the Elder (70 A.D.) included wearing a hangman's noose around the head or

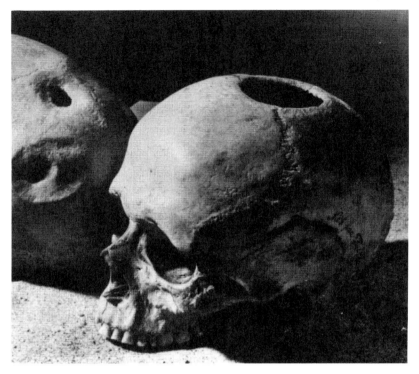

Figure 2 Neolithic skulls showing evidence of trepanation, the surgical removal of a segment of bone from the skull. Ancient man believed evil spirits caused headache and could be released by trepanation.

moss scraped off the head of a statue on a red string tied around the neck (4).

Headache as a Disorder

Many Greek physicians were more scientific about headache. Hippocrates (460–377 B.C.) first used the term *hemicrania* and recorded symptoms of aura, nausea, and vomiting (5). Hemicrania is the etymological root of migraine.

Galen (130–200 A.D.) hypothesized that migraine was related to an excess of body fluid or humor entering through the gastrointestinal system and irritating the brain. To draw off the surplus fluid, the Greeks

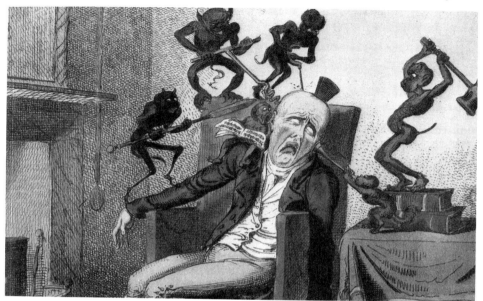

Figure 3 19-century French lithograph by George Cruikshank depicts a helpless migraineur clutching an empty pill bottle while demons inflict all manner of unspeakable pain.

advocated bloodletting and purging (2). Galen's influence dominated medical thinking for the next thousand years.

Early Headache Treatment

In *Charmides*, Plato (428–347 B.C.) describes the comprehensive treatment of headache. Socrates, playing the role of a physician, is consulted by a patient with headache. He strikes an agreement: a prescription for a pain reliever in exchange for the patient's consent to treat his soul first, "for in order to treat the eyes, you have to treat the head, and for this, you have to treat the whole body, and in order to treat the body, you have to treat the soul; neglect of this truth is the reason for the frequent failure of Greek physicians" (6, p. 661).

While most Greek physicians advocated Galen's therapies of releasing noxious substances, others experimented with early attempts at pharmacological intervention. Dioscoride found a headache cure (77 A.D.) made from the extract of a ruta plant containing a chemical (rutin) that

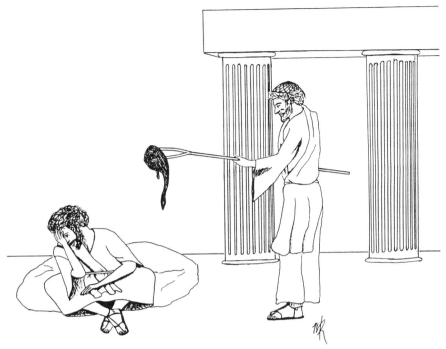

Figure 4 An early Greek physician prepares to apply an electric eel–like fish (*Torpedo ocellata*) to the head of a headache sufferer. (Courtesy of Marvin Roberts.)

lowered blood pressure. Any headache relief probably resulted from the ensuing hypotension, which collapsed painfully distended extracranial blood vessels or promoted compensatory vasoconstriction of dilated cranial vessels (7, p. 28).

A unique Greek therapy, known to the Egyptians and Hippocrates but recorded for antiquity by Scribonis Largus in 46 A.D., used a relative of the electric eel called a torpedo fish to treat headache. The fish was placed on the painful area of the head in the hope that it would "shock" away the discomfort (8).

During medieval times, illness was interpreted as divine punishment for wrong living, and suffering was considered an inevitable part of existence. Tormented individuals made pilgrimages for healing and drank concoctions brewed to cure disease. Around 800 A.D., one headache compound consisted of the pulverized head of a vulture placed in the skin of a deer and mixed with the best oil. The mixture, dabbed inside the nose, reportedly expelled "all ailments of the head" (4). An English headache tonic popular during the ninth century contained elderberry juice, cow's brain, vinegar, and goat dung. The success of these remedies may be attributed to a belief that a headache may be easier to tolerate than the body's reaction to such mixtures, or may be an example of the under-appreciated placebo response.

Novel headache remedies evolved in other parts of the world. The Incas of South America dripped coca juice, containing cocaine, into an incision in the scalp to relieve pain (4). American Indians combined extracts of willow bark and beaver testes to relieve head pain (7, p. 22); both of these substances are natural analgesics containing significant quantities of salicylatelike compounds. The gallbladder of the bear was also reported to treat headache (4).

Acupuncture for Headache

Eastern medicine devised therapies that have helped headache sufferers throughout centuries, which is why they are still widely used. The beneficial effects of acupuncture were recorded in *The Yellow Emperors Text of Internal Medicine*, dating back to between the eighth and third centuries B.C. For over 20 centuries, this text has stood as the authority on acupuncture treatment. The Chinese recognized several different types of headache, which were differentiated by energetic factors causing them (9). Treatments featured acupuncture, cupping, herbs, and attention to diet and lifestyle.

Quackery

Then, as now, headache sufferers who found no relief from reputable medical therapies fell prey to less trustworthy, pecuniary practitioners with the promise of a quick cure. Because kidney and gallbladder pain is frequently caused by "stones," these medical magicians invented the concept of "headstones" as a cause of headaches. The unscrupulous practitioner would, for a fee, pretend to remove the stones—which were surreptitiously given to him by his assistant during the operation (7, p. 30).

MODERN UNDERSTANDING OF HEADACHE

Vascular Therapy

During the 17th century, the modern understanding of headache began to take form. Thomas Willis, the father of modern neurology, wrote a treatise (1672) that described various types of headaches extending along a continuous spectrum (6, p. 665). Willis suggested that the source of pain was not the brain but rather the nerve fibers being pulled by the distended vessels (10,11). Willis' proposal became the foundation for the vascular theory of migraine. He offered many suggestions for therapy; however, few had a rational medical foundation.

In 1788, John Fothergill, a physician as well as a migraine sufferer himself, recounted the symptoms of migraine and suggested a relationship to diet: "The headache proceeds from the stomach, not the reverse." In Fothergill's account of the visual disturbances of migraine, he was the first to use the term *fortification spectra* to describe their zig-zag appearance, which to him resembled the ground plan of a typical stellate Tudor castle (5).

In 1796, Erasmus Darwin, the grandfather of Charles Darwin, suggested subjecting the headache sufferer to centrifugal force to force blood flow away from the brain. Harold Wolff, 150 years later, developed such a centrifuge. The procedure was not tolerated well by patients.

Treatment of headache through the 19th century was largely a matter of folklore and aggressive trial and error. Romberg (1853) implored physicians to take a more conservative and rational approach to headache— "We (physicians) must avoid everything that is unnecessary"—and he was critical of the practice of bloodletting (quoted in Ref. 4).

William Gowers emphasized that lifestyle modification was essential to the treatment of headache, writing in 1888, "If any error in mode of life or defect in general health can be traced, the removal of this is the first and most essential step in treatment." Gowers organized treatment into prophylactic and acute, and defined therapeutic goals for both. He proposed that bromide could be an effective prophylactic therapy at low doses, and at higher doses it could be abortive. Bromides, often in combination with Indian hemp (marijuana), became widely known as "Gowers' mixture." Interestingly, Gowers did not find early extracts of ergot useful in headache (4). The use of cannabis for acute headache therapy was also recommended by William Osler. In addition, Osler observed that forerunners of aspirin and acetaminophen, used early in headache attacks, could be effective (4).

Neurogenic Theory

Edward Liveing (1873), a London physician, challenged the vascular theory, suggesting that migraine resulted from a brain seizure or "nervous storm" (11). Liveing's belief that the origin of headache was within the central nervous system was the basis of the neurogenic theory of migraine.

Although a derivative of ergot (ergotin) was isolated in 1875, its potency for headache relief was low and the drug was poorly accepted by the medical community. But in 1925 a Swiss chemist, Rothlin, isolated ergotamine and in 1928 introduced it into clinical practice (11). Following a report by Graham and Wolff (1938), ergotamine became the preferred medical treatment for migraine.

The clinical observations and experimental approach of Harold Wolff and John Graham forged today's understanding of headache. Even though a few of their conclusions have been supplanted, their intuition and brilliance have withstood the challenge of the contemporary headache researchers.

Arnold Friedman, a major contributor to the field of headache, summarized the medical history thus: "It is astonishing how successful we have been in treating headache without really knowing what pain is or being able to define accurately how drugs can relieve it. This perhaps is our present day magic" (4).

MIGRAINE: A WINDOW TO CREATIVITY?

Even though headache is agonizing to most victims, for some the periodic disruption of the nervous system opens a window of creativity. Hildegard of Bingen, a 12th-century abbess of Rupertsberg, Germany, wrote and painted descriptions of "visions" that appeared during an aura of migraine (7, pp. 81–83) (Figures 5 and 6). In one of the accounts, Hildegard reports a display of fireworks and "a great star, most splendid and beautiful, and with its exceeding multitude of falling stars." This description parallels the phenomena now defined as scintillating scotoma. In other visions, the scene darkened, today known as negative scotoma. She also recorded images of zig-zag lines that resemble modern reports of fortification spectra.

Another migraine sufferer, Charles Lutwidge Dodgson (Lewis Carroll) relived the memories of his own auras and migraine attacks when he created the characters in his books *Through the Looking-Glass* and *Alice in Wonderland*. Carroll provides a classic account of the migraine "blind spot" when he describes Alice in a shop and wherever she looks the shelves are

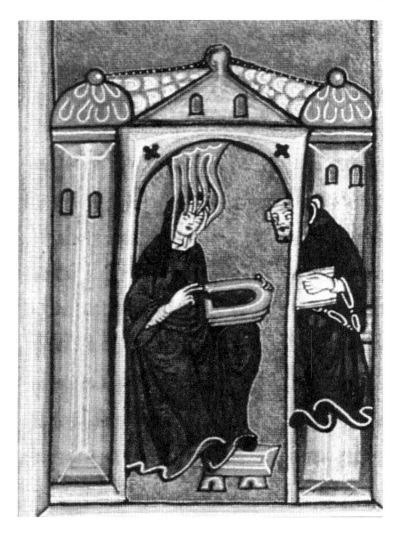

Figure 5 12th-century manuscript depicting Hildegard of Bingen recording a vision while flames from above burn at her head.

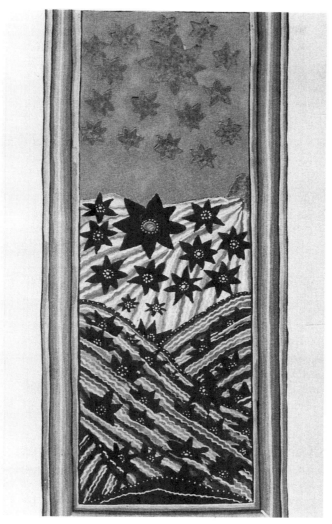

Figure 6 Flashes of radiant stars falling into an abyss are interpreted by Hildegard as being angels falling from the grace of God.

bare, although all the shelves around her were quite full. Alice grows tall or becomes short "like a telescope." Carroll's descriptions are so graphic and accurate of perceptual disturbances seen occasionally in migraine auras that these auras are now known as Alice-in-Wonderland syndrome (7, pp. 78–79).

New Mexican artist Leslie Crispan sketched a picture entitled "Death with Long Hair" that depicts a bizarre hallucination appearing to her hours before the onset of her migraine (7, p. 84). Other of her works reflect the influence of her migraine auras.

HISTORICAL VIGNETTES

Lady Anne of England was described as a gifted child, schooled in mathematics, Latin, Greek, and the philosophies. At age 12 she began having severe headaches that occurred every 3 weeks. Each bout was described as lasting 1–4 days, during which she would retire to bed in a dark quiet room, reject food and drink, and refuse visitors. Her attacks would end when she fell into a deep sleep. Over time, her headache eventually became continuous.

Anne was evaluated by many of the most prominent physicians of her time, including Sir Francis Prujean, a president of the Royal College of Physicians; William Harvey; and Thomas Willis. She was treated with all the known types of therapy and in 1660 Harvey recommended that she undergo trepanning, which she and her physician, Willis, wisely rejected. Despite all these attempts, Lady Anne did not find relief from her headache (12).

Other members of the British Royal Family also suffered headache, including Queen Mary Tudor. In one account she was described as resting "in an open litter clad in splendid blue velvet, with a jeweled diadem so heavy that its weight on the usual headache—she was having one of her bad days—was sheer agony, so that for part of the way she tried to ease the blind pain by resting her head on her hand" (13). The present Queen's sister, Princess Margaret, another migraine sufferer, is the patron of the esteemed Migraine Trust in Great Britain (14).

Charles Darwin, described as a shy, worry-ridden man, was known to suffer migraine, believed to be often precipitated by stress. In a letter to his fiancee, he complained of a "bad headache, so that I doubt whether it ever meant to allow me to be married" (quoted in Ref. 7, p. 20).

General Ulysses S Grant wrote in his diary on April 8, 1865, "I spent the night in bathing my feet in hot water and mustard, and putting mustard plasters on my wrists and the back of my neck, hoping to be cured [of headache] by morning." That day, after learning of the surrender of General Lee, he recorded in the diary, "The instant I saw the contents of the note, I was cured" (quoted in Ref. 7, p. 20).

Headaches have influenced the lives of many notable people throughout history, including Virginia Woolf, Edgar Allan Poe, Thomas Jefferson, and George Bernard Shaw. Today's list of accomplished migraine sufferers includes baseball pitcher Orel Hershiser, singer Michael Jackson, former basketball player Kareem Abdul Jabbar, and tennis champion Chris Evert.

As we close the 20th century, new medicines, advances in blood flow studies, and computer-enhanced images have boosted understanding of debilitating headaches. Physicians and patients alike are more educated about health and diseases. Neurobiology, along with discoveries in receptor biochemistry, have already provided us with medicines, that can abort a majority of migraine attacks. Perhaps in the not too distant future science will be able to answer the ancient question "What causes headache?"

REFERENCES

1. Celantano DD, Stewart WF, Lipton RB, Reed MI. Medication use and disability from severe headache: a national probability sample. Cephalalgia 1991; 11(suppl 11):105.
2. Lyons A, Petrucelli RJ II. Medicine: An Illustrated History. New York: Harry N. Abrams, 1978.
3. Thorwald J. Science and Secrets of Early Medicine. London: Thames and Hudson, 1962:300–307.
4. Edmeads J. The treatment of headache: A historical perspective. Presented at Headache: Changing Perspectives and Controversies, Scottsdale, Ariz., Feb 1–3, 1990.
5. Lance JW. Mechanism and Management of Headache, 4th ed. London: Butterworth Scientific, 1982:1–6.
6. Isler H. Retrospective: The history of thought about migraine from Aretaeus to 1920. In: Blau JN, ed. Migraine: Clinical and Research Aspects. Baltimore: Johns Hopkins University Press, 1987.
7. Murphy W. Dealing with Headache. Alexandria, Va.: Time-Life Books, 1982.
8. Tapio D, Hymes AC. New Frontiers in Transcutaneous Cutaneous Electrical Nerve Stimulation. Minnetonka, Minn.: Lec'tec, 1987:1.
9. O'Conor J, Bensky D. Acupuncture: A Comprehensive Text, 4th ed. Seattle: Eastland Press, 1985:624–626.
10. Sacks O. Migraine: Understanding a Common Disorder. Berkeley: University of California Press, 1985:1–8, 228.

11. Raskin NH. Headache, 2nd ed. New York: Churchill Livingstone, 1988:35–98.
12. Edmeads, J. The widening gap between migraine theory and therapy. Presented at John Graham Senior Clinicians Forum, June 24–27, 1993.
13. Ziegler DK. Headache public health problem. Neurol Clin 1990; 8(4):781.
14. Presented at the 9th Migraine Trust International Symposium, London, Sept 7–10, 1992.

2

Complexities of Presentation and Pathogenesis of Migraine Headache

James R. Couch, Jr.

University of Oklahoma
Health Sciences Center
Oklahoma City, Oklahoma

BACKGROUND

Migraine was first described by the ancient Greek physician Arataeus of Cappodocia, who described hemicranial headache (1). The syndrome itself became more clearly defined in the 1800s with definition of menstrual headache in women. By the late 1800s, extracts of ergot, the rye fungus, were known to be beneficial to migraineurs. Gower described migraine as one of the borderlands of epilepsy, referring to the fact that the syndrome causes periodic disability. In the 20th century, there has been a tremendous increase in the literature dealing with migraine headache. Harold Wolff started his pioneering studies of migraine in the 1930s. With very crude instrumentation, Wolff made many observations on migraine and then formulated the vascular theory of migraine, which held sway until the late 1970s (see Ref. 1 for review).

DEFINITION AND CLASSIFICATION OF MIGRAINE

Migraine has a large number of associated symptoms. There may be great diversity in expression in terms of location, type, and amount of pain, and a variable number of symptoms other than pain. For this reason, a good definition of the migraine syndrome has been long in coming. In 1988, the International Headache Society (2) developed a classification of headache as an attempt to put the whole area of headache and head pain into perspective. These were proposed as working criteria and intended to stimulate research, and this has certainly been the case. They have acquired acceptance as diagnostic criteria in lieu of a better definition and as aspects of the criteria have been confirmed with research studies. These criteria are presented below.

In the literature dealing with migraine, the terms *classic* and *common migraine* have been used to delineate migraine occurring with neurological symptoms and migraine occurring without neurological symptoms (1,3). *Common migraine* referred to migraine headache occurring without visual or other neurological symptoms. *Classic migraine* was employed to identify migraine occurring with neurological symptoms. Confusion, however, resulted from interpretation of *classic migraine*, which, in its strictest interpretation, referred to migraine headache preceded by a visual phenomenon of some type. Typically, the visual phenomena began 15 to 30 minutes prior to the headache and remitted just prior to onset of the headache. Migraine-like headaches without such phenomena were classified as common migraine, vascular headaches, or, sometimes, nonspecific headaches. With further study, it became readily apparent that neurological symptoms other than visual symptoms occurred with migraine and that these symptoms might occur at times other than immediately prior to the migraine headache. For this reason, the committee on Classification of the International Headache Society (IHS) felt that a new terminology was needed (2). The committee used *aura* to denote the group of focal symptoms associated with a migraine attack. In the new IHS criteria, then, *migraine with aura* is used to describe migraine headache occurring in association with neurological symptoms. This includes headache that was previously defined as classic migraine as well as headache with neurological symptoms occurring at times other than just before the headache or head pain. *Migraine without aura* is used for migraine without neurological or visual symptoms.

The IHS criteria subdivide migraine into two categories: 1) migraine with aura and 2) migraine without aura. Table 1 summarizes the classification of migraine and the criteria for making these diagnoses. In addition,

Table 1 Classification and Characteristics of Migraine According to the Criteria Set by the International Headache Society

---

Migraine without aura: idiopathic, chronic headache disorder occurring in attacks
1. Headache attacks lasting 4–72 hours with pain-free intervals between headaches
2. Pain characteristics (at least two necessary):
   a. Unilateral location
   b. Pulsating quality
   c. Moderate or severe intensity
   d. Aggravation by physical activity
3. Symptoms during the headache (at least one required):
   a. Nausea and/or vomiting
   b. Photophobia and/or phonophobia
4. At least one of the following:
   a. No organic neurological disorder found on history, physical, and neurological examinations
   b. History, physical, or neurological examination suggests organic disorder, but neuroimaging or laboratory procedures rule out the possibility
5. The patient must have at least 5 attacks fulfilling criteria 1 to 4 above

Migraine with aura
1. Patient must fulfill criteria 1–5 above.
2. Patient must have at least three of the following four characteristics with a headache:
   a. One or more fully reversible symptoms that are manifestations of focal hemispheric and/or brain stem dysfunction
   b. At least one aura symptom develops gradually over 4 minutes or more or symptoms may occur in succession
   c. Aura symptoms last less than 60 minutes
   d. Headache follows the aura by an interval of less than 60 minutes but may occasionally begin before the aura
3. The patient has at least two attacks fulfilling criterion 1 above

---

Source: Adapted from Ref. 2.

Table 2 Types of Migraine with Aura
Recognized by the IHS Classification

---

1. Migraine with typical aura
2. Migraine with prolonged aura
3. Familial hemiplegic migraine
4. Basilar migraine
5. Migraine aura without headache
6. Migraine with acute onset aura

Source: Adapted from Ref. 2.

the classification recognizes ophthalmoplegic and retinal migraine as potentially separate but rare subgroup of the migraine syndrome (2). Table 2 outlines the types of migraine with aura recognized by this classification.

The IHS criteria were formulated as research criteria, proposed in an effort to stimulate research to provide a better and clearer definition of the migraine syndrome, with the eventual goal of enabling more acute diagnosis and better treatment. Much of the material presented in these criteria has gained acceptance, and they have evoked a great deal of research. At present, however, there is not universal agreement on all parts of the proposed classification scheme. In addition to Tables 1 and 2, the reader is referred to the full classification as presented in *Cephalalgia* (2) for greater detail and further information.

THE MIGRAINE SYNDROME

General Description

The migraine syndrome has a number of components, which generally have been defined from various studies of large numbers of patients. In 1961, Selby and Lance (5) reported on the features of migraine in 500 patients. In a follow-up study in 1966, Lance and Anthony (67) reported on symptoms in a second cohort of 500 patients. In 1975, Couch et al. (6) reported the symptoms of a group of 235 migraineurs, and in 1991 Couch et al. (7) reported the symptoms of subjects in a group of 793 migraineurs. The results of these studies are reviewed in Table 3. The studies were based on patients seen in a headache clinic, and the criticism can be raised that they present a potentially biased outlook on the migraine syndrome. However, studies of migraine in nonclinic populations by Ziegler et al. (8),

Table 3 Breakdown (%) of Headache Symptoms in Four Major Studies

Symptoms	Selby and Lance, 1960 (5) *n* = 500	Lance and Anthony, 1966 (67) *n* = 500	Couch et al., 1975 (6) *n* = 235	Couch et al., 1991 (7) *n* = 793
Location of headache				
Unilateral only	38	68	—	48
Bilateral or mixed (unilateral/bilateral)	62	32	—	52
Non-headache symptoms				
Nausea	87	93	86	92
Vomiting	56	59	57	57
Diarrhea	—	19	—	14
Photophobia	~80	—	—	79
Phonophobia	—	—	—	62
Visual symptoms	41	—	75	57
Positive	—	—	—	37
Negative	—	—	—	20
Blurred vision	—	—	—	30
Mono- or hemiparesis	—	—	32	8
Mono- or hemisensory	33	—	36	17
Four-limb weakness	—	—	—	8
Four-limb sensory loss	—	—	—	8
Aphasia	—	—	—	18
Dizziness	72	—	35	—
True vertigo	33	—	—	11
Loss of or alteration of consciousness	19	19.4	22	17
Confusional state only	—	—	6.8	9
Difficulty thinking	—	—	—	7
Giddiness	—	—	—	13

Rasmussen and Olesen (Ref. 9, pp. 221–228), and Henry et al. (10) in adults and Mortimer et al. (11) in children have observed characteristics of migraine similar to those seen in the other studies noted above.

An additional aspect of this variability of presentation was elucidated in 1967 when Whitty and Oxon (12) described the syndrome of "migraine-sans-migraine." They described 16 patients who had transient neurological symptoms similar to those seen with migraine but did not have headache. These patients had headaches at other times, and it was postulated that these were migraine-associated neurological symptoms occurring in the absence of head pain. O'Connor and Tredici (13) expanded this concept in 1972, reporting on a group of Air Force personnel who had visual symptoms usually associated with migraine but no headache. All were young and generally under a good deal of stress. None of these cases had a prior history of headache, and none had headache in association with his episodes. The authors noted the similarity of transient visual symptoms in these patients to those associated with migraine and coined the term *acephalgic migraine.*

Fisher (4) recognized and reported a different aspect, onset of migraine with associated neurological symptoms in an older population. He studied transient neurological symptoms in older individuals and defined the syndrome of transient migrainous accompaniments. He evaluated a group of 120 patients over the age of 50 who had no prior history of migraine and were being seen for occurrence of transient neurological events. After a thorough work-up, Fisher concluded that these patients were all having transient neurological symptoms as a result of migraine syndrome and not as a result of thromboembolic transient ischemic attacks. Their work pointed out that migraine can have onset after age 50 and its symptoms can be confused with those of transient ischemic attacks.

Of note in this series, Fisher found that 50% of the patients had migraine-sans-migraine. Many of these patients were diagnosed only after an arteriogram was carried out, and the arteriogram did not allow explanation of the transient neurological symptomatology. Fisher reported that visual symptoms occurring in conjunction with other neurological symptoms were often the factor that pointed him toward a transient migrainous accompaniment.

In children, the syndrome of abdominal migraine has been described (14). In this syndrome, the child has prominent gastrointestinal symptoms of nausea and vomiting with minimal or no headache. Vertigo has also been described as a prominent component in childhood migraine by Fenichel (15) and by Watson and Steele (16).

Finally, Bruyn (17) has reviewed a number of patients who had migraine-associated fugue or dissociative states. Migraine has also been noted to be associated with changes in mood—either elation or depression.

In summary, the migraine syndrome appears to have five components:

1. Pain
2. Gastrointestinal symptoms
3. Other autonomic symptoms
4. Neurological symptoms including visual symptoms
5. Changes in mood or emotion

Extrapolating from the work of Whitty and others who have worked in the area of migraine-sans-migraine (4,12,13–16), it appears that any of the five migraine-associated components may occur with or without any of the other components.

Pain

For most people, the prominent feature of migraine is pain. The classic description of migraine headache is unilateral, usually throbbing pain (1–5). Couch et al. (6,7) reviewed reports of pain and noted that in only 48% of patients was the pain strictly unilateral or hemicranial. The remainder had bilateral pain. Over a lifetime of headache, many patients initially have unilateral headache that in later years, as headaches become more frequent, evolves to a mixture of unilateral and bilateral headache.

The pain is usually described as throbbing but may be characterized as steady aching pain, pressure pain, or even stabbing sharp pain (19). It is typically located in the frontal region and may involve the temple areas. Complaints may include retro-orbital pain, pain in the cheek or jaw, or suboccipital pain, and the pain may migrate from one area to another.

A significant number of patients complain of pain in the neck, often in the base of the neck. At times pain presents in the interscapular area and radiates upward to the suboccipital region. This type of pain may be unilateral or bilateral (1–4). A smaller number of patients will complain of pain radiating into the shoulder or arm. Pain outside of the head relates to the anatomy of the spinal trigeminal tract (see Chapters 12 and 13). Very rarely, pain is perceived along the entire side of the body, including the arm and leg. The origin of this type of pain is more difficult to explain, but a few cases have been noted by the author.

Gastrointestinal Symptoms

As noted in Table 1, gastrointestinal symptoms are very common in the migraine syndrome. Nausea, the most common, occurred in 86–93% of the patients from studies in Table 3 (4–7). Vomiting was seen in 56–59%. Patients are often unwilling to admit that they are nauseated with a headache, especially if the nausea is mild and there is no vomiting. Most patients think of nausea as occurring with vomiting and tend to ignore or forget headaches in which there was only nausea. Most patients will also have anorexia with the nausea but will seldom recognize it as such. Nausea usually begins with the headache but occasionally occurs as part of the migraine prodrome.

Diarrhea is not uncommon in migraine headache (5,7). Diarrhea occurred in 14–19% of the patients in studies reviewed in Table 3. While this symptom is often only a troublesome part of the migraine headache for many patients, occasional patients may have diarrhea as a major manifestation of migraine. This, in turn, can enhance the fluid loss and the potential for dehydration that may occur with a migraine syndrome.

Constipation may also be a symptom of migraine, but it is more difficult to document. Occasionally, patients may note severe constipation as a prodrome or as a symptom occurring with migraine.

The gastrointestinal symptoms associated with migraine may occur in the absence of head pain or in conjunction with only modest or minimal head pain. Children may display the syndrome of abdominal migraine, in which the patient has episodic vomiting but does not complain of headache (14). A pattern of migraine headache may later develop in these children. Occasional patients may also have episodic diarrhea for which no cause is found and later develop frank migraine headaches.

Other Autonomic Symptoms Associated with Migraine

Migraine has classically been associated with peripheral vasoconstriction. This was well described by Wolff in his early works (1) and later by Appenzeller et al. (20). Subsequently, the finding of diminished temperature in the hands with migraine headache has been used extensively by people interested in biofeedback as one of the parameters for developing a biofeedback therapy (21–23). In addition to coolness in the hands, patients may also complain of coolness in the feet from the peripheral vasoconstriction.

Other autonomic symptoms have included paroxysmal tachycardia, as reported by Thomas and Post (24). Migraine-associated chest pain was reported in 159 of the 684 patients studied by Briggs and Bellomo (25). In 1981, Miller et al. (26) suggested that variant angina (Prinzmetal's angina) could be seen as a feature of migraine. The nongastrointestinal autonomic features are generally thought to be related to vasospasm, although the tachycardia noted above may relate to another mechanism, possibly one of central origin.

Neurological Symptoms Associated with Migraine

The neurological symptoms are the most dramatic nonpain symptoms of the migraine syndrome. At times, these symptoms may be intense enough to suggest a stroke or transient ischemic attack (4). At other times, these symptoms are rather minor and may be elicited only by intensive questioning from the physician. Table 1, which shows the results from four different studies, presents the spectrum of migraine-associated symptoms. There is a remarkable concordance for incidence of neurological symptoms among these four studies.

The neurological symptoms can generally be divided into those that are primarily of cortical origin and those of brain stem origin. It is possible that the "brain stem symptoms" may in fact relate to areas of the cortex that represent these functions rather than to the brain stem itself. It is also possible that the brain stem and cortical symptomatology may originate from completely different but as yet undefined mechanisms.

Cortical Symptomatology

The cortical symptomatology associated with migraine includes visual symptoms, hemiparesis, hemisensory loss, and aphasic speech difficulties (4–7). The most common of these problems are the visual symptoms.

Visual Symptoms The number of patients with visual symptoms ranges from 40 to 75% (4–7). Generally, the figure in most series is approximately 50%. In the recent study reported by Couch et al. (7), visual symptoms were experienced by 57% of the 793 patients, two-thirds of whom had positive symptoms consisting of flashing lights, zigzag lines, bright lines, grids, or spots. Only one-third had negative visual symptoms consisting of black spots, grids, or heat waves.

The visual symptoms vary greatly in their manifestations. The classic visual symptomatology is the fortification spectra: a zigzag line defining a boundary (1). This boundary may enclose an area of loss of vision noted by a black spot or it may enclose an area of blurred vision. Generally, the zigzag line is in the shape of an arc or other curve. Initially, this is usually a small area, in terms of an entire visual field. Over 15–30 minutes, the arc grows larger and becomes less intense and finally moves out of the visual field entirely. The time from onset to completion of the sequence is 15 to 30 minutes in the "textbook" case of migraine with aura, i.e., "classic migraine."

Other types of visual symptomatology may include horizontal or vertical zigzag lines, straight lines, or kaleidoscopic patterns of various colors. The well-formed visual phenomena, however, are usually seen in the minority of cases. The most common visual phenomena are unformed patterns of flashing lights or twinkling stars, which may be either large circular patterns as if a flashbulb had just gone off or very tiny dots similar to stars in a night sky. They may occur over the whole visual field or only part of the visual field. They may be limited to a quadrant or a hemifield distribution, in only the central vision or in only the peripheral vision.

The negative phenomena usually consist of black spots, which may occur in the distributions noted above. Patients may note loss or blackout of peripheral vision and retention of central vision: tunnel vision. In this situation, the patient may often have positive visual phenomena in the black area constituting the walls of the tunnel.

A key feature of any migraine-associated visual phenomenon is that there is usually a sensation of movement. This may vary from feeling as if the spots are swimming or rolling around to a sensation of scintillation within the visual phenomenon itself. This is most often seen when there is a formed lined such as the fortification spectra. The patient will often describe that the fortification spectra itself has scintillation within the zigzag line. Another variation is that the patient may see scintillating geometric figures that move in a pattern or seem to change shapes with some type of periodicity. Rockets or lines moving rapidly across the visual field are not uncommon and were particularly noted by Fisher (4). Patients who have primarily negative visual phenomena may also see geometric figures composed of different shades of gray or black within the general area of loss of vision. Finally, patients occasionally report seeing circles of increased brightness or clearer vision surrounded by borders of scintillating light.

Usually the visual phenomena occur only once and will remit. In some patients, the phenomena may occur over and over again with each peak of headache intensity.

In the classic description of visual phenomena as an aura to the migraine, these symptoms occur immediately before the headache. In these patients, the visual phenomena last 15–30 minutes and usually remit just prior to the onset of the headache. With detailed questioning, however, it is very common to find patients who have brief periods of visual phenomena sometime during the headache. In an analysis of the timing of migraine-related visual phenomena, Couch (27) noted that 40% of patients had visual phenomena prior to the headache; 40% during the headache, usually occurring at the peak; and 20% both before and during the headache.

In rare cases, patients may manifest visual phenomena associated with migraine that will continue for prolonged periods of days or weeks. In these cases, the etiology of the prolonged visual phenomena is unclear. In the presence of a normal EEG, which would tend to rule out epileptiform activity or ischemia, these are postulated to be migrainous in origin.

Hemiparesis and Hemisensory Loss Hemiparesis and hemisensory loss usually but not always occur together. These symptoms are usually relatively mild, although the spectrum of symptomatology may run from minimal to quite severe.

Overall, the incidence of hemisensory loss ranges from 17 to 36% (4–7). Selby and Lance (4), in their study of 500 patients, reported that 33% of patients reported hemisensory loss, while Couch's earlier study reported this symptom in 36% (6). The later study by Couch (7), in 1991, noted hemisensory loss in only 17% of 793 patients. The hemisensory loss often involves only part of the hemibody, which is usually the arm or the arm and face. In other situations, the face alone is involved. Less commonly, the patient will note numbness over the entire side. Most patients with this symptom will note variability, with involvement of the arm or face individually at times and spread of the numbness from arm to face, or vice versa, at other times. Very seldom, patients will report numbness in only a leg. The sensory loss, like the visual aura, usually manifests a march from one area to another, often spreading from the arm to the face or from face to arm. Less commonly, spread from leg to arm will be seen.

In Fisher's report of transient migrainous accompaniments, hemiparesis and hemisensory loss were quite common (4). This series was selected because it comprised an older group of patients who had symptoms due to migraine that could be confused with symptoms of stroke or transient ischemic attack. The most common symptoms in Fisher's 120 patients were visual. However, 57 of the 120 patients reported transient paresthesias and/or paresis. Thirty-two of these 57 had associated visual symptoms; 25 did not. Of this entire series, 50% had migraine-sans-migraine (acephalgic migraine) or neurological symptoms occurring in the absence of migraine pain. Hemiparesis and hemisensory loss are frightening symptoms, and the ones most likely to be confused with those of transient ischemic attack of vascular or emboli etiology.

The sensory symptoms associated with migraine are transient and tend to involve the arm or face to a much greater extent than the leg. These symptoms are often mild, usually consisting only of paresthesia. They may occur in concurrence with other neurological symptoms such as the visual symptoms, or at times other than the visual symptoms. They may occur as an aura preceding the headache or during the headache. If they occur during the headache, it is most often either in the early part of the headache or at the peak of the headache pain. The sensory loss is most often in the arm or the face, and may spread to the leg. Seldom does a patient perceive sensory loss in the trunk.

With hemisensory loss as well as hemiparesis, which is discussed below, patients often note that it does not occur with every headache. Most patients report having these symptoms only occasionally, or perhaps with only the most severe headaches. Some patients, however, find that the sensory or motor symptoms occur with almost every headache.

The duration of the sensory loss is variable. In some patients it lasts for only a few minutes; others report that it lasts throughout the entire headache. Most patients note this and other neurological symptoms occurring either as a prodrome to the headache or at the peak of the headache. A smaller percentage of patients report that sensory loss begins before the headache and continues on into the headache. Tabulation of the timing of the occurrence has been poorly documented. In general, it would seem to follow the pattern reported by Couch (27) for occurrence of visual symptoms. Approximately 40% noted visual symptoms before the headache, 40% during the headache, and 20% symptoms before the headache but persisting on into the headache.

Hemiparesis is a symptom that usually occurs in conjunction with the hemisensory loss but may at times occur in the absence of sensory symptoms. The hemiparesis is usually mild and often a monoparesis. The patient will usually complain of minor clumsiness in an arm or leg that usually lasts for only a short period of time. Less commonly, patients will note a somewhat more prolonged hemiparesis. In rare cases, the patient will manifest hemiplegia that is transient and will clear without residua. This pattern, which may tend to recur in families, has been termed *familial hemiplegic migraine*, as reported by Rosenbaum (28) and Glista et al. (29).

Aphasia Aphasia, or dysphasia, is a relatively common syndrome in migraineurs, if the lifetime experience is taken into consideration. In the earlier study of Couch et al. (6), 35% of the patients were found to have some type of speech difficulty during the headache, but this did not distinguish between dysarthria and dysphasia. In the later study in 1991, dysphasia was noted to occur in 18.2% of 793 patients (7). In the study of transient migrainous accompaniments, Fisher (4) found speech disturbance in 17.5% of his 120 patients. O'Connor and Tredici (13), in their study of acephalgic migraine, found four patients who had prominent dysphasia and scotoma.

Aphasia or dysphasia is difficult to distinguish from other migraine-associated symptoms of confusion or disinclination to speak. Expressive aphasia, manifested by difficulty in finding words, paraphrasia, or cir-cumlocution, can be relatively easy to diagnose in the straightforward case. The dysphasia is usually mild and consists of a primarily expressive dysphasia with word-finding difficulties. Less commonly, patients will manifest more significant dysphasic problems. Many cases, however, are not straightforward, and only after taking a careful history can the examiner determine that the patient is having difficulty with finding words. This type of aphasia—expressive aphasia—was noted in 18% of 793 subjects evaluated by Couch et al. (7). As with the symptoms of hemiparesis and hemisensory loss, the aphasia is usually mild and tran-sient, and may occur before or during the headache. Aphasia may also occur as a symptom of migraine-sans-migraine. Prolonged expressive aphasia with migraine is, in my experience, a very uncommon problem.

Receptive aphasia as a symptom of migraine can be extremely dif-ficult or even impossible to differentiate from other confusional states. Confusion associated with migraine was noted by 8.7% of 793 subjects by Couch et al. (7). The patient is rarely, if ever, seen during migrainous aura of this type, and the examiner is limited to trying to make the diag-nosis from historical data. The patient with receptive aphasia usually cannot give a history that is adequate to make the diagnosis of receptive aphasia.

Posterior Vascular Distribution Symptoms

Brain Stem Symptomatology The brain stem symptoms that can be associated with migraine are vertigo, loss of consciousness, and dysarthria. Not infrequently, patients with migraine complain of numb-ness as well as weakness in both arms and both legs. This probably represents brain stem symptomatology, but the possibility of bilateral cortical involvement should be considered. Finally, tinnitus is an occa-sional complaint. It is usually difficult to determine whether tinnitus is a primary complaint or one that is secondary to medication. The symptoms of diplopia, vertigo, loss of consciousness, and dysarthria are quite easy to identify. General weakness or numbness may relate to other causes such as hyperventilation or generalized anxiety, or may be related to medica-tion. Complete loss of vision with migraine is an uncommon but well-described phenomenon. While this is usually considered an extreme example of visual symptoms associated with migraine and thought to be related to migraine-associated scotomata, the possibility exists that bilateral blindness is associated with basilar artery vasospasm in relation to a migraine headache.

Brain stem symptomatology is less common than cortical symp-tomatology. Table 1, however, shows that, in terms of lifetime occurrence, brain stem symptoms can be seen in 10–20% of patients. Fisher (4) noted that brain stem symptomatology was present in 14 (12%) of his 120 patients.

Vertigo as a concomitant of migraine headache has been reported by a number of authors. Koenigsberger et al. (30) and Fenichel (15) noted this syndrome in children. Watson and Steele (16), in a subsequent study, evaluated 43 children with migraine and reported that 15% had vertigo in association with their migraine.

In a study of adults, Kuritzky et al. (31) evaluated vertigo in three groups: nonmigraine subjects, patients with common migraine, and patients with classic migraine (migraine with aura). He noted that 10% of controls and 10% of common migraine patients had vertigo, while 42% of classic migraine patients had vertigo. In the 793 migraineurs studied by Couch et al. (7), 11% reported vertigo as an accompaniment of their migraine.

Loss of consciousness is a somewhat more difficult symptom to categorize. Its manifestations range from amnesia with personality change to syncope and falling. In 1958, Bickerstaff (32) described the syndrome of "basilar artery migraine in young women." In his series, these girls were noted to have onset of headache followed by loss of consciousness and then awakening with a more severe headache, or a pattern of loss of consciousness followed by awakening with a very severe headache. Most of the patients had a sensation of presyncope before passing out. Some passed out without warning, suggesting the possibility of an akinetic seizure. In the series of Selby and Lance (5), 18.5% of the patients had some type of loss of consciousness. Of these, approximately 25% were thought to have epilepsy, 55% had syncope, and the remaining 20% had confusional states. In the series of Couch et al. (7), 8% of the 793 patients had loss of consciousness. Confusional states, however, were not tabulated in this report.

In case series of anecdotal reports, other types of loss of consciousness have been reported. Transient global amnesia has been reported as a migraine accompaniment in two reports (33,34). These patients were generally alert, but confusion and repetitive questions were reported. Patients later had no memory for a period of time, and were usually noted to have a headache either before or after the episode of amnesia. Caplan et al. (34) reported that these patients were essentially indistinguishable from others with a transient global amnesia. Bruyn (17) reported patients with confusional state who had slurred speech, vertigo, and extensor plantar responses.

There have also been reports of migraine-associated coma (35). In these cases, patients are comatose for a period of time and recover with no sequelae. The comatose period is often preceded or followed by headache.

The etiology of episodic loss of consciousness as a symptom associated with migraine is only partially understood. A percentage of these patients would appear to have syncope, probably related to positional change in association with the autonomic and vascular instability associated with migraine. Other patients, however, seem to have a true alteration of brain function leading to either amnesia or loss of consciousness. This may represent coma related to a different mechanism such as focal, cerebral, or brain stem ischemia or spreading depression.

Emotional and Psychiatric Changes Associated with Migraine

Patients not infrequently report emotional changes in association with migraine headache. These tend to fall into two groups: 1) those occurring before the actual headache and 2) those associated with the headache.

Of the patients who suffer intermittent recurrent migraine headaches, a few will note significant changes in mood occurring 12–24 hours before the headache, and long before the classic aura to the headache. Patients who report this symptom usually note that they feel less energetic, slowed down, or even significantly depressed during this period. Occasionally, the opposite occurs; a patient may feel elated and have a burst of energy prior to the headache. This type of symptom, when it occurs, is usually fairly stereotyped. In most cases, the patient does not recognize it as a headache prodrome until the headache occurs, and only in retrospect will identify the change in mood as a prodromal symptom. Occasional patients will recognize a downward change in mood as a prodrome and may wish to get the headache "over with" so that their mood can return to normal.

A feeling of depression or depressed mood is very common during the migraine headache. In most cases it is unclear whether this is a migraine-associated symptom or simply a reaction to the pain of the headache. Often patients report a feeling of residual low-grade headache and lack of energy the day after a migraine headache, likening the "hangover" to the type induced by alcohol.

Finally, patients may feel a sense of elation, an up-mood, or even hypomanic behavior after a headache. Again, it is unclear whether this is a migraine-associated symptom or simply related to relief that the headache has passed.

THE EPIDEMIOLOGY OF MIGRAINE AND PATTERN OF OCCURRENCE

Familiarity with the epidemiology of migraine is certainly necessary to the overall understanding of this almost ubiquitous syndrome. The studies of Bille (36) in children in Scandinavia were a landmark in the epidemiology of migraine. In his group of approximately 9000 schoolchildren, he found that migraine occurred in approximately 5% of boys and girls in the prepubertal age group, with a male-to-female ratio of 1.05 to 1 (the study by Mortimer et al. (11) confirmed these figures). This ratio appeared relatively constant throughout childhood, with some subjects having onset as early as 3 years of age. Bille reported that 1% of subjects under age 7 and 5% under age 11 had migraine; Mortimer et al. noted a somewhat higher incidence in children under 8 years old. At puberty, the incidence of migraine in females doubled or tripled, while that in males fell slightly.

As indicated earlier, Epstein et al. (37) found that the onset of migraine by age was relatively constant from childhood to age 30—except for the period within 3 years of puberty, at which time the incidence was about three times the usual baseline incidence. Granella et al. (38) evaluated migraine onset in 1280 females and noted more of a bell-shaped curve, with 15% onset at <10 years, 45% onset at 10–19 years, and 24% at 20–29 years. Only 15% had onset after age 30. As noted previously, the first migraine headache can occur almost anytime during life; however, 80% of migraineurs have had their first migraine by age 40. Nevertheless, workers such as Fisher (4) have demonstrated that migraine can have its onset beyond age 50 and into later life. Stang et al. (39) looked at the incidence of migraine in Rochester, Minnesota. For males, they noted incidence of 167, 246, 151, 160, and 213 per 100,000 for ages 5–9, 10–14, 15–17, 20–24, and 25–29, respectively. For females of similar age, the incidence rates were 170, 296, 462, 689, and 573 per 100,000. After age 45, the incidence in men and women was similar but somewhat greater in women.

The reported prevalence of migraine varies, due in part to different definitions of migraine and different methods of data collection. In the early studies of Waters (40,41), populations within a circumscribed geographic area were interviewed using a standard technique, and a decision was made as to whether each patient's headache represented a migraine. In Waters' first study (40), migraine was diagnosed in 13% of women and 3% of men. In a subsequent study, of 1977 men and 2227 women, Waters suggested that 23–29% of women and 15–20% of men had migraine headaches (41). In the recent study of Stewart et al. (42), a questionnaire survey of 20,468 subjects produced an overall response rate of 63.4%. Of these, 17.6% of women and 5.7% of men had migraine by criteria compatible with the IHS classification. However, the prevalence of "severe headache" was similar to that reported by Waters (41). Stewart et al. also found that prevalence was age-specific, with the highest prevalence between 30 and 50 years for males and females. In a survey of 4204 subjects in France, 17.6% of females and 6.1% of males had "definite" or "borderline" migraine by IHS criteria (10). In a survey from Denmark consisting of a random sample of 387 men and 353 women, 6% and 23%, respectively, had migraine (9).

The Centers for Disease Control reported on prevalence of "chronic migraine" for the period 1980–1989 (43). Their report does not delineate the criteria for the diagnosis of migraine. They found that in 1989, prevalence of migraine was 2.5% for males <65 years and 1.8% for those ≥65. Prevalence for females was 5.9% for those <45, 7.6% for those 45–64, and 2.7% for those ≥65 years. This report may reflect different data from those of the earlier studies, and they may indicate only those subjects with more severe or frequent headache. It was also noted that the prevalence of "chronic migraine" had increased by 65–75% over a 10-year period. Whether this was a real increase or due to reporting bias could not be determined. With the variability noted among studies to date, it is apparent that getting complete reporting of migraine in a population would be very difficult.

Migraine is a cyclical problem (44). There have been relatively few formal studies on this because the data depend on patients' memory and the accuracy of reporting. Nevertheless, it is well known to physicians who deal with headache that patients will have marked variation in occurrence of headache at various times throughout life. It appears that migraine patients have cycles in which there will be a period with fairly frequent migraine episodes followed by periods of relatively infrequent headache. In women, it is quite common that peaks of migraine coincide with menarche and menses (5,45). The incidence of migraine is often greater shortly after than before menarche (37), and usually greater before than after menopause (42). However, many examples of the opposite of these patterns can be found.

Eighty percent of women will have relief of migraine during pregnancy (4), although about 20% will have exacerbation of migraine. A not uncommon pattern is for the patient to have exacerbation of migraine in the first trimester of pregnancy and then relative relief for the last two trimesters. Again, examples of the opposite can easily be found.

Migraine associated with menstruation, or menstrual migraine, is a relatively common problem (39,45). A few women will have migraine only in association with menstrual periods throughout their life. Usually, however, in addition to the most severe migraine headaches associated with their menstrual periods, patients will also note migraine headaches occurring at other times, often in conjunction with other stimuli (46).

Other factors that may be associated with exacerbating or triggering cycles of migraine include psychological stress, depression, "letdown" after a period of intense psychological stress, and injury to the central nervous system, for example, a severe blow producing concussion with a postconcussion (posttrauma) syndrome. Another type of injury is the meningeal inflammatory process, such as a septic or aseptic meningitis or a sterile meningeal reaction seen in subarachnoid hemorrhage.

Typically the migraine patient will note periods in which headaches occur relatively infrequently—that is, one to several times per year—at the ebb of the cycle and then very frequently at the peak of the cycle. Occasionally the pattern at the top of the cycle may be that of the chronic daily headache. The exact relationship of precipitating events to cycles of migraine is unclear and inexact, but it is not uncommon to find that a patient underwent a stressful situation such as a divorce without any difficulty, and then a second stressful situation, for example, the loss of a loved one, precipitated severe and frequent migraine headaches. Some patients may report that a past head injury seemed to precipitate a cycle of severe migraine headaches, while another head injury of equal intensity had no effect on migraine headaches.

A final problem that the physician dealing with headaches very often encounters is "limited memory" on the part of the patient. Studies by Ziegler et al. (8) and Waters (40,41) have suggested that patients tend to forget about headaches occurring more than a year previous to the interview. Patients will frequently indicate that headaches have been present for only 2 to 3 years. With careful questioning and interview, the examiner often finds that patients had earlier headaches but they were not recognized as migraine or no medical attention was sought because the patient recovered without incident. The patient may attribute these past headaches to "sinus trouble," "24-hour flu," or a "bad menstrual period." Careful questioning can elicit a history of headache remote to the present problem, producing very important information that may lead to the diagnosis of functional headache syndrome, lessening the need for testing that may be financially burdensome.

From the information given, then, it can be seen that determining the overall incidence and prevalence of migraine is a difficult task, one that is fraught with inaccuracy. It is, necessary, however, for the physician to be aware of the general nature of the incidence and prevalence of migraine to deal with the overall problem.

GENETICS OF MIGRAINE

The possibility of a genetic influence in migraine has been mentioned in medical literature for many years. Ziegler (47) reviewed this material and noted that Tissot was the first to mention such a possibility in the 18th century. In the 19th century, Liveing and Gowers both noted a hereditary disposition. In this century, the possibility of a direct hereditary mechanism has been approached through studies of monozygotic and dizygotic twins. These studies, as reviewed by Ziegler, were thorough and did not reveal a definite genetic mechanism (47).

Other family-history studies have varied greatly in their results. Allan (48) in 1930 noted a family history of migraine in 91% of his patients; Graham (49) found 80% in 1952. Friedman's study of 1000 cases in 1954 noted a 65% incidence of migraine in families (50) (but these results were criticized because family history was one of the criteria for the diagnosis of migraine). In 1960, Selby and Lance (5) reported that 55% of their patients had a history of migraine in a parent, sibling, or grandparent. In another study, Heyck (51) noted recurrent headaches in 59% of his patients but definite migraine in only 14%.

When only parents are considered, studies have noted a range of migraine occurring in a parent from a low of 27% to a high of 73%. In a study reported by Couch et al. (52) involving 382 patients, 76% had migraine in a first-degree family member and 48% had a parent with migraine.

It is quite apparent that the studies that have been done on genetics of migraine have shown a great disparity in familial incidence and have failed to produce a definite genetic mechanism. Barolin and Sperlich (53) postulated four possible mechanisms: 1) dominant in women, recessive in men, 2) dominant in both sexes, with 100% penetrance in women and 40% penetrance in men, 3) recessive with varying degrees of penetrance, and 4) polygenetic. The authors suggested that polygenetic inheritance was the most likely.

As pointed out previously, determination of cases of migraine is difficult in population studies because of variability in manifestations of the disease and in age of onset, and difficulty in obtaining information from all members of a family. It appears likely that there is some inherited tendency toward developing migraine, and that the expression of this tendency is dependent on the presence of one or more environmental factors. Finally, until some definite marker for migraine is obtained that can be reproduced in multiple studies, migraine remains a syndrome— and, as such, trying to determine any genetic predisposition or transmission will remain very difficult.

THEORETICAL BASIS OF MIGRAINE

The early work of Harold Wolff was seminal in trying to establish a pathophysiological mechanism for migraine (see Ref. 1 for review). Based on his work with tambours and a relatively primitive recording system, he and his collaborators postulated that the primary cause of migraine is vasoconstriction of the extracranial arteries in the early phases of the headache followed by vasodilation (1). They also observed tenderness over the dilated arteries, and proposed that the migraine pain emanates from the wall of the artery. Prior to Wolff's work, there had been various theories of migraine as an arterial process versus migraine as a problem related to the central nervous system. Wolff's observations swung the pendulum in favor of the arterial system as the etiology of migraine. It was proposed that the neurological manifestations of migraine related to vasoconstriction resulting in ischemia of cortex or brainstem.

Even after Wolff's work, the suggestion that migraine had its origin in the central nervous system continued to surface from time to time. In 1941 Lashley (55), a physiologist who worked with the visual system, studied his own migraine-associated scotoma. He plotted the progress of the scotoma by tracing it on paper at various stages of its development. Lashley noticed that the scotoma began as a small point and enlarged progressively until it moved to the periphery and disappeared. From his knowledge of the anatomy of the visual system, Lashley could not explain the steady enlargement of the scotoma by progressive vasoconstriction of the arterial system. He analogized his findings to a pebble dropped into a pool, with concentric rings of disturbance emanating from a central point and moving ever outward. Attempting to explain the visual aura of migraine, he postulated that some process must be initiated at a point and then move in all directions across the surface of the cerebral cortex at a rate of 2 to 3 millimeters per minute.

In 1944, Leao (56,57) described the neurophysiological phenomena of spreading depression from neurophysiological experiments with cats. He noted that application of concentrated potassium chloride to the cortex in a cat would elicit a phenomenon represented by a front of intense electrical activity followed by electrical silence or inactivity. This, in turn, represented a front of intense neural activity followed by neural silence. The depression would spread in all directions from the point at which the potassium chloride was applied, traveling at a rate of 2 to 3 millimeters per minute.

In 1958, Milner (58) repeated Lashley's observation with his own migrainous scotoma, and proposed that the progressive scotoma of migraine was due to spreading depression originating in the visual cortex. These observations rekindled interest in the possibility that migraine originates within the central nervous system.

Beginning in 1979, based on experiments with cerebral blood flow in migraine, Olesen et al. (59,60) reported the presence of spreading oligemia in the cerebral cortex. In patients who had migraine with aura, he found a spreading oligemia in the brain, and this appeared to coincide with the visual aura. The spreading oligemia would begin in the occipital region and move anteriorly at a rate of 2 to 3 millimeters per minute. Olesen noted that this did not occur in patients with common migraine, and that it did not follow the patterns of cerebrovascular distribution but moved across the cortex as if starting from a point. He postulated that the spreading oligemia would account for the march of migraine-associated scotoma and that the spreading oligemia may relate to spreading depression.

Lauritzen and his group (61) studied spreading depression in experimental animals and looked at the blood flow in areas affected by spreading depression. They found that spreading depression was associated with a decrease in cerebral cortical blood flow. This was thought to relate to the fact that the neurons became relatively inactive and essentially electrically silent, thus requiring less blood to supply metabolic needs. Lauritzen therefore proposed that the spreading oligemia was actually a manifestation of spreading depression, passively reflecting the spreading depression rather than being an intrinsically active process.

A number of criticisms of the oligemic hypothesis have been raised. In some of Olesen's cases, the migraine was triggered by use of reserpine. It has also been suggested that Olesen's results can be interpreted as showing a static area of low blood flow complicated by the occurrence of a "Compton effect," giving the appearance of a spreading oligemia when in fact the process was static (62).

Another theory of central origin of migraine was postulated by Raskin et al. (63). Working with Hosobuchi, this group looked at patients who had had lesions placed in the midbrain central gray for relief of cancer-associated pain. Some of these patients who had no prior history of migraine developed migraine-like headaches. From these observations, and review of the physiology of the raphe nuclei in the brain stem,

Raskin postulated that the raphe nuclei were the main driving force in migraine (63).

The raphe system is a phylogenetically primitive one; it is present in very early vertebrates. The raphe nuclei project both rostrally and caudally, and have an extensive distribution of nerve endings to cortical, subcortical, brain stem, and spinal neurons. Some of the raphe nuclei terminations end on a cerebral vasculature within the brain parenchyma, and their system appears to have strong effects on the cerebral microcirculation. Raskin postulated that the pain of migraine could be related to caudal projections of the raphe system whereas the neurological symptoms could relate to the rostral projections. Raskin also suggested that the dorsal raphe nucleus was the prime mover in migraine and that alterations in raphe nuclei output, especially the dorsal raphe nucleus, could trigger migraine.

The work by Moskowitz and his coworkers (65,66) on the trigemino-vascular system has provided some very interesting data and a strong hypothesis regarding the pain associated with migraine syndrome. It was noted by Wolff and his colleagues that patients with migraine developed swelling and tenderness around the superficial temporal arteries when a migraine headache occurred. They theorized that a substance released by the blood vessels caused the swelling, tenderness, and edema. In a series of experiments with cranial arteries whose afferent innervation came from the trigeminal nerve, Moskowitz and others have noted varicosities in the small nerve fibers surrounding blood vessels. These varicosities have subsequently been shown to contain substance P. Stimulation of these sensory fibers antidromically can release substance P, bradykinin, serotonin, and calcitonin gene-related peptide (CGRP). The antidromic stimulation may also activate mast cells with release of histamine. In addition, the vasodilating and protein permeability-increasing activity of substance P may activate endothelium and platelets, increasing the amount of serotonin and other factors that may be released from these blood units.

Work by Graham and Wolff in 1938 demonstrated that ergotamine can reduce the diameter of dilated vessels and diminish the edema around the blood vessels seen in some migraine headaches. It has since been shown that dihydroergotamine and sumatriptan, a specific serotonin-1 receptor agonist, can also reverse this sterile inflammation and exudation. Moskowitz has proposed that the pain of migraine is related to antidromic stimulation of trigeminal nerve fibers that end on blood vessels. This antidromic or axon-reflex stimulation causes release of serotonin substance P bradykinin and CGRP. These compounds in turn result in sterile inflammation of the blood vessel, stimulation of pain fibers, and pain. This could happen either in extracranial or intracranial meningeal vessels. This could also explain the variable location of migraine pain, which can be holocranial, hemicranial, or even focal to one area of the head.

Moskowitz further suggests that the stimulus for the pain may be spreading depression, which produces an eflux of potassium into the extracellular space in the brain. A high concentration of extracellular potassium at the meninges could stimulate the axon reflux and initiate migraine-related pain.

All the available theories explain some of the aspects of migraine but none explains the *total* syndrome. It does appear that a central origin of migraine is very likely, and that spreading depression as well as sterile neurogenetically induced inflammation will be part of the theory that is eventually developed. However, we still seem to be in the situation of the six blind men and the elephant, with different researchers having parts of the story—the final unifying mechanism has not yet been defined.

REFERENCES

1. Dalessio DJ. Wolff's Headache and Other Head Pain. 4th ed. New York: Oxford University Press, 1980.
2. Olesen, J. Classification and diagnostic criteria for headache disorders, cranial neuralgias and facial pain. Cephalalgia 1988; 8:1–96.
3. Ad Hoc Committee on Classification of Headache. Classification of headache. JAMA 1962; 179:717–718.
4. Fisher CM. Late-life migraine accompaniments as a cause of unexplained transient ischemic attacks. Can J Neurol Sci 1980; 7:9–17.
5. Selby G, Lance JW. Observations on 500 cases of migraine and allied vascular headache. J Neurol Neurosurg Psychiatry 1960; 23:23–32.
6. Couch JR, Ziegler DK, Hassanein RS. Evaluation of the relationship between migraine headaches and depression. Headache 1975; 15:41–50.
7. Couch J, et al. Migraine: a single entity or multiple syndromes. Cephalalgia 1991; 11(suppl 11):91–92.
8. Ziegler DK, Hassanein RS, Couch JR. Characteristics of life headache histories in a nonclinic population. Neurology 1977; 27:265–269.
9. Rasmussen BK, Olesen J. Migraine with aura and migraine without aura: an epidemiological study. Cephalalgia 1992; 12:221–228.
10. Henry P, et al. A nationwide survey of migraine in France: prevalence and clinical features in adults. Cephalalgia 1992; 12:229–237.
11. Mortimer MJ, Kay J, Jaron A. Childhood migraine in general practice: clinical features and characteristics. Cephalalgia 1992; 12:238–243.
12. Whitty CWM, Oxon DM. Migraine without headache. Lancet 1967; i:283–285.
13. O'Connor PS, Tredici TJ. Acephalgic migraine. Fifteen years experience. Ophthalmology 1981; 88:999–1003.

14. Prensky AL. Migraine and migrainous variants in pediatric patients. Pediatr Clin North Am 1976; 23:461–471.
15. Fenichel GM. Migraine as a cause of benign paroxysmal vertigo of childhood. J Pediatr 1967; 71:114–115.
16. Watson P, Steele JC. Paroxysmal dysequilibrium in the migraine syndrome of childhood. Arch Otolaryngol 1974; 99:177–179.
17. Bruyn GW. Migraine equivalents. In: Rose FC, ed. Handbook of Clinical Neurology. Vol 4. Amsterdam: Elsevier Science Publishing, 1986:155–171.
18. Raskin NH, Schwartz RK. Icepick-like pain. Neurology 1980, 30:203–205.
19. Lance JW. Headache. Ann Neurol 1981; 10:1–10.
20. Appenzeller O, Davison K, Marshall J. Reflex vasomotor abnormalities in the hands of migrainous subjects. JNNP 1963; 26:447–450.
21. Diamond S, Montrose D. The value of biofeedback in the treatment of chronic headache: a four-year retrospective study. Headache 1984; 24:5–18.
22. Sargent JD, Green EE, Walters ED. The use of autogenic biofeedback training in a pilot study of migraine and tension headaches. Headache 1972; 12:120–124.
23. Bruhn P, Olesen J, Melgaard B. Controlled trial of EMG feedback in muscle contraction headache. Ann Neurol 1979; 6:34–36.
24. Thomas WA, Post WE. Paroxysmal tachycardia in migraine. JAMA 1925; 84:569–570.
25. Briggs JF, Bellomo J. Precordial migraine. Dis Chest 1952; 21:635–640.
26. Miller D, et al. Is variant angina the coronary manifestation of a generalized vasospastic disorder? New Engl J Med 1981; 304:763–766.
27. Couch JR. Are visual phenomena and pain in migraine related to independent generators? Annual Meeting of American Academy of Neurology, New York, April 25, 1993, 662P:A327.
28. Rosenbaum HE. Familial hemiplegic migraine. Neurology 1960; 10:164–170.
29. Glista GG, Mellinger JF, Rooke ED. Familial hemiplegic migraine. Mayo Clin Proc 1975; 50:307–311.
30. Koenigsberger MR, et al. Benign paroxysmal vertigo of childhood. Neurology 1970; 20:1108–1113.
31. Kuritzky A, Ziegler DK, Hassanein R. Vertigo, motion sickness and migraine. Headache 1981; 21:227–231.
32. Bickerstaff ER. Basilar artery migraine. Lancet 1961; i:15–17.
33. Olivarius BF, Jensen TS. Transient global amnesia in migraine. Headache 1979; 19:335–338.
34. Caplan L, et al. Transient global amnesia and migraine. Neurology 1981; 31:1167–1170.
35. Fitzsimons RB, Wolfenden WH. Migraine coma. Brain 1985; 108:555–577.
36. Bille B. Migraine in school children. Acta Paediatr 1962; 51:13–51.
37. Epstein MT, Hockaday JM, Hockaday TDR. Migraine and reproductive hormones throughout the menstrual cycle. Lancet 1975; i:543–548.
38. Granella F, et al. Migraine without aura and reproductive life events: a clinical epidemiological study in 300 women. Headache 1993; 33(7):385–389.

39. Stang PE, et al. Incidence of migraine headache: a population-based study in Olmstead County, Minnesota. Neurology 1992; 42:1657–1662.
40. Waters WE. Community studies of the prevalence of headache. Headache 1970; 9:178–186.
41. Waters WE. Review of the epidemiology of migraine in adults. Danish Med Bull 1975; 22:86–88.
42. Stewart WF, et al. Prevalence of migraine headache in the United States. JAMA 1992; 267:64–69.
43. Prevalence of chronic migraine headaches—United States, 1980-1989. MMWR 1991; 40:331–338.
44. Whitty CWM, Hockaday JM. Migraine: a follow-up study of 92 patients. Br Med J 1968; 1:735–736.
45. Waters WE, O'Connor PJ. Epidemiology of headache and migraine in women. J Neurol Neurosurg Psychiatry 1971; 34:148–153.
46. Silberstein SD, Merriam GR. Estrogens, progestins, and headache. Neurology 1991; 41:786–793.
47. Ziegler DK. Genetics of migraine. In: Rose FC, ed. Handbook of Clinical Neurology. Vol. 4. Amsterdam: Elsevier Science Publishing, 1986:23–30.
48. Allan W. The inheritance of migraine. Arch Intern Med 1930; 13:590–599.
49. Graham JR. The natural history of migraine: some observations and a hypothesis. Trans Am Clin Climatol Assoc 1952; 4:61–74.
50. Friedman AP. Treatment of migraine in children. Neurology 1954; 4:157.
51. Heyck J. Varieties of hemiplegic migraine. Headache 1973; 12:135–142.
52. Couch JR, Bearss CM, Verhulst SJ. Effect of parental occurrence of recurrent severe headache on siblings of migraineurs. 30th Annual Meeting of the American Association for the Study of Headache, San Francisco, CA, June 1988.
53. Barolin GS, Sperlich D. Migraine families—contribution to the genetic aspect. Fortschr Neurol Psychiatr 1969; 37:521–544.
54. Graham JR, Wolff HG. Mechanism of migraine headache and action of ergotamine tartrate. Arch Neurol Psychiatry 1938; 39:737–763.
55. Lashley KS. Patterns of cerebral integration indicated by the scotomas of migraine. Arch Neurol Psychiatry 1941; 46:331–339.
56. Leao AAP. Pial circulation and spreading depression of activity in the cerebral cortex. J Neurophysiol 1944; 7:391–396.
57. Leao AAP. Spreading depression of activity in the cerebral cortex. J Neurophysiol 1944; 7:359–390.
58. Milner PM. Note on a possible correspondence between the scotomas of migraine and spreading depression of Leao. Electroencephalogr Clin Neurophysiol 1958; 10:705.
59. Olesen J, Larsen B, Lauritzen M. Focal hyperemia followed by spreading oligemia and impaired activation of rCBF in classic migraine. Ann Neurol 1981; 9:344–352.
60. Olesen J, et al. Timing and topography of cerebral blood flow, aura, and headache during migraine attacks. Ann Neurol 1990; 28:791–798.

61. Lauritzen M, et al. Persistent oligemia of rat cerebral cortex in the wake of spreading depression. Ann Neurol 1982; 12:469–474.
62. Skyhøj T, Friberg L, Lassen NA. Ischemia may be the primary cause of the neurologic deficits in classic migraine. Arch Neurol 1987; 44:156–161.
63. Raskin NH, Hosobuchi Y, Lamb S. Headache may arise from perturbation of brain. Headache 1987; 27:416–420.
64. Raskin NH. On the origin of head pain. Headache 1988; 28:254–257.
65. Moskowitz MA. The neurobiology of vascular head pain. Ann Neurol 1984; 16:157–168.
66. Saito K, Markowitz S, Moskowitz MA. Ergot Alkaloids block neurogenic extravasation in dura mater: proposed action in vascular headaches. Ann Neurol 1988; 24:732–737.
67. Lance JW, Anthony M. Some clinical aspects of migraine. Arch Neurol 1966; 15:356–361.

3

Epidemiology of Migraine

Paul Stang and Jane T. Osterhaus

Glaxo Inc. Research Institute
Research Triangle Park, North Carolina

INTRODUCTION

Headache is one of the most common presenting symptoms to health care facilities, accounting for close to 10 million outpatient visits per year in the United States (1). Migraine headaches are among the more debilitating headache types seen in clinical practice. Although it is a highly prevalent condition, relatively little consensus has been achieved on the number of people affected, the level of disability, and the economic impact of this disease. This is probably due to difficulties in identifying migraine sufferers, lack of uniformity of the application of diagnostic criteria, variations in study designs, and gender bias in that migraine is predominantly an affliction of females.

Migraine headache presents many challenges in diagnosis and research. It is defined by a cluster of symptoms reported by the patient for which no laboratory test exists to confirm the diagnosis. It is understandable, therefore, that it is often misdiagnosed, ignored, or considered to be secondary to another condition. This not only makes epidemiological studies difficult, but also impedes the recognition of migraine as a separate and distinct clinical entity. Basic biochemical and biological research has been ongoing for many years, and recent advances in technology have created the opportunity to identify the particular biochemical and neurochemical receptor pathways of the disorder (see Chapters 2 and 9).

This chapter reviews the basic epidemiology, economic impact (including utilization of services), and quality of life data available for migraine. It is hoped that the reader will gain some broad insights into the breadth and impact of migraine on the population.

EPIDEMIOLOGY

Prevalence and incidence—epidemiological measures of disease frequency—provide the broad foundation in our understanding the distribution, demographics, and determinants of migraine in the population. Prevalence, a measure of the number of patients with the disorder in a given time period, is a cross-sectional measure of disease frequency and can be based on headache occurring during a particular day, week, month, or year, or, as in lifetime prevalence, reflect whether the patient has ever suffered a migraine headache. Prevalence estimates are usually obtained from cross-sectional sampling techniques, through interviewer-administered questionnaires, mail or telephone surveys, or retrospective estimates generated through patient data pools or records. Incidence, on the other hand, reflects the number of new migraine cases arising in a given period. Incidence estimates are more difficult to obtain because they necessitate following a population over a long period of time, or performing repeated prevalence estimates over a long period to identify new cases as they arise.

Many epidemiological studies of migraine were conducted prior to the availability of the 1988 International Headache Society (IHS) criteria and are reviewed in detail elsewhere (2). Most suffer from biases in the design, identification of the sample population, or high variability in the ascertainment of migraine. Table 1 provides an overview of the current published estimates of migraine prevalence and incidence based on IHS criteria. There is some variability in these estimates despite the fact that the same diagnostic criteria are used, most of which is probably due to different methods of identifying cases. Epidemiological studies are also important, as they form the foundation for determining the impact of the disease;

consequently, economic studies are only as good as the epidemiological studies on which they are based.

Identification and Diagnosis of Migraine Sufferers

There has been an evolution in the classification of migraine headache from a fairly loose system—1964 ad hoc criteria (3)—to the more rigorous 1988 IHS criteria (4). The 1988 diagnostic criteria have had a positive impact on epidemiology studies because they are relatively rigid. These criteria have been used in many research settings (see Table 1); however, it has recently been suggested that the criteria are too restrictive and may exclude as many as 5% of clinical migraine (5).

Various case ascertainment or identification methods have also been used in epidemiological studies over the past years, creating methodological problems in comparing the results. Identifying migraine patients in

Table 1 Published Population-Based Epidemiology Studies Based on 1988 IHS Criteria

Ref.; country	Method of collecting data	Prevalence or incidence	Results	
			Males	Females
Pryse-Phillips et al., 1993 (48)— Canada	Random-dialing telephone survey and interview of 24,159 households in Canada	Lifetime prevalence	10.0%	23.0%
Stewart et al., 1992 (23)— U.S.	Mailed questionnaire to panel of 15,000 households representative of the U.S.	Annual prevalence	5.7%	17.6%
Henry et al., 1992 (49)— France	Face-to-face interviews with a representative sample of 4204 aged ≥ 15 years (rates include "borderline migraine")	Lifetime prevalence	6.1%	17.6%
Rasmussen et al., 1992 (50)— Denmark	1000 randomly selected residents of western Copenhagen county	Annual prevalence	6.0%	15.0%
Stang et al., 1992 (21)— Olmsted County, U.S.	Review of all Olmsted County residents' medical records with any headache diagnosis; identified initial visit for headache 1979–1981; all ages	Incidence of medically detectable migraine	137 per 100,000	294 per 100,000

a clinical interview provides a great deal of latitude in the use of probing questions and clinical judgment; the technique is neither infallible nor reproducible (6,7). Comparisons of research ascertainment and clinical interview (8,9) have generally found poor agreement between the two. Further variability may manifest, as different methods of ascertainment are used in research studies. Nikiforow (10) found that subjects more readily reported by questionnaire symptoms occurring less frequently than they would in clinical interviews, potentially increasing the likelihood that migraineurs would be identified in questionnaire studies. Inconsistency has also been described among physicians in their diagnosis of migraine. Weeks and Rapoport (11) presented 50 headache patients' histories to 13 U.S. and 17 non-U.S. headache specialists and found low levels of agreement among neurologists (57%), nurses (67%), and internists (58%) for the U.S. headache specialists (all neurologists) and 65% for those outside the U.S. In part, the poor agreement between raters may be due to the poor specificity of the diagnostic protocol.

Ascertainment of migraine can be addressed only in highly developed record systems (e.g., the Rochester Epidemiology Project) or by obtaining component symptoms directly from patients via questionnaire or interview. Rates based solely on self-report of physician diagnosis underestimate the true extent of the disorder, as subjects must have sought medical attention and must accurately recall and report the diagnosis. This is particularly important because it has been shown in many studies that only a portion of migraineurs actually consult physicians for their headache, with consultation rates ranging from less than 40% in the U.S. (12) to 56% in Denmark (13), to over 80% in Canada (14). Additionally, even among those who do seek medical care, many escape diagnosis as migraineurs, as the likelihood of a migraineur receiving a clinical diagnosis of migraine may be as low as 45% (7).

Questionnaires and non-physician interviews have also been shown to have a great deal of variability associated with them. Bias often arises when patients are asked to recall events remote from the date of inquiry and in those studies that have limited their questions to the patient's most recent headache. This approach ignores the fact that patients often suffer from many different types of headache. An alternative is to ask a patient to describe his "typical headache"; however, the resulting report may be of an amalgam of symptoms experienced by the individual in different types of headache on separate occasions which are not per se representative or diagnostic of any one headache type. Patients who experience both migrainous and nonmigrainous headaches then create an interesting clinical and research problem. It is this difficulty in bridging research epidemiology with clinical reality that has led to some differences in estimates of frequency and impact.

Migraine headaches do not occur in isolation; some studies (7,15) have shown that as many as 60% of identifiable migraine patients actually suffer from a mixture of migraine and tension-headache symptoms, with a high level of disability. The presence of tension-headache features probably decreases the likelihood that migraine will be diagnosed by the clinician (7). There are many questions about the underlying pathophysiology of these two disorders and how over time they may represent a continuum of the same clinical entity. The fact that tension headache is so common in the general population suggests that, by chance alone, it will co-occur with migraine at least as frequently.

Finally, research epidemiology has the problem of intraindividual variability in the way headaches are experienced. Circadian rhythms may distinguish the headache types, but this is probably of little diagnostic value in the individual; migraine tends to occur between 6 A.M.. and noon, while tension headaches predominate later in the day (16). The impact that headache has on patient functioning varies. This could be grossly conceived as severity or dysfunction; however, severity scales of chronic intermittent disorders often depend on frequency of attacks, or fail to include measures of impairment more sensitive than time missed from work. The fallacy is that clinical disability does not depend on attack frequency; a patient who experiences relatively infrequent migraine (e.g., one per month) may be totally disabled for that day, while a patient who experiences several migraines a month may not be severely impaired during each attack. Severity indices have been suggested (17–19); however, their application in a clinical setting has been sparse. Recent work by Von Korff and colleagues (17,20) has shown that a graded chronic pain dysfunction score may be a more important predictor of long-term outcome than clinical diagnosis. Graded chronic pain dysfunction predicts headache pain days, depression, activity limitation, and narcotic analgesic use. Based on this work, one could argue the need to assess migraine patients not only by clinical signs and symptoms but also, crucially, by measuring functional impact.

DEMOGRAPHIC FEATURES OF MIGRAINE

Gender and Age

It is widely accepted that migraine is a disorder that disproportionately affects females. All IHS-based prevalence and incidence studies (Table 1) have shown a female preponderance across most age ranges. The gender discrepancy is less apparent in those under age 15 years, which has helped substantiate the role of female sexual maturation and its associated hormonal milestones in the genesis of migraine. Little attention has been given to migraine in children, in part because of the difficulties in diagnosis and patient reporting. However, 16% of the Olmsted County, Minnesota, incident cohort were under the age of 15 years at the time of their first migraine visit (21), and over half of the 12–29-year-old migraineurs in the Washington County study (22) were believed to have the onset of their migraines at age 15 years or less.

Race

Little work has appeared that allows comparison of migraine prevalence across racial groups. In the American Migraine Study (23), the adjusted prevalence rates among black females was 20% lower than in white females, while the adjusted rate in black males was half that of white males. The 1989 National Health Interview Survey (24) reported significantly higher prevalence of self-reported migraine among whites than among blacks. Data from a population-based prevalence study of Mexican-Americans (25), when compared to the American Migraine Study (23), reveal that the prevalence in Hispanic females is slightly higher than that in U.S. white females (21.1% vs. 17.6%) and nearly identical in Hispanic and white males (6.1% vs. 5.7%). Interestingly, the rates of migraine in Mexican-Americans born in Mexico appear to be twice as high as those in Mexican-Americans born in the United States (26).

Income/Socioeconomic Status

Two recent U.S. prevalence studies (23,24) have shown that the prevalence of migraine is higher in households with lower incomes. These data challenge the commonly held notion that migraine is a disease of the privileged and wealthy, as it is those of higher income who seek medical attention (12,27). Some authors (27,28) believe that these data reflect a "downward drift" in that the effects of the migraine may be responsible for relegating the sufferer to a lower economic status or that the environment of lower economic stations (poor access to care, stress, social adversity, higher exposure to precipitating factors) contains factors that may predispose to migraine (social causation).

Inheritance

Genetics may also play a role in the frequency and distribution of migraine. There appears to be a strong familial component of migraine, as family history in first-degree relatives is highly likely (25,29–32). Good reviews of the genetics of migraine have been published elsewhere (31,32).

Migraine Comorbidities

Epidemiology can also address the second great class of problem: whether migraine and other medical conditions are associated (Table 2). Comorbidities can increase disability, utilization of health care services, or a patient's risk of other adverse outcomes. Clearly, this also has economic implications because the patient may be using resources and experiencing events due to conditions occurring in concert with his migraine. Psychiatric comorbidities, especially depression, are commonly associated with migraine and magnify the impact on the patient in both humanistic and financial terms. Physical comorbidities, including stroke, cardiovascular disease, hypertension, preeclampsia, and seizure disorder, have been shown to be more prevalent among migraineurs. The relationship of migraine to these comorbid conditions has tremendous public health impact because the onset of migraine is characteristically in the first three decades of life while the onset of many of these more devastating diseases occurs some 20 years later. Conceivably, migraine could be used as a marker to identify patients who are at higher risk and most likely to benefit from early intervention, aggressive screening, and possible prevention.

IMPACT

When considering the impact of migraine on a patient, one must consider three kinds of costs: direct, indirect, and humanistic. Direct costs are those incurred within the health care system due to the provision of health care services, including the cost of physician visits, laboratory tests, medications, and hospitalization. Indirect costs are those associated with the condition but not directly related to the provision of health care services, for example, lost productivity, time missed at work, and curtailed leisure activities. Human costs are health-related declines in quality of life and satisfaction, and restriction of choices. Such information may be used to compare chronic conditions, as well as to measure the personal value of an

Table 2 Conditions Associated with Migraine

Condition	Magnitude of association: migraine vs. no migraine	Ref.
Psychiatric		
Depression	OR = 4.22; 4.1 males, 4.9 females	51
	Adj OR = 2.5 (no hx panic)	51
Nonbipolar major depression	OR = 2.9 (of migraine in depressives vs. controls)	52
Depression (major) and panic	Adj OR = 25.2	51
Sleep disorders	OR = 1.9 females, 6.9 males	29
Panic disorder	Males RR = 6.96 risk of migraine attack in previous week among those w/wo panic attack	53
	Females RR = 3.70 risk of migraine attack in previous week among those w/wo panic attack	53
	OR = 6.05; 6.2 males, 5.5 females	51
	Adj OR = 9.5 (no hx MDD)	51
Panic syndrome	Males RR = 4.25 risk of migraine attack in previous week among those w/wo panic syndrome	53
	Females RR = 2.38 risk of migraine attack in previous week among those w/wo panic syndrome	53
Suicide	Adj OR = 2.7 (of suicide in migraineurs w/o aura, no MDD)	54
	Adj OR = 4.3 (of suicide in migraineurs w/ aura, no MDD)	54
	Adj OR = 10.9 (migraineurs w/o aura plus MDD)	54
	Adj OR = 23.2 (of suicide in migraineurs w/ aura plus MDD)	54
	Adj OR = 1.6 (of suicide in migraineurs w/wo auras vs. nonmigraineurs)	55
	Adj OR = 3.0 (of suicide in migraineurs w/ aura vs. nonmigraineurs)	55
Medical: cardiac and vascular		
Angina	PR = 4.0 of migraine in pts w/wo angina	56
Cerebrovascular disease	OR = 3.1	57
	OR = 2.6 (migraine with aura)	58
	OR = 1.1–1.7	59
	OR = 1.97–2.48	60
Hypertension	PR = 1.26 (mothers of migraineurs)	61
	PR = 1.07 (fathers of migraineurs)	61
	RR = 1.7; 1.7 females, 1.8 males	62
Mitral valve prolapse	RR = 0.97 (7/19; 16/43) hemiplegic vs. nonhemiplegic migraineurs	63
	PR = 9.8 (of MVP in complicated migraine vs. controls)	64

Table 2 (Continued)

Condition	Magnitude of association: migraine vs. no migraine	Ref.
	PR = 2.2 (of MVP in classic migraine vs. controls)	64
	PR = 1.8 (of MVP in common migraine vs. controls)	64
	PR = 2.1 (of definite and possible MVP in migraineurs vs. controls)	65
	PR = 1.7 (of MVP in migraineurs w/o stroke vs. nonmigraineurs w/o stroke)	66
	PR = 0.3 (of MVP in migraineurs w/ stroke vs. nonmigraineurs w/o stroke)	66
Myocardial infarction	OR = 2.4	57
	PR = 1.11 (mothers of migraineurs)	61
	PR = 0.91 (mothers of migraineurs)	61
	RR = 1.3; 1.3 females, RR = 1.3 males	62
Peripheral vascular disease (Raynaud's)	PR = 4.3	67
	PR = 1.5 (in classic vs. common migraine)	67
	OR = 5.4 of migraine in Raynaud's vs. controls	68
	PR = 2.14 for chest pain in Raynaud's and migraine vs. Raynaud's alone	68
	PR = 4.28 for chest pain in Raynaud's and migraine vs. migraine alone	68
	PR = 3.53 for chest pain in Raynaud's and migraine vs. no migraine, no Raynaud's	68
Medical: other		
Asthma	Crude RR = 1.95 (in children given mom with migraine and no asthma vs. mom w/o migraine or asthma)	69
	Crude RR = 3.59 (in children given mom with migraine and asthma vs. mom w/o migraine or asthma)	69
	Crude RR = 1.8 in children given mom with migraine and no asthma vs. mom without migraine or asthma	69
Preeclampsia and hypertension of pregnancy	OR = 1.7–2.4	70
Seizure disorder	OR = 1.2–3.6	71
Lupus erythematosus	PR = 3.0 (of classic migraine in lupus pts vs. controls)	72

OR = odds ratio: the odds of having migraine given this disorder divided by the odds of not having migraine given this disorder; PR = prevalence ratio: ratio of the prevalence of a disorder among migraineurs to the prevalence of the disorder among those without migraine; RR = relative risk: ratio of the risk of disorder among those with migraine to those without migraine; Adj = adjusted—incorporation of or "controlling" the other effects of other variables on the magnitude of an association, usually using regression models; MDD = major depressive disorder.

intervention to treat a condition. A thorough review of the patterns of health care utilization by migraineurs appears elsewhere (33).

Entry to the health care system governs the direct costs of migraine. Because many migraine patients never seek formal medical attention for their disease, the direct costs for migraine-related services are attributable only to those who do seek care. The entire spectrum of health care use by the migraineur is thus often overlooked. Because of the possible effect of comorbid disease, it is important to examine the aggregate use of health care by the migraine patient in addition to the services used specifically for headache. Additionally, even many of those who do seek medical care escape diagnosis as migraineurs (6,7).

Direct Costs and Utilization of Health Care Services

The direct costs of migraine-related health care services appear to be relatively small. In the United Kingdom, it was estimated that the National Health Service spent approximately 5 pounds per migraine sufferer per year, of which medications represented 68%, physician visits 25%, and hospitalizations 7% (34). In France, the mean medical cost of migraine was estimated as being 3.8 times that of nonmigraineurs (FF469 vs. FF123 for 6 months per patient) (35).

Outpatient Costs

To appreciate the true spectrum of health care use, it is important to identify the migraineur at the time he or she first seeks medical attention for headache and follow their subsequent use of services. The Olmsted County study (36) captured utilization data for all residents whose initial visit for migraine occurred between 1979 and 1981 and followed them for 3 years in the comprehensive medical record. The highest utilization of health care services among migraineurs occurred during the 12 months subsequent to the initial migraine visit. After that initial year, the use of services, including physician visits, decreased precipitously to levels about the same as before the diagnosis of migraine: Headache-related visits to general practitioners dropped 75% and neurology visits decreased 80% in the 13–39 months after the initial migraine visit. Over 50% of the cohort initially presented to family practitioners and internists, while 16% initially sought care in the emergency department; 32% of the cohort were referred to a neurologist, with males referred more frequently than females (36). Once in the health care system, 40% of newly identified migraineurs in Olmsted County, Minnesota, had some type of diagnostic procedure performed during the year after they were diagnosed (CT scan, x-rays, lumbar puncture, or EEG). Medication prescribed depended on the clinical setting: Narcotics were more often administered and prescribed in the emergency room than in general outpatient settings. Over the 3 years evaluated, medication switching was common (37).

In a study of 202 migraineurs in Great Britain (38), 4% reported that they consulted their physician every month, 10% consulted every 3–6 months, and 16% consulted their physician once per year or less. Overall, the consultation rate for migraine in the United Kingdom has been reported to be 12.8 consultations per 1000 patients (34). In contrast, data from 648 migraine clinical trial patients revealed that 91% of the subjects had had at least one outpatient visit for migraine in the prior year and 7.6% reported at least 12 visits (39).

Of interest is data from Georgia Medicaid (40), an entitlement program that provides unrestricted access to medical care (similar to the U.K. system). Of the 7509 migraineurs who were followed for 22 months, 40% had only one outpatient visit for migraine, 20% had two outpatient claims. Use of technology was somewhat higher, with over 33% undergoing CT scan and 21% undergoing x-rays or EEG. These data from prevalence population samples highlight the importance of determining the use of health care services from the onset, as clearly patients' use of medical services is relatively low overall and prevalent cases may have already had extensive contact with medical professionals prior to being sampled.

Use of migraine-specific health care services is only a portion of the direct costs that should be considered. Total volume of health care use reflects the impact of comorbidities, many of them psychiatric, which contribute to the total burden of the disease. The best information to date can be gleaned from a study using data from a managed care organization (MCO) data base comparing the utilization of health care services by 1336 migraineurs to that by 1336 age- and gender-matched controls (41). Overall, the migraineurs generated 70% more claims than did the controls (57,622 vs. 33,772). Similarly, the migraineurs generated twice as many psychiatric care claims as the controls did (1210 vs. 642). The average monthly medical claim for migraine patients was $186, versus $112 for the control group. Physician services were used more by the migraine group, even though just a small fraction of the visits were attributed to migraine.

The emergency department (ED) is a common source of medical care for migraineurs because some rely on emergency departments as their primary source of treatment. Only 16% of patients initially presented to the ED for their incident migraine encounter in Olmsted County, while 22% had at least one ED visit during the first 12 months after initially seeking care for their migraine (36). Data from Canada (42) reveal that 14%

of migraineurs had used the ED for headache care. Osterhaus et al. (39), in their study of 648 clinical trial patients, found that 15% of the migraine ED users accounted for 60% of the visits, with almost half having had at least one visit in the prior year. In a study of ED use in a staff model HMO's walk-in emergency department (43), 323 visits were made by 152 migraine patients over a 5-month period, with 36% of the patients having repeat visits (mean of 4.2 repeat visits). The majority (85%) of these patients received both an injectable narcotic and an antihistamine as treatment. Migraineurs in the United Health Care MCO generated almost four times the volume of ED claims that their nonmigraine counterparts did (1992 vs. 513), 50% of which were headache-related (41).

Hospitalization of a migraineur is infrequent but expensive, and no data are available on the relative numbers of hospitalizations for diagnostic workup, headache management, and analgesic detoxification. Migraine was the principal discharge diagnosis for only 0.11% of U.S. hospital discharges in 1987; however, the migraineur was hospitalized for an average of 4 days at a mean cost of $2215 (44). About 5% of the migraineurs in Olmsted County were hospitalized in the first 3 years after initial diagnosis, most of which occurred in the first year (36). Only 8% of the self-reported migraineurs in the National Health Interview Survey (24) reported ever being hospitalized, a result similar to that reported in a clinical trials population (39). Rates from Denmark are substantially lower; only 2% reported a migraine-related hospitalization (13).

While direct costs may not seem large, additional research to further characterize the distribution of direct costs among migraineurs and the impact of therapies would be valuable. The relationships between migraine-specific health care costs, the effect of comorbidities on direct costs, and the natural course of the disease and utilization over time warrant further research.

Indirect Costs

Indirect costs of migraine must be examined to appreciate the full impact of the disorder on productivity and leisure. The National Health Interview Survey in 1989 (24) gave a striking picture on restricted-activity days among working males with self-reported migraine. Among this group of males, over 108,000 restricted-activity days were experienced in a 2-week period due to migraine. Similarly, among working females with migraine, over 581,000 restricted-activity days occurred in a 2-week period. Of more interest is that among homemakers it was estimated that 1.4 million restricted-activity days occurred in a 2-week period. These are probably gross underestimates as they are based on self-report of migraine.

When a worker experiences restricted activity or total loss of a day, the costs of the disease begin to affect those who depend on the migraineur, especially employers and family. School-aged children (6–18 years old) are not immune from impairment either—over 329,000 school days are lost per month due to migraine among the 970,000 self-reported migraineurs in the United States (24), days on which a parent may also have to stay home from work to care for the child.

Rasmussen et al. (13) estimated that the total loss of workdays per year due to migraine in Denmark was 270 days per 1000 persons. In the United Kingdom, approximately 19.7 million working days per year are lost due to migraine (45). The U.S. labor costs of migraine were estimated based on a survey of people who met IHS criteria for migraine and had participated in a clinical trial designed to assess the efficacy of an antimigraine compound (sumatriptan) (39). Although these patients represent a clinical trial population, most (89%) of the employed respondents reported that job performance was adversely affected by migraine, and over 50% reported missing an average of 2 days of work per month due to their headaches. Additionally, working migraineurs reported working approximately 5 days per month at reduced productivity due to their migraines. The annual cost of lost time to a U.S. employer due to migraine has been estimated to range from $3000 to 3600 per year for female employees and $5500 to 6800 per year for males. Extrapolated to the U.S. working population, the aggregate cost to employers of migraine headache ranges from $6.5 to 17.3 billion. These figures reflect the substantial impact of this relatively common disorder.

The indirect costs of migraine are substantial and crucial to an estimate of the burden of migraine on society. Although these data are more difficult to obtain and interpret, they provide insight into how migraine truly affects the daily life of the sufferer and what toll that has on the population. To complete our understanding of the impact of this disorder, we need to examine how migraine affects the individual on a more humanistic basis. Data on quality of life are even more complex because these data are difficult to obtain and perhaps more difficult to interpret since the results cannot be translated into tangible losses of time or money.

Quality of Life

Standard, validated health-related quality of life terms may be used to compare migraineurs with sufferers of other chronic diseases, and with the healthy population (46). A cross-sectional mail survey of 845 migraine patients contained a standardized questionnaire, which was self-administered by migraine patients several months after they had been in a single-dose, placebo-controlled clinical trial. The Medical Outcomes Study (47) and the U.S. population without chronic disease were used as comparator groups. Eight scales from the MOS SF-36 health survey were evaluated: limitations in physical activities due to health problems, limitations in usual role activities due to physical problems, bodily pain, general health perceptions, vitality, limitations in social activities due to physical or emotional problems, limitations in usual role activities due to emotional problems, and general mental health.

Functioning and well-being in the MOS SF-36 scales were strongly affected by migraine (Figure 1). Patients who perceived their migraines as "very severe" reported significantly lower quality of life than did those patients who reported their migraines as "severe" or "moderate" in the four dimensions of physical functioning, role disability due to physical health problems, pain, and social disability. Role disability due to emotional problems and vitality were not significantly affected by migraine severity. Compared to age- and sex-adjusted population norms from a

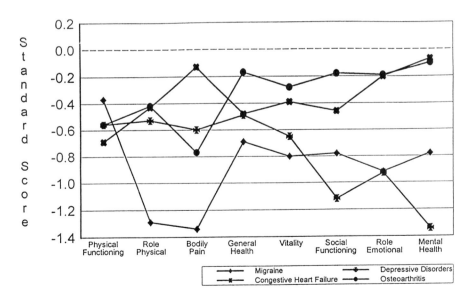

Figure 1 MOS SF-36 quality of life scores for migraine and other chronic conditions. Dashed line indicates national well norm.

healthy population, migraineurs scored significantly lower on all eight health-status scales.

The quality of life in the migraine population was worse than that for patients with other chronic conditions in several dimensions (46) (Figure 1). Role-physical and bodily pain scores were significantly lower in the migraine group than in patients with congestive heart failure, depressive disorder, or osteoarthritis, demonstrating that the physical morbidity associated with migraine is at least comparable to that of other chronic conditions. General health perception scores in the migraineur population were comparable to those of patients suffering from congestive heart failure or depressive disorder. For the three MOS SF-36 scale scores most sensitive to mental health outcomes (mental health, emotional role disability, and social functioning), the magnitude of the differences between the migraine population and the general population were second only to those for the MOS sample with depressive disorder, suggesting that migraine sufferers also have a substantial mental health burden. Migraine, therefore, appears to be a condition of physical morbidity and consequent social and role limitations. The human cost of migraine in a relative and an absolute sense is considerable.

CONCLUSION

Migraine is a common disorder whose demographics, frequency, and impact can now be realized through high-quality epidemiological and economic studies. Significant morbidity has been attributed to migraine. The annual cost of migraine to a U.S. employer is estimated to be as high as $3600 per female migraineur and $6800 per male due to days worked at reduced productivity and days missed from work. Housewives bear a large proportion of the burden; migraine also affects children, resulting in a notable amount of missed school days. Migraines have been shown to affect patients' ability to function and their sense of well-being. Relative to the healthy population and to patients with other chronic conditions, the burden of migraine in quality of life terms is profound.

REFERENCES

1. Schappert SM. National Ambulatory Medical Care Survey: 1989 Summary. National Center for Health Statistics. Vital Health Statistics 1992; 13(110).
2. Linet MS, Stewart WF. Migraine headache: epidemiologic perspectives. Epidemiolog Rev 1984; 6:107–139.

3. Headache Classification Committee of the International Headache Society. Classification and diagnostic criteria for headache disorders, cranial neuralgias, and facial pain. Cephalalgia. 1988; 8(suppl 7):19–28.

4. Ad Hoc Committee on the Classification of Headache. Classification of Headache. JAMA 1962; 179:127–128.

5. Michel P, Dartigues JF, Henry P, et al. Validity of the International Headache Society criteria for migraine. Neuroepidemiology 1993; 12:51–57.

6. Stang PE, Yanagihara T, Swanson JW, Guess HA, O'Fallon WM, Beard CM, Melton LJ. A population-based study of migraine headaches in Olmsted County, MN: Case ascertainment and classification. Neuroepidemiology 1991; 10:297–307.

7. Stang PE, Von Korff M. The diagnosis of headache in primary care: factors in the agreement of the clinical and standardized diagnosis. Headache 1994; 34:138–142.

8. Rasmussen BK, Jensen R, Olesen J. Questionnaire versus clinical interview in the diagnosis of headache. Headache 1991; 31:290–295.

9. Lipton RB, Stewart WF, Solomon S. Questionnaire versus clinical interview in the diagnosis of headache (letter). Headache 1992; 32:55–56.

10. Nikiforow R. Features of migraine: comparison of a questionnaire study and neurologist-examined random sample. Cephalalgia 1981; 1:157–166.

11. Weeks RE, Rapoport AM. A critical look at reliability of headache diagnosis (abstract). Ann Neurol 1987; 22:148–149.

12. Lipton RB, Stewart WF, Celentano DD, Reed ML. Undiagnosed migraine headaches: a comparison of symptom-based and reported physician diagnosis. Arch Intern Med 1992; 152:1273–1278.

13. Rasmussen BK, Jensen R, Olesen J. Impact of headache on sickness absence and utilisation of medical services: a Danish population study. J Epidemiol Community Health 1992; 46:443–446.

14. Edmeads J, Findlay H, Tugwell P, et al. Impact of migraine and tension-type headache on lifestyle, consulting behavior and medication use: a Canadian population survey. Can J Neurolog Sci 1993; 20:131–137.

15. Rasmussen BK, Jensen R, Schroll M, Olesen J. Interrelations between migraine and tension-type headache in the general population. Arch Neurol 1992; 49: 914–918.

16. Solomon GD. Circadian variation and the frequency of migraine. Cleveland Clin J Med 1992; 59:326–328.

17. Von Korff M, Ormel J, Keefe FJ, Dworkin SF. Grading the severity of chronic pain. Pain 1992; 50:133–149.

18. Celentano DD, Stewart WF, Lipton RB, Reed ML. Medication use and disability among migraineurs: a national probability sample survey. Headache 1992; 32:223–228.

19. Jacobson GP, Ramdan NM, Aggarwal S, Newman CW. The development of the headache disability inventory (abstract). Cephalalgia 1993; 13(suppl 13): 124(P66).

20. Von Korff M, Wagner EH, Dworkin SF, Saunders KW. Chronic pain and the use of ambulatory health care. Psychosom Med 1991; 53:61–79.
21. Stang PE, Yanagihara T, Swanson JW, Guess HA, O'Fallon WM, Beard CM, Melton LJ. The incidence of migraine headaches: A population-based study in Olmsted County, MN. Neurology 1992; 42:1657–1662.
22. Stewart WF, Linet MS, Celentano DD, et al. Age- and sex-specific incidence rates for migraine with and without visual aura. Am J Epidemiol 1991; 134:1111–1120.
23. Stewart WF, Lipton RB, Celentano DD, Reed ML. Prevalence of migraine headache in the US. JAMA 1992; 267:64–69.
24. Stang PE, Osterhaus JT. Impact of migraine in the United States: data from the National Health Interview Survey. Headache 1993; 33:29–35.
25. Turner LC, Molgaard C, Horvath, C, Rothrock J, Stang PE. Prevalence of migraine among Mexican-Americans in San Diego, California, USA: Survey II (abstract). VIth International Headache Congress Paris, August 26–29, 1993. Cephalalgia 1993; 13(suppl 13): 49(P6).
26. Molgaard C, Morton D, Stanford P, Turner LC, Rothrock J, Stang PE. Prevalence of migraine among Mexican-Americans in San Diego, California: Survey I (abstract). Headache 1993; 33:278–279.
27. Stewart WF, Lipton RB. Migraine headache: epidemiology and health care utilization. Cephalalgia 1993; 13(suppl 12):41–46.
28. Celentano DD, Stewart WF, Lipton RB. Race, socioeconomic status and migraine headache: social causation or social selection. In press.
29. Turner LC, Molgaard C, Horvath C, Rothrock J, Golbeck A, Stang PE. Neural shift theory of migraine: a case-control study (abstract). 1993 XVth World Congress of Neurology. Can J Neurolog Sci 1993; 20(suppl 4):S226.
30. D'Amico D, Leone M, Macciardi F, et al. Genetic transmission of migraine without aura: a study of 68 families. Ital J Neurolog Sci 1991; 12:581–584.
31. Russell M, Olesen J. The genetics of migraine without aura and migraine with aura. Cephalalgia 1993; 13:245–248.
32. Merikangas KR. Genetic epidemiology of migraine. In: Sandler M, Collins GM, eds. Migraine: A Spectrum of Ideas. New York: Oxford University Press, 1990:40–50.
33. Stang PE, Osterhaus JT, Celentano DD. Migraine: Patterns of health care utilization. Neurology. In press.
34. Blau JN, Drummond MF. Migraine. London: Office of Health Economics, 1991.
35. Chicoye A, Auray JP, Duru G, Lamure M, Michel P, Milan JJ, and the GRIM. The burden of migraine in France. Fifth International Conference on System Science in Health Care. Prague: Omnipress Publishing, 1992:1554–1559.
36. Osterhaus JT, Stang PE, Yanagihara T, Swanson JW, Beard CM, O'Fallon WM, Melton LJ. Use of diagnostic procedures associated with incident migraine headaches among Olmsted County, Minnesota residents 1979–1981. Presented at the International Society for Technology Assessment in Health Care, Vancouver, Canada, June 1992.

37. Osterhaus JT, Stang PE, Yanagihara T, Swanson JW, Beard CM, O'Fallon WM, Melton LJ. Prescription drug use of newly diagnosed migraine headache sufferers in Olmsted County, Minnesota (abstract). Neurology 1992; 42(suppl 31):260–261.

38. Rawlins E. Epidemiology of migraine. In: Proceedings of the European Headache Federation. Bremen, Germany: European Headache Federation, 1992:6.

39. Osterhaus JT, Gutterman DL, Plachetka JR. Health care resource use and lost labour costs of migraine headaches in the US. PharmacoEconomics 1992; 2(1):67–76.

40. McMillan JA, Martin BC, Jankel CA. Migraine-related utilization and costs in a Medicaid population. Presented at the Annual Meeting of Association for Health Services Research, Chicago, 1992.

41. Clouse JC, Osterhaus JT. Healthcare resource utilization by migraineurs in an HMO setting (abstract). Presented at the 27th Annual Meeting of the American Society of Hospital Pharmacists, Orlando, Florida, midyear meeting, 1992.

42. Edmeads J, Findlay H, Tugwell P, et al. Impact of migraine and tension-type headache on life-style, consulting behavior and medication use: a Canadian population survey. Can J Neurolog Sci 1993; 20:131–137.

43. Kaa KA, Carlson JA, Osterhaus JT. Emergency department and drug utilization by migraine and asthma patients in a Health Maintenance Organization (abstract). Presented at the 27th Annual Meeting of the American Society of Hospital Pharmacists, Orlando, Florida, midyear meeting, 1992.

44. Elixhauser A, Andrews RM, Fox S. Clinical classifications for health policy research: discharge statistics by principal diagnosis and procedure. Division of Providers Studies research note 17, Agency for Health Care Policy and Research publication 93-0043. Rockville, MD: Public Health Service, 1993.

45. Wells N. The cost of migraine to society. Poster presentation at the 1st International Conference of the European Headache Federation, Bremen, Germany, June 24–27, 1992.

46. Osterhaus JT, Townsend RJ, Gandek B, Ware JE. Burden of migraine headache measured in quality of life terms. Headache. In press.

47. Stewart AL, Greenfield S, Hays RD, et al. Functional status and well-being of patients with chronic conditions: results from the Medical Outcomes Study. JAMA 1989; 262(7):925–930.

48. Pryse-Phillips W, Findlay H, Tugwell P, et al. A Canadian population survey on the clinical, epidemiological and societal impact of migraine and tension-type headache. Can J Neurolog Sci 1992; 19:333–339.

49. Henry P, Michel P, Brochet B, et al. A nationwide survey of migraine in France: prevalence and clinical features in adults. Cephalalgia 1992; 12: 229–237.

50. Rasmussen BK, Jensen R, Schroll M, Olesen J. Epidemiology of headache in a general population—a prevalence study. J Clin Epidemiol 1991; 44:1147–1157.

51. Breslau N, Davis G. Migraine, major depression and panic disorder: a prospective epidemiologic study of young adults. Cephalalgia 1992; 12:85–90.

52. Merikangas KR, Risch NJ, Merikangas JR, Weissman MM, Kidd KK. Migraine and depression: association and familial transmission. J Psychiatr Res 1988; 22:119–129.
53. Stewart WF, Linet MS, Celantano DD. Migraine headaches and panic attacks. Psychosom Med 1989; 51:559–569.
54. Breslau N. Migraine, suicidal ideation, and suicide attempts. Neurology 1992; 42:392–395.
55. Breslau N, Davis G, Andreski P. Migraine, psychiatric disorders, and suicide attempts: an epidemiologic study of young adults. Psychiatry Res 1991; 37: 11–23.
56. Miller D, Waters DD, Warnica W, Szlachcic J, Kreeft J, Theroux P. Is variant angina the coronary manifestation of a generalized vasospastic disorder? N Engl J Med 1981; 304:763–766.
57. Merikangas KR. Comorbidity of migraine and other conditions in the general population of adults in the United States. Cephalalgia 1991; 11(suppl): 108–109.
58. Henrich JB, Horowitz RI. A controlled study of ischemic stroke risk in migraine patients. J Clin Epidemol 1989; 42:773–780.
59. Chen TC, Leviton A, Edelstein S, Ellenberg JH. Migraine and other diseases in women of reproductive age: the influence of smoking on observed observations. Arch Neurol 1987; 44:1024–1028.
60. Buring J, Herbert P, Manson J, et al. Migraine and risk of stroke in the Physician's Health Study (abstract). Am J Epidemiol 1991; 134:719.
61. Couch JR, Hassanein RS. Headache as a risk factor in atherosclerosis-related diseases. Headache 1989; 29:49–54.
62. Leviton A, Malvea B, Graham J. Vascular diseases, mortality, and migraine in the parents of migraine patients. Neurology 1974; 24:669–672.
63. Pfaffenrath V, Pollmann W, Autenrieth G, Rosmanith U. Mitral valve prolapse and platelet aggregation in patients with hemiplegic and non-hemiplegic migraine. Acta Neurol Scand 1987; 75:253–257.
64. Lanzi G, Grandi AM, Gamba G, Balottin U, Barzizza F, Longoni P, Fazzi E, Venco A. Migraine, mitral valve prolapse and platelet function in the pediatric age group. Headache 1986; 26:142–145.
65. Spence JD, Wong DG, Melendez LJ, Nichol PM, Brown JD. Increased prevalence of mitral valve prolapse in patients with migraine. Can Med Assoc J 1984; 131:1457–1460.
66. Rothrock JF, Dittrich H, Meyerhoff B, Swenson MR. Migraine, stroke, and mitral valve prolapse. Neurology 1988; 38:296.
67. Zahavi I, Chagnac A, Hering R, Davidovich S, Kuritzky A. Prevalence of Raynaud's Phenomenon in patients with migraine. Arch Intern Med 1984; 144:742–744.
68. O'Keeffe ST, Tsapatsaris NP, Beetham WP Jr. Increased prevalence of migraine and chest pain in patients with primary Raynaud disease. Ann Intern Med 1992; 116:985–989.

69. Chen TC, Leviton A. Asthma and eczema in children born to women with migraine. Arch Neurol 1990; 47:1227–1230.

70. Marcoux S, Berube S, Brisson J, Faboa J. History of migraine and risk of pregnancy-induced hypertension. Epidemiology 1992; 3:53–56.

71. Lipton RB, Ottman R. Co-morbidity of migraine and epilepsy (abstract). Neurology 1993; 43:A331.

72. Isenberg DA, Meyrick-Thomas D, Snaith ML, McKeran RO, Royston JP. A study of migraine in systemic lupus erythematosus. Ann Rheum Dis 1982; 41:30–32.

4

Impact of Migraine

Richard B. Lipton

*Albert Einstein College of Medicine
and Montefiore Medical Center
Bronx, New York*

Walter F. Stewart

*Johns Hopkins School of Public Health
Baltimore, Maryland*

INTRODUCTION

Integrating epidemiological studies with clinical observations of migraine provides primary-care physicians with a more comprehensive view of the disease state (16). By evaluating the scope, distribution, and care-seeking pattern of the migraine population, primary-care physicians can more effectively understand their role in headache care.

Most people with migraine are not seen within the health-care system (12). Population-based studies are therefore required to examine migraine prevalence, headache-related disability, and patterns of health-care utilization. These studies can help identify the reasons for which people consult or lapse from medical care for their headache disorders. They also portray the impact of migraine on the lives of individual sufferers.

A critical prelude to the study of migraine is the development of a reliable and valid case definition. The International Headache Society (IHS) criteria, published in 1988 (17), have provided a uniform case definition for epidemiological research. Although it is still being validated and extended (1,2,11,18–20,25), this case definition has been used widely in recent epidemiological studies in several countries (3–7).

In this chapter, we consider the scope and definition of the migraine problem, pattern of consultation, the impact of migraine on individuals and society, and treatment implications for primary-care physicians.

Migraine and other headache disorders inflict an enormous burden on individuals, which ultimately translates into direct and indirect costs to society. The magnitude of these costs provides one measure of the possible benefits of effective diagnosis and treatment. Analyzing the sources of the costs is an essential prelude to devising interventions that will limit them.

The societal impact of migraine is determined in part by its high prevalence and long duration of illness. The American Migraine Study (4,15) evaluated over 20,000 U.S. residents between the ages of 12 and 80, selected to be representative of the U.S. population. Estimates from this study indicate that there are more than 23 million Americans who currently have migraine, and that more than 11 million experience significant levels of headache-related disability.

Migraine typically begins in childhood or adolescence (8), and attacks often continue to occur throughout early adult life, middle age, and beyond (4–7). The fact that migraine attacks frequently recur for decades in large part explains its high prevalence (see Chapter 4). Clinic-based studies underestimate the prevalence of migraine because many people with severe headache are not diagnosed or treated (9,12).

As noted above, a significant proportion of headache sufferers experience frequent disabling attacks. But the impact of migraine is not limited to the time of attack. If attacks interfere with school performance, disrupted education may have serious long-term consequences. Missed work may lead to unemployment or underemployment. Family and social life, as well as psychological well-being, may be impaired. In evaluating the impact of migraine, all these factors must be taken into account.

The primary purpose of this review is to describe the extent of the migraine problem and its impact on society. By extension, we consider intervention strategies that may mitigate the impact of migraine. We begin with the epidemiology of migraine, describing the scope and distribution of the problem. We next consider the short- and long-term impact of migraine on the individual and the direct and indirect costs. Finally, we propose several intervention strategies.

SCOPE OF THE PROBLEM

Although migraine is a very common condition overall, its prevalence varies considerably by age and gender (4,15,36). Prevalence estimates range from 11 to 28% in females and from 5.3 to 19% in males (36). Prevalence also varies by age in both males and females, increasing from age 12 to 40 and falling thereafter (Figure 1) (15). The prevalence is highest between 25 and 55 years of age—and thus is most common during the years of peak productivity (15). Although data are limited, the incidence of migraine without aura peaks at about age 10 in boys and age 15 in girls (37). Because migraine sufferers begin to experience attacks early in life, headache-related disability may interfere with educational achievement for many people, setting up a lifetime of underachievement.

Migraine produces a broad array of symptoms that vary from attack to attack and among individuals (14). Migraine sufferers report that seeking pain relief is the main reason for medical consultation (6,13). Other

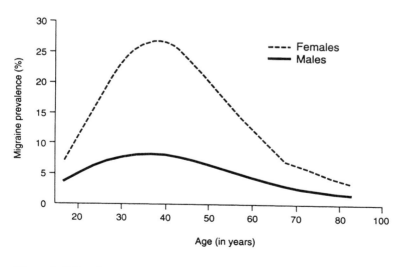

Figure 1 Migraine prevalence by age. Prevalence increased from 12 to 38 years of age in both females and males; the peak was considerably higher among females. (From Ref. 15.)

important aspects of the attack include pain location; sensitivity to movement, light, sound, and odors; and aura, nausea, and photophobia.

As a heterogeneous disorder, migraine produces varying degrees of disability (14). Figure 2 shows disability data from the American Migraine Study (4,15). In this study, people were asked about the impact of severe headaches on their ability to work, study, or enjoy life. About one-third of subjects reported severe disability or the need for bed rest. Over 85% of migraine sufferers reported at least some headache-related disability.

The impact of migraine on the individual is reflected by the frequency and degree of disability associated with the attacks (14). Among current migraine sufferers, 59% of females and 50% of males experience one or more attacks per month (4); 25% are struck by four or more severe attacks per month (4,15).

Severe attacks often interfere with daily activities, preventing the suffer from performing at home, work, or school (13). Pain may be exacerbated by routine physical activity (17); pain that is tolerable with bed rest may become excruciating with movement. For some, intractable nausea or

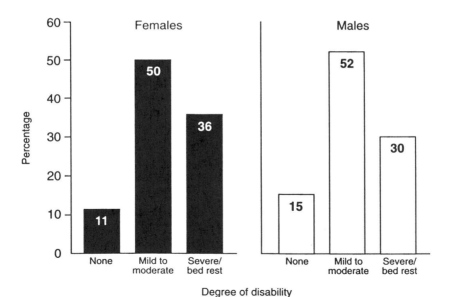

Figure 2 Gender-specific degree of disability for migraine. One-third reported severe disability. (From Ref. 15.)

vomiting may be as disabling as the pain. Sensitivity to light or sound may lead to restricted activity and limit social interaction. At times, the aura may impair vision or disrupt motor or somatosensory function. Thinking may become confused, disturbing efficiency and competency on the job or at home (13).

To obtain information about individual attacks, we asked subjects with migraine in Washington County, Maryland, specific questions about their most recent headache (14,29). Not surprisingly, as pain intensity increased, disability increased as well. Almost everyone with headache-related disability rated his pain as 5 or greater on a scale of 0 to 10 (14). There appears to be a pain threshold that must be exceeded before disability occurs—but many people with high pain intensity deny headache-related disability. Thus, moderate or even severe pain is not in and of itself always sufficient to cause disability.

The most painful headaches were more likely to be associated with nausea/vomiting, visual aura, numbness/tingling, and other neurological symptoms (14). Most people reported disability from symptom complexes; very few people reported disability from only a single feature of migraine or tension-type headache. The tendency of symptoms to occur together may account in part for the relationship between pain severity and disability. For example, in individual attacks, nausea was highly associated with visual and somatosensory aura. The disability of migraine may be determined by factors other than pain, such as attack duration, length of illness, and extent of social support.

An individual with disabling migraine may have to leave school, take a less demanding job, or actually lose a job because of an inability to function (13,14,22). Frustrated in their social roles, spouses may feel guilty about canceled plans. Parents may feel inadequate because they are at times unavailable to their children. When work is missed or plans are broken, migraine may not be accepted as a legitimate reason for failing to fulfill obligations. Others may consider the migraine sufferer weak or lazy rather than physically ill. Individuals selected for clinical trials who meet IHS criteria for migraine (27) often have significant dysfunction related to their illness. The development of appropriate measures of life disruption resulting from migraine is an area of active research.

SOCIOECONOMICS: CAUSE OR CONSEQUENCE

In the United States, data from the American Migraine Study (4,15) demonstrated that the prevalence of severe migraine is inversely related to household income. Figure 3 shows that the prevalence of migraine falls, in

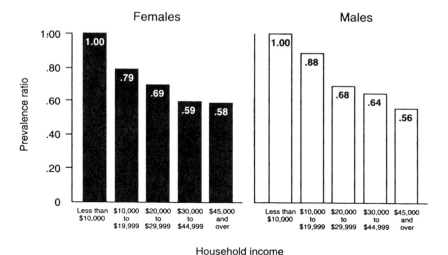

Figure 3 Prevalence ratio of migraine by income. Ratio decreased with increasing income. Ratio adjusted for age, race, and geographic location. (From Ref. 15.)

both males and females, as household income rises. For example, the prevalence ratio of 0.58 for females with household incomes greater than $45,000 per year indicates that the prevalence of migraine in the highest-income group is 58% of the prevalence of the lowest-income group. A similar relationship to household income has been reported using data from the National Health Interview Survey for low- and middle-income households (21).

There are two possible explanations for this notable association between income and migraine prevalence in the United States (4,15,22): social causation and social selection. A social-causation model suggests that conditions associated with low income—for example, the stress of low income, poor diet, or poor access to health care—might lead to a higher prevalence of migraine.

Conversely, in a social-selection model, frequent disabling migraine attacks and the resulting disruptions in education or work are seen as the cause of lower income. Over the course of their lifetime, migraine sufferers may drift downward economically. The social-selection hypothesis is supported by the observation that severe headaches are associated with higher levels of unemployment (23,24) and by the patterns of migraine prevalence in disadvantaged groups (22).

The social-causation and social-selection hypotheses are not mutually exclusive; both may contribute to the relationship between migraine and income. For example, if stress or exposure to dietary precipitants is greater in lower-income groups, both the incidence of new cases and the duration of illness may be greater. Low-income migraine sufferers, with poor access to medical care, may be more likely to misuse over-the-counter medication (9). If overuse of these remedies prolongs the duration of the disease through the mechanism of medication rebound (25,33) (see Chapter 5), migraine prevalence will be greater. In the higher-income groups, good access to health care may decrease the duration of illness through effective treatment.

While our understanding of the impact of migraine on individuals has improved substantially in the last decade, relatively little is known about the long-term effects of migraine on functional status and psychological well-being. Of special importance is impairment during attacks and its effect on productivity in the workplace. Longitudinal studies that assess the age of onset of migraine-related disability, the occurrence of comorbid conditions, and impairment of performance in the workplace would improve our understanding of the impact of migraine.

METHODS OF MEASURING ECONOMIC IMPACT

Health economists differ on the most appropriate methods for estimating the cost of illnesses such as migraine (26). A conservative approach focuses only on the direct costs, which consist primarily of medical-care expenditures. For migraine, this is likely to underestimate the true cost of disease, as many people with disabling migraine are not currently being appropriately diagnosed and treated. More importantly, this method fails to capture the indirect costs associated with missed work and leisure due to headache-related disability.

A second approach is to simply describe the epidemiology of the illness in terms of disability, pain, and diminished quality of life, without attempting to translate these consequences of the illness into economic terms. This approach does not provide the necessary quantitative information for a cost-benefit analysis of treatment. A third strategy is to capture the total cost of illness (COI). This type of assessment considers the directly measurable costs associated with medical care, the indirect costs associated with lost productivity, and the less tangible factors related to quality of life (26). COI studies go well beyond the usual measures of prevalence and disability and can help establish research and treatment priorities (26).

Quantification of indirect costs may be problematic (26). For example, these measures assign more importance to the suffering of high-income individuals than to that of low-income individuals. Moreover, it is not clear how best to assess a lost workday; its value may actually be less than the wages for that day, if other workers compensate for the absence or the migraine sufferer makes up the lost time through increased productivity or extra, unpaid work hours. On the other hand, the cost of impairment at work may exceed wages for the day, if, for example, a physician with migraine makes a serious diagnostic error or an assembly-line worker produces defective products.

Direct Costs

The cost of health care for migraine is difficult to estimate. In population-based studies that identify migraine sufferers based on reported symptoms, about one-third of migraineurs have received a medical diagnosis and most headache sufferers are not currently consulting physicians (9,10). In contrast, studies that utilize self-report to identify migraineurs find much higher rates of health-care use. At least three factors may contribute to this pattern. First, people who are aware that they have migraine may be more likely to utilize the health-care system. Second, people who consult physicians for headache may be more likely to receive and remember a specific headache diagnosis. Third, medically diagnosed cases experience higher levels of disability, providing a motive to seek and utilize health care (9).

For example, in a study that used self-reported diagnosis (21), about 85% of females and 77% of males sought medical attention for headache; high rates of care-seeking in this study may occur because migraineurs who had been diagnosed by a doctor were overrepresented in the migraine case group. In the American Migraine Study (10), 66% of sufferers had ever consulted a doctor for headache but only 16% of migraineurs were currently consulting a doctor for headache. In a study of migraineurs who participated in a clinical trial, almost 50% reported using emergency health-care services within 1 year of an interview (27). In a more representative sample, 19.5% of female and 13.4% of male migraineurs reported utilizing emergency services (28). In the study of clinical trial participants, the average cost of health care per migraine sufferer was $817 (27).

Indirect Costs

Migraine leads to substantial losses of productivity. Linet et al. (29) reported that 10.6% of females and 4.5% of males had missed all or part of a day of work or school because of headache (of any type) within the 4 weeks preceding a telephone interview. Two recent studies have used different methods to assess the economic cost of missed work. The first (27) used subjects with IHS migraine who participated in clinical trials. These subjects may not be representative of migraine sufferers in general, as participation in clinical trials may be associated with severe disease. The migraineurs in this study who missed work were absent an average of 2.2 workdays per month. Migraineurs went to work despite migraine symptoms that impaired their function another 5.8 days per month. Of the employed respondents in the study, 89% reported that migraine adversely affected their job performance.

Using data on migraine prevalence from the National Center for Health Statistics (NCHS), in this study the lost-labor cost due to migraine in the United States was estimated to be $5.6–17.2 billion per year. The NCHS figures for prevalence are low in comparison with those of population-based studies that ascertain migraine case status by direct interview. This might lead to an underestimation of economic impact. On the other hand, because participants in clinical trials were used, increased frequency and severity of attacks may lead to an overestimation of economic impact. It is difficult to determine how these factors interact.

In a second study (21), NCHS data were utilized to estimate both prevalence and disability. This study estimated that the cost of missed labor was $1.2 billion per year in the United States. This number is almost certainly an underestimate, for two reasons. First, only people who knew they had migraine were included, so may people with migraine were missed. Second, only employed individuals were included, so the cost of missed housework or schoolwork was not captured. Although the exact cost of missed work due to migraine is not known and more precise estimates would be useful, it is likely that the costs exceed $1.5 billion per year.

OPPORTUNITIES FOR TREATMENT AND IMPLICATIONS FOR PRIMARY CARE

With changes in the understanding of migraine have come opportunities to more effectively treat this disorder. New acute treatments rapidly relieve pain and restore normal function (30). To the list of effective preventive drugs, new agents such as divalproex sodium (31) and selective serotonin reuptake inhibitors (32) have shown promise. Perhaps even more importantly, emerging evidence suggests that misuse of some acute treatments may increase headache frequency and limit the benefits of prophylactic drugs (25,33). Avoiding medication overuse decreases medication costs, lessens side effects from polypharmacy, and improves outcome.

The effects of optimal treatment on the impact of migraine require further study. From an intuitive point of view, control of migraine pain should enhance quality of life, decrease work absenteeism, improve function at work, and decrease the use of emergency-department services. However, longitudinal studies demonstrating long-term benefits of treatment have not yet been completed, and they present challenging methodological problems.

To date, epidemiological studies reveal that migraine is a highly prevalent, underdiagnosed clinical disorder that has a significant impact on the lives of sufferers and on society in general. Efforts to improve the diagnosis and treatment of migraine must begin in the primary-care setting. Not only do most migraine sufferers seek help first from the primary-care physician, many others with migraine who do not consult for headache are evaluated for other problems in the primary-care setting.

The challenge to the busy primary-care physician is to identify and effectively treat the migraine sufferers who most need care. In a population-based study (29), 90% of males and 95% of females reported at least one unprovoked headache within the year preceding an interview. Because headache is a ubiquitous symptom, the question "Do you have headaches?" often elicits a long description of mild, tension-type headaches that respond well to over-the-counter medications and are of little consequence. Practitioners quickly learn not to ask about headache unless it is a chief complaint for the visit. Instead, we suggest asking a question more likely to identify headaches of consequence, for example, "Do you have headaches that interfere with your ability to work, study, or enjoy life?" An affirmative answer warrants further discussion, and the respondent will often benefit from medical care.

Tools are available to assist diagnostic screening for headache disorders in the primary-care setting, such as symptom checklists and diagnostic guides that identify features of secondary headaches and serve as aides to the diagnosis of migraine or other primary headache disorders. Self-administered measures of headache severity or headache impact can help identify the headache sufferers most in need of care (23,24,34). Within a diagnostic category, headaches span a range of pain intensity, disability, frequency, and duration (14). We are currently developing a self-administered Migraine Impact Measure intended for use in primary-care settings (34).

PUBLIC-HEALTH SIGNIFICANCE

The public-health significance of migraine has recently been reviewed (35). Several key features of migraine epidemiology underscore its significance as a public-health concern. Migraine is highly prevalent and underdiagnosed. Most migraineurs experience frequent severe attacks; 25% of female migraineurs have four or more severe attacks per month, 35% have one to three severe attacks per month, and 40% have one or fewer severe attacks per month (4,15). Male migraineurs experience a similar pattern. The attacks often cause disability and disrupt functional ability and, as reviewed, have a significant economic impact. Although there are many effective treatments available, future research must assess whether screening and treating migraine more aggressively will limit its impact in a cost-effective manner. For the practitioner, more effective treatment of migraine provides an important opportunity to limit pain and suffering and improve quality of life for individual patients.

REFERENCES

1. Lipton RB, Stewart WF, Merikangas K. Reliability in headache diagnosis. Cephalalgia 1993; 13(suppl 12):29–33.
2. Merikangas KR, Frances A. Development of diagnostic criteria for headache syndromes: lessons from psychiatry. Cephalalgia 1993; 13(suppl 12):34–38.
3. Rasmussen BK, Jensen R, Schroll M, Olesen J. Epidemiology of headache in a general population—a prevalence study. J Clin Epidemiol 1991; 44:1147–1157.
4. Stewart WF, Lipton RB, Celentano DD, Reed ML. Prevalence of migraine headache in the United States. JAMA 1992; 267:64–69.
5. Henry P, Michel P, Brochet B, Dartigues JF, Tison S, Salamon R. A nationwide survey of migraine in France: prevalence and clinical features in adults. Cephalalgia 1992; 12:229–237.
6. Pryse-Phillips W, Findlay H, Tugwell P, Edmeads J, Murray TJ, Nelson RF. A Canadian population survey on the clinical epidemiology and societal impact of migraine and tension-type headache. Can J Neurol Sci 1992; 19:333–339.
7. Breslau N, Davis GC. Migraine, physical health and psychiatric disorder: A prospective epidemiologic study in young adults. J Psychiatr Res 1993; 27:211–221.
8. Linet MS, Stewart WR. Migraine headache: epidemiologic perspectives. Epidemiol Rev 1984; 6:107–139.
9. Lipton RB, Stewart WF, Celentano DD, Reed ML. Undiagnosed migraine: a comparison of symptom-based and self-reported physician diagnosis. Arch Intern Med 1992; 152:1273–1278.
10. Lipton RB, Stewart WF. Health care use for migraine. 1994. Submitted.

11. Rasmussen BK, Jensen R, Olesen J. A population-based analysis of the diagnostic criteria of the International Headache Society. Cephalalgia 1991; 11: 129–134.
12. Stang P, Osterhaus JT. Healthcare utilization for migraine. Neurology 1994. In press.
13. Edmeads J, Findlay H, Tugwell P, et al. Impact of migraine and tension type headache on life-style, consulting behavior and medication use. Can J Neurol 1993; 20:131–137.
14. Stewart WF, Schecter A, Lipton RB. Migraine heterogeneity: disability, pain intensity, attack frequency and duration. Neurology 1994. In press.
15. Lipton RB, Stewart WF. Migraine in the United States: Epidemiology and health care use. Neurology 1993; 43(suppl 3):6–10.
16. Lipton RB, Silberstein SD, Stewart WF. An update on the epidemiology of migraine. Headache 1994. In press.
17. International Headache Society. Classification and diagnostic criteria for headache disorders, cranial neuralgias, and facial pain. Cephalalgia 1988; 8(suppl 7):1–96.
18. Ottoman R, Hong S, Lipton RB. Validity of family history data on severe headache and migraine. Neurology 1993; 43:154–160.
19. Granella E, D'Alessandro R, Mazoni GC, et al. Inter-observer reliability of the IHS classification for primary headaches. Presented at the 9th Migraine Trust International Symposium, 1992. Abstracts, pp. 4–5.
20. Solomon S, Lipton RB, Newman LC. Evaluation of chronic daily headache comparison to criteria for chronic tension-type headache. Cephalalgia 1992; 12:365–368.
21. Stang PE, Osterhaus JT. Impact of migraine in the United States: data from the National Health Interview Survey. Headache 1993; 33:29–35.
22. Celentano DD, Stewart WF, Lipton RB. Race, socio-economic status and migraine headache: Social causation or social selection. 1994. Submitted.
23. Von Korff M, Ormel J, Keefe F, Dworkin SF. Grading the severity of chronic pain. Pain 1992; 50:133–149.
24. Von Korff M, Stewart WF, Lipton RB. Assessing headache severity: New directions. Neurology 1994. In press.
25. Silberstein SD, Lipton RB, Solomon S, Mathew NT. Classification of daily and near daily headaches. Proposed revisions to IHS criteria. Headache 1994; 34:1–7.
26. DeLissovoy G, Lazarus SS. The economic cost of migraine: The present state of knowledge. Neurology 1993. In press.
27. Osterhaus JT, Gutterman DL, Plachetka JR. Headache resources and lost labour costs of migraine headaches in the U.S. Pharmacoeconomics 1992; 2:67–76.
28. Celentano DD, Stewart WF, Lipton RB, Reed ML. Medication use and disability among migraineurs: A national probability sample. Headache 1992; 32:223–228.
29. Linet MS, Stewart WF, Celentano DD, Siegler D, Sprecher M. An epidemiologic study of headache among adolescents and young adults. JAMA 1989; 261:2211–2216.

30. Cady RK, Wendt JK, Kirchner JR, Sargent JD, Rothrock JF, Skaggs H. Treatment of acute migraine with sumatriptan. JAMA 1991; 265:2831–2835.
31. Saper J, Mathew NT, Silberstein S, et al. Safety and efficacy of divalproex sodium in the prophylaxis of migraine headache. Neurology 1993; 43:401.
32. Adly C, Straumanis J, Chesson A. Fluoxetine prophylaxis in migraine. Headache 1992; 32:101–104.
33. Mathew NT. Transformed migraine. Cephalalgia 1993; 13(suppl 12):78–83.
34. Lipton RB, Amatniek J, Ferrari MD, Gross M. Migraine: identifying and removing barriers to care. Neurology 1994. In press.
35. Ziegler DK. Headache: Public health importance. Neurology 1990; 8:781–791.
36. Stewart WF, Simon D, Schecter A, Lipton RB. Population variation in migraine prevalence: A meta-analysis. J Clin Epidemiol 1994. In press.
37. Stewart WF, Linet MS, Celentano DD, Van Natta M, Ziegler D. Age- and sex-specific incidence rates of migraine with and without visual aura. Am J Epidemiol 1991; 34:111–1120.

5

Migraine Transformation and Chronic Daily Headache

Ninan T. Mathew

Baylor College of Medicine
and Houston Headache Clinic
Houston, Texas

INTRODUCTION

Chronic daily headache (CDH) is a widespread clinical problem, but little data are available as to the actual incidence and prevalence of this disorder. Approximately 40% of patients seen in the major headache clinics fall under the category of CDH. Various other terms have been given to this condition, including chronic tension headache, migraine with interparoxysmal headache (MIH), transformed migraine, evolutive migraine, mixed headache syndrome, and tension-vascular headache.

Traditionally, migraine and tension-type headache have been considered distinct entities. It was assumed that distinct peripheral mechanisms are involved in the pathogenesis of these two conditions, namely, vasculature in migraine and musculature in tension-type headache. Historically, clinicians have used the term chronic tension headache to characterize low-grade daily or almost-daily chronic headache disorder that is without migrainous features and clearly and not necessarily associated with provocation by stress or other emotional factors. Based on the old concept, it was traditional to diagnose any non-descript daily or near-daily headache as "tension headache." Increasing clinical opinion supports the view that migraine and tension headaches are physiologically related entities with a wide spectrum of clinical expression, which may reflect a complex interaction of central (neurotransmitter centers of the brain), cephalic vascular, and myogenic elements.

The dichotomy between the tension headache and migraine has been challenged by observations of various authors (1–3), which led Raskin and Appenzeller (4) to describe primary headache disorders as a "clinical continuum," with classic migraine at one end of the spectrum and chronic tension headache on the other end. The concept of transformation of episodic migraine into a CDH was first introduced in 1982 (5). Thirty-nine percent of patients seen at the Houston Headache Clinic were found to suffer from CDH. Based on clinical history, various categories of CDH are recognized. Table 1 shows the common varieties of CDH. Table 2 shows the breakdown of CDH from the literature.

MIGRAINE, CHRONIC TENSION-TYPE HEADACHE COMPLEX

Overlap among the clinical features of migraine and chronic tension-type headache (CTH) and the coexistence of these two conditions are well accepted. In large clinical populations, patients with CTH that meets the IHS criteria (6) form only a small proportion of those with CDH (Table 2).

Table 1 Classification of Chronic Daily Headache (CDH)

1. Chronic tension-type (CTH)

2. Migraine, chronic tension-type headache complex
   A. Transformed migraine
      Drug-induced
      Non-drug-induced
   B. Evolved from tension-type
      Drug-induced
      Non-drug-induced

3. New daily persistent headache (NDPH)

4. Posttraumatic headache

Table 2 Breakdown of Types of CDH

Authors	Total cases	Sex (%) Male	Sex (%) Female	Chronic tension-type (CTH)	Migraine tension-type headache complex Transformed migraine	Migraine tension-type headache complex Evolved from tension-type
Mathew et al., 1987 (7)	630	26	74	84 (14%)	487 (77%)	57 (9%)
Manzoni et al., 1987 (8)	250	24	76	57 (22.8%)	178 (71.2%)	8 (3.2%)
Manzoni et al., 1991 (9)	58	11	89	4 (7%)	44 (75%)	9 (15.5%)
Solomon et al., 1992 (10)[a]	100	28	72	66 (66%)[b]	34 (34%)[c]	—

[a]Reported that the majority evolved from migraine, but no figures given. Pointed out the need for separate classification for CDH.
[b]Met IHS criteria for CTH.
[c]Met IHS criteria for migraine.

The rest, the majority, are patients who exhibit a different category of mixed migraine, CTH syndrome, with different natural history, clinical profile, and perpetuating factors.

Transformed Migraine

The term transformed migraine was first introduced in 1987 by Mathew et al. (7) to describe a common, daily or near-daily headache condition that characterized 77% of their CDH patients. In two separate series Manzoni et al. (8,9) reported that 71 and 75%, respectively, of their patients transformed their headaches into a chronic daily pattern from a distinct pattern. Solomon et al. (10) also recognized chronic daily headaches, and mentioned that the majority of their 100 cases transformed from episodic migraine, although actual percentages were not given.

Typically the patient gives a history of distinct attacks of migraine with or without aura starting in the teens or early twenties, which eventually become more frequent. In addition, they develop interparoxysmal tension-type headache which also become more frequent, eventually leading to a daily or near-daily headache. Women in this group may show definite exacerbations of their migraine perimenstrually. Many of the headaches retain certain characteristics of migraine while others are indistinguishable from chronic tension-type. Patients may suffer from a migraine one day and a tension-type headache the next.

Manzoni et al. (8,9) analyzed the evolutionary pattern of transformed migraine (Table 3). It should be noted that the majority maintained migraine attacks in addition to developing tension-type headache daily or near daily. Others did not fit the temporal profile of migraine, but developed continuous headache with many migrainous features. In general, the transformed-migraine group showed a higher incidence of family history of headache, more neurological and GI symptoms, aggravation during menstruation, and relief during pregnancy compared to patients with other forms of daily headaches, particularly CTH.

In our series of 489 patients with transformed migraine, 444 (90.8%) had episodic migraine without aura to start with, and the rest (9.2%) had migraine with aura (7). There were 21 cases in whom we could document the transformation from migraine with aura to migraine without aura, and then to CDH. In patients with established CDH, there were instances where they had attacks of migraine with aura even though most of the severe headaches were migraine without aura.

In transformed migraine, severe headaches tended to be predominantly unilateral in 58% of patients and predominantly frontal or frontotemporal in 54% of patients. The chronic low-grade headaches also tended to be on the same side and at the same site as the severe headaches.

Table 3 Natural History of Transformed Migraine

Manzoni et al., 1987 (7); N = 178	118/178	Maintained migraine attacks and developed interparoxysmal tension-type headache Frequency of migraine was more than 1/week in only 35 patients
	60/178	Lost the distinct migraine attacks and developed either a "steady" (41) or a "fluctuating" (19) pattern
Manzoni et al., 1991 (8); N = 44	28/44	Maintained migraine attacks and developed interparoxysmal tension-type headache
	16/44	Lost the distinct migraine attacks and developed a continuous headache which exhibited most of the features of migraine, except the temporal profile

Migraine, Chronic Tension-Type Headache Complex Evolved from Episodic Tension-Type Headache

A relatively small percentage of patients in the migraine, CTH headache complex give a history of evolution of the chronic headache from episodic tension-type headache (Table 2). The figures varied from 3 to 15%. The frequency of headaches with migrainous features is significantly less in this group compared to transformed migraine. Manzoni et al. (9) also found a subset of patients who developed CDH from the onset, without a history of previous migraine or tension-type headache.

Transformational Factors

Table 4 lists the probable factors that influence transformation of episodic headaches to chronic daily form. Analgesic/ergotamine overuse, comorbidity such as depression, anxiety, abnormal personality profile, and stress appear to top the list. Drug-induced and non-drug-induced varieties are clearly identifiable. There may be a group of patients who evolve into a chronic daily headache spontaneously, as a course in the natural history of

Table 4 Probable Factors in the Development of CDH from Episodic Headache (%)

	Mathew et al., 1982 (5); N = 80	Manzoni et al., 1987 (8); N = 250	Manzoni et al., 1991 (9); N = 58	Solomon et al., 1992 (10); N = 100
Analgesic/ergotamine overuse	52	59	67	50
Abnormal personality profile including depression	70.5	—	39.7	—
Stress	67	22	44	—
Traumatic life events	13	9	—	—
Hypertension	10	1.5	3.8	—
Nonheadache medications including sex hormones	—	1.5	3.8	—
Percentage with identifiable factors	—	78	—	—
Percentage without any identifiable factors	—	22	—	—

the disease. Manzoni et al. (9) reported that in 22% of patients no apparent transformational factors could be found.

CHRONIC TENSION-TYPE HEADACHE

In our experience, chronic tension-type headaches form the second major group of CDH. Diagnostic criteria for CTH is well described in the new international headache classification (6) (Table 5). Two clinical types of chronic tension-type headache may be recognized: those associated with pericranial muscle tenderness and/or increased electromyogram (EMG) level and those without pericranial muscle tenderness and with normal EMG level. Those with muscle disorder show tenderness of the cervical muscle as well as the pericranial muscles. There is usually a correlation between pericranial muscle tenderness and tenderness of paravertebral muscles of the thoracic and lumbar regions, indicating a generalized muscle problem in them. However, there is no evidence that it is related to fibromyalgia.

Schoenen et al. (11) measured the pericranial EMG levels, pressure pain thresholds, and exteroceptive silent periods (ES$_2$) in 32 patients with CTH. Twenty-three (72%) were classified as CTH with disorder of the pericranial muscles (2:2:1 of IHS classification) and nine (28%) as CTH unassociated with disorder of pericranial muscles (2:2:2 of IHS classification). There was no correlation between the pericranial muscle abnormalities and severity of headache, anxiety, response to biofeedback therapy, or duration of ES$_2$, thereby indicating that the division of the disorder into two subtypes may be artificial. Pericranial EMG is of no pathogenetic, diagnostic, or prognostic significance, and the significance

Table 5 Chronic Tension-Type Headache: Diagnostic Criteria

A. Average headache frequency ≥15 days/month (180 days/year) for ≥6 months fulfilling criteria B–D listed below.
B. At least two of the following pain characteristics:
    1. Pressing/tightening quality
    2. Mild or moderate severity (may inhibit but does not prohibit activities)
    3. Bilateral location
    4. No aggravation by walking stairs or similar routine physical activity
C. Both of the following:
    1. No vomiting
    2. No more than one of the following: nausea, photophobia, or phonophobia

of increased pericranial muscle tenderness is not clear. On the other hand, pericranial/muscle tenderness may be found in migraine and mixed migraine/tension-type headache (migraine 17%, mixed headache 41%, and tension-type 63%) (12).

Sometimes, episodic tension-type headache transforms into the chronic variety. The others start out as a chronic variety with no change in character. Headaches are usually diffuse, bilateral, and pressing/tightening in quality and mild to moderate in severity. The posterior aspects of the head and neck are involved in the majority. Rarely, any one of the following symptoms may occur: photophobia, phonophobia, or mild nausea. Vomiting is not a feature of chronic tension-type headache. In an epidemiological study undertaken in Denmark, Rasmussen et al. (13) reported that the severity of tension-type headache increased significantly with its frequency. Therefore, CTH tends to be more severe than the episodic variety. Tension-type headaches in migraine sufferers were significantly more frequent and severe in Rasmussen and colleagues' survey of the general population (13). They found the prevalence of CTH in males

Table 6 Comparison of Features of Transformed Migraine and Chronic Tension-Type Headache

Transformed migraine	CTH
Headache: >15 days/month, 180 days/year	Headache: >15 month, 180/year
Previous history of distinct migraine attacks	No history of distinct migraine attacks
Increased incidence of headache in family	Positive family history less prominent
Retains migrainous characters to a significant degree, intermittently or continuously	Migrainous features absent or very insignificant
Increased neurological and GI symptoms	Neurological and GI symptoms minimal
Menstrual aggravation	No particular aggravation during menstruation
More relief during pregnancy	Less relief during pregnancy
Excessive intake of analgesics	Excessive intake of analgesics
Responds to antimigraine therapy	Response to antimigraine therapy occurs, but less striking
Behavioral and psychological factors prominent	Behavioral and psychological factors prominent

to be 2% and in females 5%. Table 6 compares and contrasts the CTH with transformed migraine.

NEW DAILY PERSISTENT HEADACHE (NDPH)

It is not uncommon to see patients who give a history of a fairly rapid onset of a persistent headache that continues on a daily basis (14). These patients do not have a history of a previous migraine or tension-type headache, nor do they give a history of trauma or psychological stress. The patients may distinctly remember the "onset event" or the day or time when the headache started. Epstein-Barr virus–induced immune changes have been implicated as an etiological factor (15). In an unpublished series of NDPH we found serological evidence of active Epstein-Barr viral infection in nine of 10 cases. Other features of chronic fatigue syndrome are seen in only a few. Whether the headache is a monosymptomatic manifestation seen in association with serological evidence of Epstein-Barr viral infection is not clear. The disease is usually self-limiting, but it is not uncommon to see patients continuing to have daily headache for a long period of time. Follow-up of these patients is not adequate to have any reliable data as to the ultimate prognosis. Further research is needed.

BEHAVIORAL AND PSYCHOGENIC ABNORMALITIES IN CDH

The question of whether CTH unassociated with pericranial muscle disorder should be considered psychogenic has not been settled. Bakal and Kaganow (16) reported that CTH patients with low EMG values also experienced more diffuse, nonspecific pain. They may also show other features of psychogenic pain (APA DSM-III 1980) such as "systematic time pattern," as evidenced by such statements as "my pain usually starts at the same time every day."

CTH patients exhibit more anxiety and depression than normal controls, and significantly greater repressed anger (17). They had more life events, higher inadequacy, social inadequacy, and "injuredness" (criticism and distrust of others) (18).

Depression and Type-A Behavior Scales

The scores of CDH patients on behavioral scales including the Zung Depression Scale (19), the Beck Depression Scale (20), and type A behavior pattern as measured by Friedman and Rosenman (21) are tabulated in

Table 7 Scores on Behavioral Scales in CDH

Type of CDH	Zung Depression Scale	Beck Depression Scale	Type A behavior pattern (Friedman and Rosenman)
Chronic tension-type headache ($N = 84$)	53 ± 9.9^a	11 ± 8.6^a	42 ± 4.7
Transformed migraine ($N = 489$)	52 ± 10.8^a	13 ± 10.3^a	50 ± 9.2^a
Control			
Episodic common migraine ($N = 100$)	34 ± 4.2	8 ± 2.4	42 ± 4.8

$^a p < 0.01$.
Source: Modified from Ref. 7.

Table 7. It should be noted that CDH patients (both CTH and transformed-migraine groups) showed significantly higher depression scores compared to episodic-migraine patients. In addition, transformed-migraine patients had elevated type A behavioral pattern scores (21).

MMPI Scales

The MMPI profile types (cluster membership) have no specificity for headache types and do not discriminate CTH from other chronic headaches (22,23). All chronic headache groups show considerable abnormality in the MMPI profile (23).

Based on the MMPI, an abnormal personality profile was found in 61% of patients with CDH compared to 12.2% of patients in the episodic-migraine group ($p < 0.01$). Fifty-six percent of patients showed elevations of scales I (hyperchondriasis), II (depression), and III (hysteria), with the majority showing a typical V configuration. Thus, "neuroticism" was found to be significantly higher in CDH patients. There was no statistical difference between the various types of CDH. Twenty-one percent also showed various combinations of elevated scores of 6, 7, 8, and 9. Such scores were more often seen in the most persistent and intractable cases.

EXCESSIVE USE OF SYMPTOMATIC MEDICATIONS IN CDH

The CDH group, in general, overused symptomatic medications. Seventy-three percent of the CDH patients used excessive amounts of analgesics, sedative/caffeine/analgesic combinations, or ergotamine on a daily basis. The use of daily symptomatic medication is more common in patients with transformed migraine (87.2%) than in those with CTH (67%) (7). There are two groups of patients in the transformed-migraine type of CDH: one in whom there is clear-cut excessive use of symptomatic medications and another, smaller group whose headache is unrelated to excessive use of medications. In the latter group, it appears to be a natural transformation of an episodic migraine to a chronic daily problem.

Withdrawal of daily symptomatic medications, the institution of a low-tyramine, low-caffeine diet, the initiation of prophylactic antimigraine therapy, and biofeedback and behavioral therapy caused significant improvement in 76% of CDH patients followed for a 6-month period (7). Based on these data and our previous experience (5), we proposed that the majority of CDH patients represent a continuum of the migraine process, influenced and perpetuated by a number of factors such as excessive use of symptomatic medications, abnormal personality profile, depression, stress, and traumatic life events (Figure 1). We further proposed that the diagnosis of a separate entity of tension-type headache

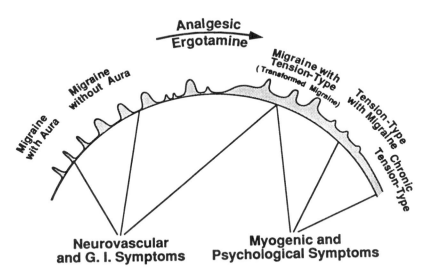

Figure 1 Graphic representation of migraine, tension-type headache spectrum. Frequent analgesic/ergotamine use may transform episodic migraine into chronic headache. Neurovascular and GI symptoms are more common in episodic headache, whereas myogenic and psychological symptoms are prominent in the chronic varieties.

is not justified in these patients under those circumstances, as the underlying biological abnormality appears to be common to both entities.

DRUG-INDUCED HEADACHE

It is obvious from clinical observations that some of the symptomatic
medications used for immediate relief of headache may in fact perpetuate
headaches, if used frequently in excessive quantities. Two main forms of
drug-induced headache occur as a result of medications used for headache
relief: analgesic-rebound headache and ergotamine-rebound headache.

Analgesic-Rebound Headache

The fact that analgesics may increase the tendency for headache and
perpetuate chronic headache was recognized in the early 1980s. Kudrow
(24) studied the paradoxical effect of frequent analgesic use in 200 patients
with daily headaches. He found that the analgesic overusers treated with
amitriptyline had a mean improvement of only 30% if they continued to
use analgesics, compared to 72% in those who stopped their analgesics.
Isler (25) studied 235 migraine patients who were overusing analgesics
at the rate of 30 or more tablets per month; many were also taking
ergotamine. He found that these patients had twice as many headache
days per month as those who took fewer than 30 tablets. He concluded
that their chronic headaches were a direct consequence of overuse of
medications designed for acute relief; restriction of these medications to
once per day or less was recommended.

Rapoport et al. (26) studied the question of analgesic rebound in 70
patients with daily headaches who were consuming 14 or more analgesic
tablets per week. Sixty-six percent of the sample improved considerably 1
month after discontinuing their analgesics, and a total of 81% were significantly improved at the end of the second month. Maximum improvement was shown in those who were given either cyproheptadine or
amitriptyline after discontinuing analgesics. Dichgans et al. (27) observed
the effects of abrupt withdrawal of mixed analgesics in 52 patients with
chronic headaches. The patients developed withdrawal symptoms but
later improved markedly for long periods of time.

Table 8 lists the common daily symptomatic or immediate-relief
medications consumed by a group of 200 patients (28) with chronic daily
headache. Table 9 shows the pattern of consumption of these medications;
22% of patients took more than three or more preparations concomitantly.
The prescription medications that were most commonly overused for

Table 8 Daily Symptomatic or Immediate-Relief Medications

Medications	No. of tablets per week		Patients	
	Average	Range	No.	%
Butalbitol/aspirin or acetaminophen/caffeine with or without codeine	30	14–86	84	42
Natural or synthetic codeine-containing preparations	28	10–84	80	40
Aspirin or acetaminophen with caffeine	42	14–108	50	25
Ergotamine with or without phenobarbital	15 mg	6–42 mg	44	22
Acetaminophen	52	15–105	34	17
Propoxyphene	26	14–56	32	16
Nasal decongestants and antihistamines	14	6–30	24	12
Aspirin	28	10–64	8	4

Source: Ref. 28.

immediate relief were those containing butalbital, caffeine, and an analgesic combination with or without codeine. Many patients combined ergotamine with analgesics or analgesic/sedative/caffeine combinations.

Clinical Features

The characteristic features of analgesic-rebound headaches are a self-sustaining, rhythmic headache-medication cycle characterized by daily or near-daily headache, and an irresistible and predictable use of pain

Table 9 Pattern of Consumption of Symptomatic Medications

No. of preparations of symptomatic medications consumed concomitantly	Patients ($N = 200$)	
	No.	%
1	70	35
2	86	43
3	44	22

Source: Ref. 28.

medication as the only means of relieving headache attacks. The other characteristics are varying severity, location, and type of headache. It has a tendency to be precipitated by the slightest physical or intellectual effort. Most of the time, it is difficult to distinguish it from the primary headache disorders—such as tension and migraine—for which the medications are consumed. The majority of those with a history of migraine exhibit some of the features of migraine during some of the daily headache attacks, although they rarely show the typical and distinct pattern of migraine attacks. Drug-induced headache can be throbbing. Accompanying symptoms are very striking in drug-induced headache and include asthenia, nausea, restlessness, irritability, memory problems and difficulty in intellectual concentration, and behavioral abnormalities such as depression and neurotic behavioral patterns.

Sleep Abnormalities Difficulty in initiating and maintaining sleep and early-morning awakening with severe headaches are very common in patients with analgesic-rebound headaches. This was observed in 71% of our patients (28). Predictable early-morning (between 2:00 and 6:00 A.M.) headache occurred in 46%. There is usually a correlation between predictable early-morning headache and high intake of butalbital, caffeine, or ergotamine. The majority of patients would take their analgesic or ergotamine tablets in the early-morning hours when they woke up with a headache in order to get some relief.

Tolerance Tolerance to symptomatic medications including analgesics, analgesic sedatives, caffeine preparations, narcotics, nasal decongestants, and vasoconstrictor analgesic combinations such as isometheptene mucate (Midrin) develops, resulting in gradually increasing frequency of consumption and total quantity of medications. Analgesic medications may be consumed in anticipation of headache or long before the actual attack occurs. Fear of an impending severe headache leads to unnecessary consumption of symptomatic medications. This phenomenon is not the fault of the patient—there is no reliable way for a patient to predict which of the minor headaches will lead to a severe episode.

Withdrawal Headache and Related Symptoms Abrupt cessation of analgesics may result in increased intensity of headache, accompanied by nausea, abdominal cramps, diarrhea, restlessness, sleeplessness, and mental anguish. These symptoms are especially common in patients who consume butalbital and caffeine/analgesic combinations. Seizures have been reported in certain instances. Increased headache intensity may start within 24 to 48 hours, and in most cases it may subside in 5 to 7 days.

Headache Improvement After Withdrawal of Analgesics The most striking feature of analgesic-rebound headache is the continued improvement in headache frequency and severity, general well-being, and reduction in irritability, depression, and lethargy after the initial withdrawal period is over. In our series of 200 patients, mere discontinuation of symptomatic medications resulted in 52% improvement in the headache index (28). Addition of prophylactic medications, after discontinuation of daily analgesics, resulted in a 78% improvement over a 12-week period.

Concomitant Prophylactic Agents From our study (28), it is clear that daily excessive symptomatic medications nullify the beneficial effects of concomitant prophylactic agents. Of our 200 patients, 58 used prophylactic antimigraine medications such as beta-blockers, calcium channel blockers, methysergide, and tricyclic antidepressants in different combinations. Yet they continued to have daily headache. Withdrawal of daily symptomatic medication enhanced the effect of prophylactic medications in this series of patients.

The striking clinical features by which one suspects analgesic-rebound headache are the occurrence of daily headache in spite of taking large quantities of pain medications and the fact that the daily headaches are relieved temporarily, only by the medication in question. There are some patients whose headaches are controlled well with a regular dose of analgesic medication, and, as long as they take the medication, they do not suffer from daily headaches. Without the presence of daily predictable headache, diagnosis of analgesic rebound is not valid.

Ergotamine-Rebound Headache and Dependency

Modern therapeutic use of ergotamine goes back to the 1930s. In 1955, Lippman (29) characterized the ergotamine-rebound headache as a dull, daily, usually constant head pain resulting from prolonged use of ergotamine derivatives. Acute migraine would result if ergotamine was withheld. Although a number of papers appeared subsequently on this important subject, the practicing physicians were not widely aware of its clinical significance. Saper and Jones (30) presented evidence in support of ergotamine-rebound headache as a state of dependency on ergotamine tartrate. Invariably, there is a predictable headache/medication cycle occurring with a background of daily or near daily use of ergotamine. These headaches are promptly relieved by ergotamine, which is characteristically the only means of headache relief. Frequently, usage exceeds natural frequency of migraine. Frequency of migraine is variable, with an irregular pattern of occurrence that may vary from month to month and week to week. In its natural state, migraine rarely occurs more than once or twice a week, and usually considerably less. Ergotamine-rebound headache has an unnatural frequency and usually occurs daily or near-daily.

All cases reported in the literature show an increasing pattern of usage of ergotamine, and weekly total dosage frequently exceeds safety limitations. In the majority of cases, weekly doses exceed 10 mg, with some patients taking as many as 10 to 15 mg per day. Surprisingly, peripheral ischemia, and other signs of ergotism (31), are rarely exhibited by these patients. Therefore, ergotamine rebound should be distinguished from ergotamine toxicity.

Discontinuation of ergotamine invariably results in a predictable, protracted, and extremely debilitating headache accompanied by nausea, vomiting, at times diarrhea, and other physical and mental complaints. Restlessness and sleeplessness are not uncommon. This withdrawal headache usually starts within 72 hours following discontinuation of the drug and may last for another 72 or more hours once the headache begins. Spontaneous improvement after discontinuation of medication is common. The prophylactic medications that previously have been largely without benefit become more effective when ergotamine is discontinued.

How To Recognize Ergotamine Rebound Headache

In patients with ergotamine headache, a migraine type of headache occurs on an almost-daily basis. As the effect of previous doses of ergotamine wanes, the headache gradually escalates until the next dose of ergotamine is taken. As time passes, psychological dependency on ergotamine intensifies, and patients take ergotamine in anticipation of headache. Sleep disturbances and depression also occur. The headache itself is strikingly sensitive to ergotamine but will generally not respond to alternative symptomatic or preventive medications that would otherwise be expected to have beneficial effect. Because migraine is characteristically a variable disorder rarely occurring more than once or twice a week, a migraine-like headache occurring more than two to three times a week that is selectively responsive to ergotamine while refractive to other symptomatic or preventive medications should alert the physician to the possible presence of ergotamine-rebound headache. Anticipation of headache and resulting apprehension lead to use of ergotamine even before a headache attack occurs. Other patients may attempt to treat low-grade headaches with ergotamine, resulting in excessive use. Also, patients, heeding the advice of their physicians to take ergotamine as early as possible in the course of headache, tend to use ergotamine before the exact nature of the headache or its full manifestations become apparent. All this leads to excessive and frequent use of ergotamine.

Critical Dose for Rebound Headache: How Much Is Too Much?

There are no clear data on the subject of a critical dose of analgesics or ergotamine in migraine. In clinical practice, one may see an occasional patient develop a drug-induced chronic daily headache taking 0.5 to 1 mg of ergotamine four or five times per week or one or two tablets per day of butalbital/caffeine/analgesic combination. But the majority of patients with chronic drug-induced headache far exceed the above dosage.

The question of a critical dose was studied by Sholz et al. (32), who concluded that the daily "dosage at risk" for ergotamine is between 3 and 4 mg. Many clinicians believe that frequency of usage of ergotamine is more critical and do not recommend its use for more than two times per week. Sholz et al. (32) also reported that acetaminophen and salicylic acid may have a critical daily dosage, 1000 mg per day. It should be noted that Rapoport et al. (26) found analgesic headache in their patients who were consuming aspirin or acetaminophen alone. Although Sholz et al. (32) were not able to come up with a critical level for barbiturate (most of the preparations contain a short-acting barbiturate such as butalbital), most of their patients were taking 500 mg or more per day. Whether or not chronic daily intake or critical single cumulative dosage plays the crucial role remains to be clarified.

MECHANISMS OF CHRONIC HEADACHES INCLUDING DRUG-INDUCED HEADACHE

Clinical observations and laboratory findings indicate that the traditional concepts of migraine pain as vascular in origin and tension-type headache pain as myogenic is inadequate to explain the complexities of chronic headache, especially chronic daily headache. It is well documented (34–37) that myogenic nociceptive mechanisms operate in migraine patients as well as patients with tension-type headache. Conversely, patients with chronic tension-type headache often develop migraine-like episodes (38). The presence of interictal nondescript headaches in approximately 50% of patients with migraine (34), and the transformation of episodic migraine into chronic daily headache (5), indicate that relative dominance of vascular and myogenic mechanisms may vary from time to time in chronic headaches.

A great deal of evidence has accumulated in recent years of the occurrence of a central (usually facilitating) mechanism in both migraine and tension-type headache (39,40). In migraine, central serotonergic neurotransmission may be perturbed, resulting in an increased firing rate of dorsal raphe nuclei (DRN), which have important ascending projections to the visual cortex, subcortical structures such as suprachiasmatic nuclei of hypothalamus and retina (39,41). A central factor in tension-type headache was demonstrated by Schoenen et al. (40), when they reported diminished or absent exteroceptive silent periods (ES$_2$) in the temporal and masseter muscles of patients with chronic tension-type headache, indicating a lack of inhibition by the brain stem inhibitory interneurons on the myogenic nociceptive mechanisms.

Experimental studies have shown a convergence of somatovisceral afferents upon trigeminal nucleus caudalis neurons and upper cervical spinal cord with projection onto thalamus (42). Trigeminal nucleus caudalis neurons are affected by descending inhibitory influences as well as facilitatory influences. The so-called "on-cells" in the ventromedial medulla facilitate nociceptive reflex responses such as "tail-flick response," and probably exert similar effects on cephalic areas (43). Trigeminal nucleus caudalis neurons may be viewed as an integrator of central vascular and myogenic inputs. Impulses transmitted from the trigeminal caudalis neurons to the thalamus and higher centers undergo further modulation, thus adding to the complexity of the headache mechanisms.

A *vascular-central-myogenic (VCM) model* (44) for pain in migraine may explain many of the clinical features of migraine. According to this model, headache intensity is determined by the sum of nociception from the cephalic arteries and pericranial myofacial tissues converging upon trigeminal nucleus caudalis neurons, which is influenced by central effects, which are usually facilitatory. Vascular input predominates over myofacial input in migraine, and the central influences are fundamental and probably trigger migraine attacks. The relative importance of vascular, central, and myogenic factors vary between patients and in the same patient with time. Long-term potentiation of nociceptive activation and secondary sensitization of central nervous system neurons to input from wider areas and nonnociceptive stimuli are relevant in the development of chronic headache.

On the other hand, in tension-type headache a *myofacial-central-vascular (MCV) model* (44) is more appropriate, as nociception may be predominantly myofacial in approximately 50% of patients with tension-type headache, in which the vascular component is of less importance. Central facilitation probably plays an important and dominant role in tension-type headache, also explaining the type of tension-type headache without the disorder of pericranial muscles.

The *VCM and MCV models* explain much of the complexity of the clinical picture of migraine and tension-type headache and their tendency to overlap and change into one another. They also explain why muscles are tender in migraine, why trigger-point injections may ameliorate migraine attack, and why chronic tension-type headache may be associated with episodes of pulsating pain. Moreover, these models provide the rationale for multimodal treatment strategies for migraine and tension-type headache, and may also be useful in explaining the disorder to patients. Sensitization of the trigeminal nucleus caudalis neurons due to frequent vascular input in patients with frequent migraine may explain the development of chronic daily headache in that category of patients.

The mechanism of analgesic-rebound headache is not known. Evidence suggests that analgesic-rebound headache may be restricted to those with primary headache disorders, especially migraineurs. Relapses of migraine may occur in migraineurs who have been placed on analgesic for other ailments (25). Lance et al. (45) reported that chronic overuse of analgesic does not cause increased headache in nonheadache sufferers; they studied a group of patients who were taking daily analgesics for arthritis. This finding was confirmed by Bowlder et al. (46), who also reported that no difference exists between the various types of analgesics in their ability to induce chronic headache. Therefore, it appears that there is an inherent abnormality in the primary headache population that predisposes them to drug induced headache. As Lance et al. (45) postulated further, suppression or down-regulation of an already partly suppressed or abnormal antinociceptive system due to excessive symptomatic medication is a possible explanation for the analgesic-rebound headache in migraine sufferers. Recently, Hering et al. (47) reported reduction in the whole-blood 5-HT in a group of patients with analgesic-induced chronic daily headache. 5-HT levels significantly increased after analgesic withdrawal and correlated with clinical improvement. Activation of "on-cells" in the ventromedial medulla described by Fields and Heinricher (43) resulting in nociception may be one of the mechanisms by which frequent use of analgesics perpetuates further nociception. The on-cells were shown to be activated in naloxone-induced morphine withdrawal in animals (43). Alteration in the density and function of postsynaptic neuronal receptors as a result of chronic use of medications may be another explanation for the refractory headache these patients develop. Attempts have been made to therapeutically "up-regulate" the "down-regulated" central opioid system by chronic administration of naloxone in patients with chronic headache (48).

MANAGEMENT OF CHRONIC HEADACHES

A multimodality approach is essential for satisfactory results. A combination of pharmacological and behavioral intervention is necessary. Essential principles are:

1. Discontinuation of the offending medications
2. Attempts to break the cycle of continuous headache by pharmacotherapeutic agents such as intravenous dihydroergotamine (49,50) or subcutaneous sumatriptan (51)
3. Initiation of prophylactic pharmacotherapy
4. Concomitant behavioral intervention, which includes biofeedback therapy, individual behavioral counseling, family therapy, physical exercise, and dietary instructions
5. Adequate instructions about ill effects of medications with special focus on analgesics
6. Continuity of care

The multimodality approach to treatment outlined above can be taken with either outpatients or inpatients. Indications for hospitalization would include:

1. Status migrainosus with nausea, vomiting, and dehydration associated with excessive narcotic/analgesic/ergotamine use
2. Chronic refractory headache with extreme narcotic or barbiturate habituation
3. Chronic refractory headache with severe psychiatric comorbidity such as depression and panic disorder
4. Refractory headache with associated medical problems such as uncontrolled hypertension or renal, gastric, or hepatic disease

Withdrawal of Analgesics/Narcotic/Ergotamine

In a hospitalized patient, offending medications can be discontinued abruptly, bearing in mind the possibility of withdrawal reactions. Usual withdrawal reactions are increased headache, restlessness, sleeplessness, excessive sweating, and diarrhea. These can be counteracted to a significant degree by use of a clonidine skin patch 0.2 mg. Serious withdrawal reactions such as seizure can occur, specifically with abrupt withdrawal of butalbital-containing medications. In the hospital, such emergencies can be tackled effectively; it is unwise to ask a patient to stop butalbital abruptly as an outpatient. An inpatient protocol for butalbital withdrawal is recommended by Sands (52).

Breaking the Cycle of Headache

In the hospital a heparin lock is used to administer I.V. fluids for rehydration and administration of antiemetics and dihydroergotamine (DHE). Various protocols are available for I.V. dihydroergotamine (49,50). Unlike ergotamine, DHE does not appear to cause rebound headache and therefore can be substituted with repeated injections for 48–72 hours.

Side effects of DHE limit its use to some degree. Leg pain and cramps, severe nausea, and vomiting in spite of using metoclopramide or phenothiazine are major drawbacks. The claim that DHE is a minimal arterial constrictor is not substantiated by any hard data. There are instances of transient ischemic attacks and migrainous strokes developing in patients who were on DHE in the hospital (53). Angina can also occur. In general, DHE is contraindicated in 1) patients with migraine with prolonged aura (complicated migraine) or those with *frequent* migraine with aura and 2) those who are heavy smokers or have other risk factors for stroke and vascular diseases such as severe diabetes, hyperlipidemia, hypertension, and positive anticardiolipin antibody. In spite of these limitations, DHE is useful in the majority of patients to break the cycles of headaches.

Sumatriptan

Diener et al. (54) successfully used sumatriptan subcutaneously while withdrawing analgesics in patients with drug-induced headache. Sumatriptan can be given repeatedly without any major side effects. It is devoid of side effects such as nausea and vomiting which are very frequent with DHE. In fact, sumatriptan by itself may ameliorate nausea and vomiting (51). It is conceivable that sumatriptan administered in repetitive doses will become the drug of choice in breaking the cycle of refractory migraine. As with DHE, one has to be careful in using sumatriptan in patients with high risk for stroke and vascular disease.

Prophylactic Pharmacotherapy

Simultaneously with analgesic/ergotamine withdrawal, adequate combination of prophylactic pharmacotherapy can be started. Most of the patients in this category require copharmacy using one antimigraine agent and an antidepressant. Any of the agents used for prophylaxis of migraine can be used in chronic headache. Tricyclics are still the antidepressants of choice as they have an analgesic effect in addition to the antidepressant and sleep-enhancing properties, both of which are helpful to the chronic refractory headache patients. Fluoxetine (Prozac), which should theoretically be useful, as it is a specific 5-HT uptake inhibitor, has not yet been shown to have any antimigraine or analgesic effect. However, because of the lack of sedation and anticholinergic side effect, many patients prefer fluoxetine to amitriptyline.

Valproate (Depakote) has been found to be particularly useful in the prophylactic management of chronic daily headache (55). Double-blind placebo-controlled studies have reported significant benefit with valproate as a prophylactic agent in patients with migraine (56). The usual dose is 500–1000 mg/day to keep the blood level above 50 mg/ml—an occasional patient may require up to 2000 mg/day.

Hepatic toxicity, which was a major concern when valproate was used in infants and young children for seizure control, is not a problem in adults in the headache age group. Certainly it should not be used in patients with active liver disease. Asthenia, tremor, weight gain, and hair loss occur in some patients. Valproate can be combined with antidepressants.

Behavioral Therapy

Behavioral therapy alone, using biofeedback, relaxation, or a combination of the two, gives only less than a 50% improvement (57). The general experience is that when pharmacotherapy and behavioral therapy are combined, the improvement is more than with one modality alone.

Behavioral therapy should include not only relaxation or biofeedback, but also short-term cognitive stress-management therapy and individual counseling. Family counseling may also be important, if a great deal of family stress is recognized.

PROGNOSIS OF CDH; PERSISTENT INTRACTABLE CDH

The prognosis of CDH was studied by a long-term follow-up of 489 patients for an average period of 42 months (range, 18 to 72 months) (58). Of these, 38 patients (8%) were lost for follow-up. Of the remaining 451 patients, 140 (31%) showed significant recurrence of their headaches in spite of continuing efforts to use prophylactic medications, dietary control, behavioral treatment, and avoiding analgesics, sedatives, and daily ergotamine. Most of these 140 patients continued to have periodic exacerbations of headache with episodes of status migrainosus and low-grade daily headache. They continued to need some symptomatic medications or showed a tendency to use prescribed substitute medications such as isometheptene in excessive quantities. They were frequent visitors to the headache clinic compared to patients who showed improvement. Repeated hospitalization was necessary in some. Ninety-two patients (20%) were not able to work, and the rest were relatively unproductive in their work. Many of them had to change their jobs frequently because of absenteeism.

Higher Incidence of Behavioral Abnormalities in Intractable CDH

In persistent intractable CDH, the behavioral, psychological, and neuroendocrine features were strikingly different from those of the CDH patients who showed improvement (Table 10). The MMPI was abnormal in 100% of intractable cases. High scores of hypochondriasis, depression, and hysteria (scores 1, 2, and 3) were consistent, and combinations of high scores of 6, 7, 8, and 9 were seen in 56% of patients with intractable CDH. The other features of interest were high incidence of alcoholism among parents and the high incidence of physical, emotional, and sexual abuse in the intractable group compared to those who were treated successfully. The depression scale of the Zung and Beck Depression Inventory were also higher in the intractable group compared to the improved group.

Table 10 Behavioral, Psychological, and Neuroendocrine Features of Intractable CDH

	Patients with intractable CDH ($N = 140$) (31%)		Improved CDH group ($N = 311$) (69%)	
	No.	%	No.	%
Abnormal MMPI	140	100[a]	158	48
Alcoholism among parents	82	58[a]	51	17
Physical, emotional, sexual abuse	74	52[a]	26	8
Positive dexamethasone suppressive test	42	30[a]	34	11
Zung Depression Scale	62 ± 9.9[a]		51.2 ± 8.8[a]	
Beck Depression Scale	16 ± 6.6[a]		12.2 ± 8.9	

[a]$p < 0.01$.

Neuroendocrine Abnormalities

Dexamethasone Suppression Test (DST)

Martignoni et al. (59) reported an abnormal response to the DST in 40% of patients with CDH. This is in keeping with the hypothalamus-pituitary-adrenal axis hyperactivity similar to that observed in patients with mood disorders (60). In our series of patients, the intractable group had a statistically higher incidence of abnormal DST (30%) compared to those who showed improvement (11%), indicating that in the more chronic persistent cases the neuroendocrine abnormalities are more pronounced.

Clonidine Test

In addition to possible derangement in the hypothalamus-pituitary-adrenal axis, chronic headache patients also display poor responsiveness to clonidine, which suggests a deranged central noradrenergic activity as well (61), similar to that reported in depressed patients (62).

From our experience, it is obvious that there is a group of CDH patients whose headaches do not improve significantly even after symptomatic medications are discontinued, trigger factors removed, prophylactic medications instituted, and behavioral approaches used. Approximately 31% of our patients are intractable, and they appear to have a persistent neurobehavioral disorder as evidenced by continuing headache and continuing behavioral and neuroendocrine abnormalities. Further investigations are necessary to study these patients more extensively.

REFERENCES

1. Ziegler DK, Hassanein RS, Couch JR. Headache syndrome suggested by statistical analysis of headache symptoms. Cephalalgia 1982; 2:125–134.
2. Waters WE. Epidemiological enigma of migraine. Int J Epidemiol 1973; 2:189–194.
3. Kaganov JA, Bakal DA, Dunn BE. The differential contribution of muscle contraction and migraine symptoms to the problem of headache in general population. Headache 1981; 21:157–163.
4. Raskin NH, Appenzeller O. Headache. In: Major Problems in Internal Medicine. Vol. 19. Philadelphia: W.B. Saunders, 1980.
5. Mathew, NT, Stubits E, Nigam MR. Transformation of episodic migraine into daily headache: analysis of factors. Headache 1982; 22:66–68.
6. Classification and diagnostic criteria for headache disorder, cranial neuralgias and facial pain. Cephalalgia 1988; 8(suppl 7):1–96.
7. Mathew NT, Reuveni U, Perez F. Transformed or evolutive migraine. Headache 1987; 27:102–106.

8. Manzoni GC, Micieli G, Granella F, Martignoni E, Malferrari G, Nappi G. Daily chronic headache: classification and clinical features: observation on 250 patients. Cephalalgia 1987; 7(suppl 6):169–170.

9. Manzoni GC, Sandrini, Zanferrari C, Verri AP, Granella F, Nappi G. Clinical features of daily chronic headache and its different subtypes. Cephalalgia 1991; 11(suppl 11):292–293.

10. Solomon S, Lipton RB, Newman LC. Clinical features of chronic daily headache. Headache 1992; 32:325–329.

11. Schoenen J, Pasqua VD, Sianard-Gainko J. Multiple clinical and paraclinical analysis of chronic tension-type headache associated or unassociated with disorder of pericranial muscles. Cephalalgia 1991; 11:135–139.

12. Iverson HK, Langemark M, Anderson PG, Hansen PE, Olesen J. Clinical characteristics of migraine and episodic tension-type headache in relation to old and new diagnostic criteria. Headache 1990; 30:514–519.

13. Rasmussen BK, Jensen R, Schroll P, Olesen J. Interrelations between migraine and tension-type headache in the general population. Arch Neurol 1992; 49: 914–918.

14. Vanast WJ: New daily persistent headaches. Definition of a benign syndrome. Headache 1986; 26:318.

15. Vanast WJ, Diaz-Mitoma F, Tyrrell DLJ. Hypothesis: chronic benign daily headache is an immune disorder with a viral trigger. Headache 1987; 27:138–142.

16. Bakal DA, Kaganow JA. Muscular contraction and migraine headaches: a psychophysiological comparison. Headache 1977; 17:208–215.

17. Hatch JP, Schoenfeld LS, Boukros NM, Seleshi E, Moore PJ, Cyr-Provost M. Anger and hostility in tension type. Headache 1991; 31:302–304.

18. Passchier J, Schouten J, Van Der Donk J, Romunde LKJ. The association of frequent headaches with personality and life events. Headache 1991; 31: 116–121.

19. Zung WWK. A self-rating depression scale. Arch Gen Psychiat 1965; 12:63–70.

20. Beck AT, Ward CM, Mendelsohn M, et al. An inventory for measuring depression. Arch Gen Psychiatry 1961; 5:561–571.

21. Friedman M, Rosenman R. Type A Behavior and Your Heart. New York: Knopf, 1974.

22. Robinson ME, Geisser ME, Dieter JN, Swerdlow B. The relationship between MMPI cluster membership and diagnostic category in headache patients. Headache 1991; 31:111–115.

23. Kurman RG, Hursey KG, Mathew NT. Assessment of chronic refractory headache. The role of the MMPI-2. Headache 1992; 32:432–435.

24. Kudrow L. Paradoxical effects of frequent analgesic use. In: Critchley M, Friedman A, Gorini S, Sicuteri F, eds. Advances in Neurology. Vol 33. New York: Raven Press, 1982:335–341.

25. Isler H. Migraine treatment as a cause of chronic migraine. In: Rose FC, ed. Advances in Migraine Research and Therapy. New York: Raven Press, 1982:159–164.

26. Rapoport AM, Weeks RE, Sheftell FD, Baskin SM, Verdi J. Analgesic rebound headache: theoretical and practical implications. Cephalalgia 1985; 5(suppl 3): 448–449.

27. Dichgans J, Diener HO, Gerber WD, et al. Analgetika-induzierter dauerkopf-schmerz. Dtsch Med Wschr 1984; 109:369–373.

28. Mathew NT, Kurman R, Perez F. Drug induced refractory headache: clinical features and management. Headache 1990; 30:634–638.

29. Lippman CW. Characteristic headache resulting from prolonged use of ergot derivatives. J Nerv Ment Dis 1955; 121:270–273.

30. Saper JR, Jones JM. Ergotamine dependency. Features and possible mechanisms. Clin Neuropharmacol 1986; 9:244–256.

31. Anderson PG. Ergotamine headache. Headache 1975; 15:118–121.

32. Sholz E, Diener HC, Geiselhart S. Does a critical dosage exist in drug-induced headache? In: Diener HC, Wilkinson M, eds. Drug-induced Headache. Berlin: Springer-Verlag, 1988:29–43.

33. Hay KM. Pain thresholds in migraine. Practitioner 1979; 222:827–833.

34. Oleson J. Some clinical features of the acute migraine attack. An analysis of 750 patients. Headache 1978; 18:268–271.

35. Lous I, Olesen J. Evaluation of pericranial tenderness and oral function in patients with common migraine, muscle contraction headache and "combination headache." Pain 1982; 12:385–393.

36. Jensen K, Tuxen C, Olesen J. Pericranial muscle tenderness and pressure-pain threshold in the temporal region during common migraine. Pain 1988; 35:65–70.

37. Tfelt-Hansen P, Lous I, Olesen J. Prevalence and significance of muscle tenderness during common migraine attacks. Headache 1981; 21:49–54.

38. Langemark M, Olesen J, Loldrup O, Bech P. Clinical characterization of patients with chronic tension headache. Headache 1988; 28:590–596.

39. Raskin NH, Hosobuchi Y, Lamb S. Headache may arise from perturbation of brain. Headache 1987; 27:416–420.

40. Schoenen J. Tension-type headache: Pathophysiologic evidence for a disturbance of "limbic" pathways to the brain stem. Headache 1990; 30:314–315.

41. Raskin NH. Headache. 2d ed. New York: Churchill Livingstone, 1988.

42. Goadsby PJ, Zagami AS, Lambert GA. Neural processing of craniovascular pain: a synthesis of the central structures involved in migraine. Headache 1991; 31:365–371.

43. Fields HL, Heinricher MM. Brainstem modulation of nociceptor-driven withdrawal reflexes. Ann NY Acad Sci 1989; 563:34–44.

44. Olesen J. Clinical and pathophysiological observations in migraine and tension-type headache explained by integration of vascular, supraspinal and myofascial inputs. Pain 1991; 46:125–132.

45. Lance E, Parkes C, Wilkinson M. Does analgesic abuse cause headaches de novo? Headache 1988; 28:61–62.

46. Bowlder I, Kikan J, Gansslen-Blumberg S, et al. The association between analgesic abuse and headache—coincidental or causal? Headache 1988; 28:494.

47. Hering R, Catarci T, Glover V, Patichis K, Whitmarsh TE, Steiner TJ. 5-HT in migraine patients with analgesic induced headache. 9th Migraine Trust International Symposium, London, Sept. 1992.
48. Nicolodi M, Sicuteri F. Chronic naloxone administration, a potential treatment for migraine, enhances morphine-induced miosis. Headache 1992; 32:348–352.
49. Raskin NH. Repetitive intravenous dihydroergotamine as therapy for intractable migraine. Neurology 1986; 36:995–997.
50. Silverstein SD, Schulman EA, Hopkins MM. Repetitive intravenous DHE in the treatment of refractory headache. Headache 1990; 30:334–339.
51. Cady RK, Wendt JK, Kirchner JR, et al. Treatment of acute migraine with subcutaneous sumatriptan. JAMA 1991; 285:2831–2835.
52. Sands GH. A protocol for butalbital, aspirin, and caffeine (BAC) detoxification in headache patients. Headache 1990; 30:491–496.
53. Ganji S, Williams W, Furlow J. Bilateral occipital lobe infarction in acute migraine. Clinical, neurophysiological and neuroradiological study. Headache 1992; 32:360–365.
54. Diener HC, Haab J, Peters C, Ried S, Dichgans J, Pilgrim A. Subcutaneous sumatriptan in the treatment of headache during withdrawal from drug-induced headache. Headache 1991; 31:205–209.
55. Mathew NT, Ali S. Valproate in the treatment of persistent chronic daily headache: an open label study. Headache 1991; 31:71–74.
56. Hering R, Kuritzky. Sodium valproate in the prophylactic treatment of migraine: a double-blind study versus placebo. Cephalalgia 1992; 12:81–84.
57. Holroyd KA, French DJ. Recent developments in the psychological assessment and management of recurrent headache disorders. In: Goreczny AJ, ed. Handbook of Recent Advances in Behavioral Medicine. New York: Plenum Press. In press.
58. Mathew NT, Kurman R, Perez F. Intractable chronic daily headache. A persistent neurobehavioral disorder. Cephalalgia 1989; 9(suppl 10):180–181.
59. Martignoni E, Facchinetti F, Manzoni GC, Petraglia F, Nappi G, Genazzani AR. Abnormal dexamethasone suppression test in daily chronic headache sufferers. Psychiatr Res 1986; 19:51–57.
60. France RD, Krishnan KRR, Trainor M, Palton S. Chronic pain and depression. IV DST as a discriminator between chronic pain and depression. Pain 1987; 28:39–44.
61. Martignoni E, Facchinetti F, Rossi R, Sances G, Genazzani AR, Nappi G. Neuroendocrine evidences of deranged noradrenergic activity in chronic migraine. Psychoneuroendocrinology 1989; 14:357–363.
62. Siever LJ, Uhde TW, Jimerson DC, et al. Differential inhibitory noradrenergic responses to clonidine in 25 depressed patients and 25 normal control subjects. Am J Psychiatry 1984; 141:733–741.

6

Diagnosis of Headache

Roger K. Cady

Shealy Institute for Comprehensive Health Care
Springfield, Missouri

INTRODUCTION

Physicians evaluating headache are confronted with a wide range of diagnostic possibilities. This can be simplified by dividing headaches into primary and secondary disorders. Primary headache disorders are those in which headache *is* the medical condition. Secondary headache disorders are those in which headache is a symptom of another pathological process. The presence of a headache can herald a wide variety of medical conditions ranging from life-threatening disease to trivial complaints. Consequently, accurate diagnosis is essential.

The headache patient is often approached with an exhaustive medical evaluation. However, an underlying cause for most headaches is rarely discovered. It is estimated that only 0.004% of acute headaches are symptoms of a serious underlying disease (1). While physicians need to be vigilant in approaching the headache patient, it is important to balance diagnostic studies with common sense and clinical judgment. It is frequently noted in the headache patient that after completion of in-depth diagnostic investigations, the headache, along with its associated fears and disability, remains intact.

INTERNATIONAL HEADACHE SOCIETY DIAGNOSTIC CRITERIA

In 1988, the International Headache Society (IHS) set forth a comprehensive guide for headache and facial pain classification (2). Instrumental in standardizing headache diagnosis, this detailed classification is easily modified and applicable to the needs of a busy physician. The IHS criteria provide consistent diagnostic standards that show a high degree of correlation with primary care physician diagnosis (3,4). See Appendix.

IHS nomenclature has replaced the time-honored migraine terms *classic* and *common* with *migraine with aura* and *migraine without aura*, respectively. It also provides diagnostic criteria for tension headache that are more consistent with current pathophysiology and accounts for analgesic, menstrual, posttraumatic, and other common headache syndromes.

THE DIAGNOSTIC APPROACH

The single most important tool for evaluation of headache is the patient's history. Since no objective measurement of headache exists, the essence of diagnosis rests in the ability of the physician to dissect, extract, and organize relevant features of the patient's presentation into a diagnostic scheme. Patients may present for evaluation with their own agenda. They may have diagnosed their own headache or associated headache symptoms with other life events. They may withhold certain information, fearing that it would be interpreted as a psychological complaint or a symptom of a serious illness. Headaches may be viewed by the patient as a fact of life or as a life-threatening event. These factors, combined with the fact that each patient has a unique language for expressing pain and suffering, make taking a history a diagnostic challenge.

Physicians, too, may allow their own beliefs to cloud the diagnostic scheme. Some may perceive headache as an unrewarding disorder to treat and may be reluctant to pursue diagnosis. Others may view headache as a disorder with few adequate treatments, reenforcing the message that headache is something their patients will simply have to learn to live with. Concerns about medication misuse and drug-seeking can influence a physician's comfort with headache patients. Further, because medical training traditionally emphasizes headache as a symptom rather than a primary disorder, physicians may feel their responsibility to the patient is finished when completed diagnostic studies fail to demonstrate underlying pathology.

These influences are reflected in a recent patient survey in which nearly three-quarters of headache patients reported dissatisfaction with their medical encounter for headache treatment, and nearly a third perceived a physician bias as the basis for their dissatisfaction (5).

The value of the physician–patient relationship is paramount to successful diagnosis and treatment. A valued patient will provide more complete and relevant information than one met with bias and skepticism. An investment of time and sincerity early in the therapeutic relationship with the headache patient reaps rewards in successful ongoing management.

TAKING THE HEADACHE HISTORY

Perhaps the two most essential aspects of accurate diagnosis are a practical understanding of headache pathophysiology and good rapport with the patient. Headache investigators have recommended open-ended questions as a means of elaborating significant headache symptomatology (6). Asking whether a patient knows when a headache is about to begin may elicit symptoms of prodrome or aura. Asking what a patient does during a headache may provide information and insight into a patient's coping skills and how medication is being used. A diary helps uncover precipitating factors and medication usage.

Key historical facts include the following:

1. Age of onset
2. Frequency and duration of symptoms
3. Location of headache pain
4. Time of onset
5. Associated symptomatology
6. Aggravating or alleviating factors
7. Medication use

This is the initial basis for defining diagnosis and initiating management (Table 1). Over time, however, these facts may change, necessitating reevaluation of the patient. This is especially true whenever there has been a significant change in headache symptomatology or treatment response.

Age of Onset

Most primary headache disorders begin in adolescence or early adulthood. Many migraineurs can recall headaches beginning in childhood. Statistically, females after the age of menarche begin to experience migraine

Table 1 Types of Headache and Their Characteristics

	Age of onset	Frequency	Duration	Site
Migraine	Childhood through early adulthood	Rarely greater than 1/wk	4–72 hr	Unilateral in 2/3 of cases
Tension	Early adulthood	Variable	30 min to weeks	Bilateral
Mixed and transformed headaches	20–40 yrs	Near daily	Nearly continuous	Bilateral
Drug-associated	Adulthood	Near daily	Related to drug use	Diffuse bilateral
Cluster	20–40 hrs	1–6/day during active cluster period	30 min to 3 hr	Always unilateral
Chronic paroxysmal hemicrania	Early adulthood	Daily, with 75 attacks/day	1–2 min up to 30 min	Always unilateral

more frequently than males, and the prevalence ratio increases for women through the third and fourth decade, with a peak gender ratio of 3:1 (7). After menopause, the gender ratio decreases, but a predominance among females persists throughout adult life, suggesting that factors other than hormonal influences account for the higher prevalence of headaches in women. The prevalence of tension headache in childhood is not well defined. Typically, these headaches begin during a period of stress in late adolescence or early adulthood. Episodic tension headaches do not cause the same degree of disability as other primary headache disorders and are not as frequently a primary complaint as other, more debilitating headache syndromes. Nonetheless, tension headache frequently occurs in association with other types of headache, which can lead to confusion and inappropriate medication use. The prevalence of tension

Time of onset	Associated phenomena	Aggravating factors	Clinical presentation	Medication
Variable, with early A.M. onset common	GI; hypersensitive to light and sound; muscle tenderness	Multiple precipitating factors	Pain, disability; withdrawal from activity	Prescription meds often desired
Later afternoon	Anorexia; muscle tenderness	Stress; fatigue	Rest; mild disability	Mild analgesic
Variable	IBS; sleep disturbances; depression	Mental or physical activity	Variable, depending on symptoms	Overuse of medication common
Related to period of drug abstinence	Memory impairment; medication-related symptoms	Withdrawal of offending drug	Severe headache with drug withdrawal	Specific drug required for relief
1–3 hr after onset of sleep	Ipsilateral autonomic dysfunction	Vasodilators, EtOH	Pacing; agitation; hyperactive	70% response to O_2
Daytime	Ipsilateral autonomic dysfunction	Movement of head	Similar to cluster	Response to indomethacin

headache increases until the third or fourth decade of life, and then declines.

Cluster headache usually begins between early adulthood and midlife, although rare instances of cluster occurring in childhood have been reported (8). Cluster may produce a stereotypical headache picture, but when evaluated early in the first cluster cycle, a complete diagnostic evaluation may be required.

Headaches that begin later in adult life should be viewed with a greater degree of suspicion and evaluated aggressively (9). If the onset of the initial headache is after age 40, the physician should be alerted to the possibility of underlying pathology. New primary headache is rare in the elderly, and its presence should alert the physician to pursue detailed diagnostic evaluations.

Frequency, Intensity, Duration, and Therapeutic Responsiveness

The frequency of headache attacks, as well as the intensity and duration of each attack, are key features of historical information. Consistency of a headache pattern for over a year suggests a primary headache disorder. However, inquiry as to why a patient is currently seeking medical attention may uncover valuable information about a recent change in headache symptomatology or specific fears and concerns the patient may have. Headaches of recent onset or with a significant change in clinical presentation require in-depth evaluation. The overall aim is to arrive at a working diagnosis acceptable to the patient and physician, consistent with headache characteristics, leading to a logical choice of treatment. Response to a given therapy should not confirm diagnosis; conversely, nonresponse to therapy should alert the physician of the possible need to reassess the working diagnosis.

Duration of headache attacks and frequency of attacks assist in differentiating acute and chronic headache syndrome. Episodic headaches should be clearly identifiable as having distinct endpoints, while chronic daily or near-daily headaches and analgesic-rebound headaches will have fluctuation of headache intensity with the underlying headache pattern remaining intact. Episodic migraine attacks typically last 4–72 hours. Daily or near-daily headaches are not migraine. Cluster headache is a less common episodic headache, with individual attacks lasting 15 minutes to 3 hours. These attacks occur up to several times a day, for periods of weeks to several months. Lastly, tension headache may also be episodic, with attacks lasting minutes to days, with or without easily identifiable times of onset or offset of attacks.

Chronic tension defines a headache lasting more than 15 days per month, and chronic cluster is diagnosed when the cluster period exceeds 12 months. Episodic patterns may convert into chronic patterns or vice versa. Occasionally chronic headache begins de novo.

Site

Migraine is often thought of as a unilateral headache, but it is actually bilateral in approximately 40% of cases (10). Migraine may begin as an ill-defined diffuse head pain that over time localizes to one area of the head or may present with a localized pain of abrupt onset. As the migraine progresses, it may progress into a more global headache. There is often muscle tenderness in the head and neck area. The most frequent sites of headache in migraine are frontal, periorbital, temporal, and occipital (11). Unilateral pain that occurs on different sides of the head during a single attack, or from attack to attack, suggests a benign headache disorder and is fairly common in migraine.

Tension-type headache is generally bilateral, diffuse, and constant. Although it is often described in a headband or nuchal distribution, tension headache can occur in any part of the cranium. Muscle tenderness in the neck and shoulder area is often noted, but this offers little diagnostic differentiation from migraine. However, palpation of tender points within these affected muscles may radiate pain into the head. This classifies these areas as "trigger points" (12) and may have important management implications.

Cluster headache is unilateral; frequently periorbital, temporal, or frontal; and well localized, and pain is of rapid onset. Instances of cluster headache being localized elsewhere in the head or even the neck have been described (13).

Other headache disorders may have characteristic locations; for example, glaucoma is retro-orbital, temporal arteritis is often intraocular with tenderness over the temporal artery, and trigeminal neuralgia is confined to the distribution of a branch of the trigeminal nerve.

Time of Onset

Time of onset may be valuable in identifying different headache types. Cluster headache characteristically awakens an individual one to two hours after going to sleep. Migraine may also awaken an individual, but more commonly this occurs in the early morning shortly before the normal time of awakening. Tension headache rarely awakens one but begins later in the afternoon or early evening. Analgesic- or caffeine-associated headaches often begin in the early morning as blood levels of the offending drug decline over night.

Associated Phenomena

Migraine has systemic manifestations—typically, gastrointestinal symptoms such as anorexia, nausea, and vomiting; neurological symptoms such as aura and irritability to sensory input (light, sound, touch, and odors); and musculoskeletal complaints of pain and stiffness. The headache pain is commonly aggravated by a change in position or routine activity.

By contrast, cluster headache is associated with autonomic dysfunctions on the ipsilateral side of the head. Nasal congestion, conjunctival injection, lacrimation, facial swelling, and a partial Horner's syndrome (ptosis and miosis) are common.

Tension headache is associated with more subtle systemic manifestations. One may note anorexia, but nausea is uncommon. Photophobia or phonophobia may be present but are mild to moderate and, by IHS definition, not presently concomitantly (2, pp. 29–30). Muscle stiffness and tenderness are frequently noted. Fatigue and sleep disturbances are common. Headache pain is not significantly worsened by routine activity (2, pp. 29–30).

The presence of fever, arthralgia, weight loss, or other systemic symptomatology is indicative of secondary headache disorders. Careful screening of systemic symptomatology is necessary in all headache patients.

Aggravating and Alleviating Factors

Patients with migraine will characteristically seek rest in a dark, quiet environment to avoid sensory stimulation and relieve their headache. Most will desire medication to relieve their pain (14). Conversely, cluster patients find it difficult to find a position of comfort and are agitated and hyperactive and pace restlessly. They too desire medication. Those with tension-type headaches are usually able to function in a relatively normal fashion but will frequently prefer rest.

Headaches associated with increased intracranial pressure are commonly exacerbated by physical exertion, straining, or sexual intercourse. The individual avoids a "head-low" position because an increase in intracranial pressure increases the head pain. This posturing can, on occasion, be noticed in migraine. Numerous headache types are named according to initiating or aggravating factors, for example, ice cream headaches, aviation headaches, postcoital headaches, and exertional headaches.

Medication Use

Accurate history of medication usage is essential in all headache patients. Most patients during migraine or cluster attacks desire symptomatic medication. However, the inappropriate use of symptomatic medication can perpetuate headache and increase the likelihood of adverse reactions. In addition, headache can be a side effect of medications used for migraine prophylaxis or for the treatment of other medical conditions.

Chronic daily or near-daily headaches may evolve out of episodic migraine. Mathew et al. (15) have suggested that this headache pattern constitutes a separate diagnosis entity called transformed migraine.

Transformed migraine is associated with a positive family history of migraine, identifiable migraine-precipitating factors, especially menstruation, and migraine-associated GI and neurological symptomatology. These headaches are often associated with excessive use of symptomatic medication (16).

Medications can produce symptoms that obscure diagnosis or intensify headache-associated symptoms. Misunderstanding by patients of how or when to use medication can lead to poor efficacy and unnecessary side effects. Careful histories of what prompts medication usage in a given patient provide insights into coping strategies and a valuable opportunity for education.

FAMILY AND SOCIAL HISTORY

A good family and social history is of considerable value when evaluating a headache patient. A positive family history of migraine is noted in approximately 70% of migraineurs and 40–50% of the tension-headache population but is conspicuously absent in cluster. In addition, family histories are often positive for depression, sleep disturbances, alcoholism, and other illnesses associated with disturbances in serotonin metabolism.

Patterns of illness behavior, medication use, and coping skills are often learned from families. Exploration of how headaches affect the family provides insight into these coping patterns, as well as family-related distress due to the chronic headache syndrome. It is also of value to gently inquire about childhood abuse since it is often associated with chronic unremitting headaches. When important psychological issues are suspected, involving a skilled psychologist or psychiatrist in patient management is of value.

THE PHYSICAL EXAMINATION

The physical examination of the headache patient is important and is easily incorporated into headache evaluations. Typically taking less than 10 minutes, the screening exam provides diagnostic reassurance to the physician and patient.

Physical examination begins during the initial contact with the patient. Is the patient mentally alert and coherent? Is the gait pattern normal? Does the patient appear ill? The measurement of vital signs, including blood pressure and temperature, and assessment of current usage of medication, alcohol, and illicit drugs are vital to patient evaluation.

Seat the patient in the exam room. Observe and palpate the head for signs of trauma, areas of tenderness, and adequacy of temporal artery pulses. Assess cranial nerves by noting facial and pupillary asymmetry, ocular motion, or fundoscopic changes. The oral cavity should be examined for dental pathology; ascertain that the tongue is midline and the palate moves symmetrically. Temporomandibular joints can be palpated while the patient opens and closes his mouth.

Palpate the neck for the presence of lymphadenopathy, thyromegaly, and auscultate over the carotids. Assess cervical motion to determine the presence of meningeal irritation and structural abnormalities of the cervical spine. Palpate the neck, particularly in the suboccipital and sternocleidomastoid area, for significant "trigger points."

Screen for muscle weakness by testing the quality and symmetry of the biceps, triceps, and hand grip in the upper extremities, and leg extension, flexion, and ankle and toe dorsiflexion in the lower extremities. Assess sensation to light pinprick in the face, hand, and foot. Test deep-tendon reflexes of the arms, knees, and ankles, and note the Babinski response.

Examine the ears, throat, lungs, heart, and abdomen for evidence of systemic disease. Screen for postural abnormalities, especially in the chronic headache syndromes. During this examination, attention should be paid to skeletal asymmetry, scoliosis, muscle spasm, and trigger points in the neck, upper back, and shoulders (see Chapters 13 and 14).

Headache Danger Signs

Headache can occasionally be a symptom of catastrophic and life-threatening proportion. Therefore, it is essential that physicians exercise appropriate care in evaluating headache patients. No single sign or symptom differentiates primary and secondary headaches. Table 2 reviews some of the "danger signs" that may alert the physician to the possibility of a more serious disorder. It is prudent to pursue diagnostic studies or consultation when atypical features of headache are noted.

DIAGNOSTIC INVESTIGATIONS

Diagnostic investigations available for evaluation of headache are useful in ruling out secondary headache and other pathology rather than confirming the diagnosis of primary headache. These studies can be overutilized as well as underutilized. They assist in the headache diagnosis only by ruling out a serious condition masquerading as a benign headache

Table 2 Headache "Danger Signs" Suggesting the Need for Further Evaluation

Onset of headache after age 40
Onset of new or different headache
"Worst" headache ever experienced
Onset of subacute headache that progressively worsens over time
Onset of headache with exertion, sexual activity, coughing, or straining
Headache associated with change in neurological evaluation
  Drowsiness, confusion, memory impairment
  Weakness, ataxia, loss of coordination
  Sensory loss associated with headache
  Asymmetry of pupillary response, deep tendon reflexes, or Babinski response
  Signs of meningeal irritation
  Progressive visual or neurological changes
Abnormal medical evaluation
  Fever
  Hypertension
  Chronic malaise, myalgia, arthralgia
  Weight loss
  Tender, poorly pulsatile temporal arteries
  Abnormal medical examination

disorder. Conversely, when used inappropriately they can add risk and considerable cost to the diagnostic process.

If a physician or patient is not comfortable with the apparent diagnosis or danger signs are noted during evaluation, further studies are warranted. The specific nature of these studies is ultimately dictated by the clinician's judgment. Of specific value in headache evaluation are: 1) blood studies, 2) lumbar puncture, 3) radiographic imaging, and 4) electroencephalography (EEG).

Blood Studies

A CBC can screen for some infectious etiologies of headache and may suggest other underlying pathology. An elevation of the white blood cell count, in the clinical presentation of an infectious disease, requires prompt evaluation. Leukocytosis can be seen with volume depletion, pain, stress, and tobacco usage (17, pp. 63, 507–508), but an infectious etiology should be excluded before these conditions are accepted as an explanation. The presence of chronic anemia may suggest underlying malignancy, collagen vascular disease, blood loss from medication usage, or other chronic illness and requires appropriate investigations.

A raised erythrocyte sedimentation rate (ESR), especially in patients over the age of 50 presenting with an initial or new headache complaint, can warn of temporal arteritis. The ESR may also be elevated by systemic infections, inflammatory conditions, collagen vascular disease, occult malignancies, and multiple myeloma (17, p. 623). ESRs are nonspecific and must be viewed in the context of the presenting clinical picture.

Lumbar Puncture

Lumbar puncture is indicated to confirm or exclude infectious etiologies of the central nervous system or subarachnoid hemorrhage. It is an essential diagnostic study in acute infectious processes such as meningitis. Cerebral spinal fluid should be analyzed for the presence of cells, cell types, glucose, protein, and bacterial or fungal pathogens. Cultures should be obtained if infectious etiologies are considered. More specific testing is indicated by clinical indications.

Lumbar puncture can detect early subarachnoid hemorrhage and may be positive before imaging studies such as a CT scan. It is important to rule out significant elevation of CNS pressure or space-occupying lesions before proceeding with a lumbar puncture, as herniation can occur with rapid decompression. Fundoscopic examination and a noncontrast CT scan should be done prior to lumbar puncture if these conditions are suspected.

Radiographic Evaluation

As more sensitive imaging studies have become widely available, standard radiographic studies of the skull and cervical spine are less frequently indicated. However, they are of value in headache patients with histories of significant head or neck trauma. In the posttraumatic headache patient, it is valuable to obtain oblique views of the cervical spine as well as flexion and extension views to assess ligamentous injury. Muscle spasm associated with acute injury may prevent detection of significant ligamentous injury; repeat exams may therefore be necessary.

Computerized tomography (CT) is useful in revealing space-occupying lesions, such as brain tumors or subdural or epidural hematomas, or in cases of significant head trauma, or hydrocephalus. Enhancement with contrast is useful in evaluation of vascular lesions and bleeding. A normal structural study is often useful in excluding secondary headache syndromes as well as reassuring some patients. Repeated studies are indicated by significant change in clinical presentation and should not be performed without clear indication.

Cerebral angiography is the study of choice to rule out structural vascular etiologies of headache (18). It is highly sensitive for aneurysms and hemangiomas, but less risky and more cost-effective procedures should be sought first. Few neurosurgeons routinely recommend surgery on aneurysms that have not bled. However, awareness of aneurysms should prompt aggressive management of hypertension.

The role of magnetic resonance imaging (MRI) in headache is currently being delineated. Certainly, MRIs are becoming more widely utilized. They do not utilize x-rays but apply a strong magnetic field to align hydrogen atoms. When the field is released, the hydrogen atoms assume their random distribution and emit a minute radio signal that is computer-enhanced to create detailed images of internal structure.

MRIs may provide a more enhanced definition of brain structures than the CT scan and are more sensitive in areas such as the posterior fossa (19, pp. 37–48). Recent techniques utilizing contrast make it more sensitive in detecting vascular pathology. The plaques of multiple sclerosis may also be detected by MRI.

Electroencephalography

EEG changes are relatively common in migraine but are generally non-specific, with high numbers of false-positive and false-negative studies. EEGs are indicated in evaluation of loss of consciousness (20) and in investigation of seizure disorders, but their routine use in headache investigation is not generally warranted.

CONSULTATION

The need for consultation varies considerably from physician to physician and is dependent on many factors, including the physician's training, experience, motivation, and skill in diagnosis of headache. The complexity of the clinical presentation of the patient, and the patient's and/or physician's need for reassurance, may also justify consultation. Consultation is generally warranted when the history or examination suggests the possibility of ominous disease or when coexisting with the headache are complicated medical conditions that may complicate patient management. Psychological factors or psychiatric illness coexisting with headache may require consultation. This is particularly true when patterns of medication misuse and abuse are noted. Patients with chronic daily headaches or other complex management issues generally require multidisciplinary management. Referral to headache specialists can provide this level of care.

THE PRIMARY HEADACHE DISORDERS: CLINICAL FEATURES

Primary headache disorders are one of the most common complaints encountered in general medical practice (21). Despite their prevalence, they are underdiagnosed and often inadequately treated (22). The diagnosis of a primary headache disorder is made, for the most part, on clinical grounds because no specific diagnostic test is available to confirm its presence. However, specific clinical criteria for the diagnosis of primary headache syndromes are obtainable through a careful history, physical exam, and clinical judgment. Laboratory and imaging studies are primarily utilized to rule out other pathology and secondary headache disorders.

Although the understanding of headache disorders has undergone significant advancement, the basic mechanism of primary headache remains poorly defined. Primary headache disorders do not represent a single disease. They are a variety of clinical syndromes that may be interrelated. Management of these disorders depends largely on clinical judgment, educated therapeutic trial and error, and persevering patience from both the patient and the physician.

MIGRAINE

The syndrome of migraine can be divided into five distinct phases (23). Not all patient presentations will demonstrate these phases, but awareness of this full spectrum of migraine is valuable for diagnosis.

Phase 1: Prodrome

Within the 24–48-hour period preceding the onset of headache, 50–80% of migraineurs experience a prodrome (23, p. 5), suggesting subtle alterations of normal CNS activity. Typically, the prodrome begins insidiously and may include change in mood, altered sensory perception, food craving (particularly simple carbohydrates), excessive yawning, dysphasia, and/or memory dysfunction (23, p. 6). Some patients may not volunteer their personal prodrome experiences, fearing that it will suggest a psychiatric disease.

Phase 2: Aura

An aura represents focal neurological disturbances preceding the onset of headache (2, pp. 19–28). Usually, an aura develops gradually over 5 to 20 minutes and lasts less than 1 hour. An aura resolves within 60 minutes prior to or shortly after the onset of the headache (2, pp. 19–28). Most commonly, auras are visual in nature and are frequently characterized by flashing lights or shimmering zig-zag lines in the visual field or visual distortion. Changes in visual acuity, such as the sensation of looking through a window covered with rain, are also common. Sensory changes of pins and needles or numbness around the lip or hand are common. Auras may at times be profound, such as hemiparesis or vivid hallucinations.

Phase 3: Headache

The headache phase of migraine is characterized by unilateral pulsating pain of moderate to severe intensity, lasting 4 to 72 hours (2, pp. 19–28). The attack may begin abruptly or build gradually over several hours and is frequently accompanied by gastrointestinal disturbances, including anorexia, nausea, and vomiting. The headache is intensified by routine activity. In addition, there is an aversion to sensory stimulation, especially light and sound, so that many migraineurs seek rest in a dark, quiet environment.

Despite this classic picture of migraine, in approximately one-third of migraine attacks the headache is bilateral and may not throb. Muscle tenderness in the head and neck frequently accompanies the headache phase of migraine and may persist between attacks.

Phase 4: Headache Termination (Resolution)

The mechanisms by which the body regains normal homeostasis and terminates the migraine cycle are poorly understood. Restoration of serotonin metabolism probably plays an important role. The headache may end abruptly with vomiting, or with an intensely emotional experience. However, more commonly, the headache resolves over a period of several hours, often during sleep or rest.

Phase 5: Postdrome

Following headache resolution, most migraineurs experience a 24–48-hour period during which they feel drained, fatigued, and tired. They often report muscle aches and changes in mental clarity. Emotions may range from depression to euphoria. These changes range considerably in intensity and resolve insidiously.

TENSION-TYPE HEADACHE

Tension headache is very common—it is probably experienced by most people at some point during their lifetime. Frequently associated with fatigue and stress, these headaches generally respond to simple treatment measures such as rest or simple analgesics. Tension headaches occur more frequently in women and often have a familial association. Typically beginning in early adulthood as episodic events, tension headaches may evolve into a chronic disorder and occur on a daily or near-daily basis for many years. Tension headaches are classified as episodic if they occur on fewer than 15 days per month and chronic if they occur more often (2, pp. 19–28).

Tension-type headaches are generally bilateral and consist of a dull, aching, steady-pressure type of pain. Headaches may be associated with a recognizable period of stress, but as the condition becomes more chronic, this association is less clear. Individual headaches may last from 30 minutes to several days (2, pp. 19–28).

Tension headaches do not generally cause the significant disability associated with migraine or cluster headaches. Routine physical activity does not worsen the headache. Tension headaches may be associated with anorexia, but other gastrointestinal disturbances such as nausea are uncommon. Mild photophobia or phonophobia may be present, but, according to IHS criteria, they should not occur simultaneously. The presence of muscle tenderness, if any, offers little diagnostic value since it is also common in migraine. Tension-headache pain rarely awakens one from sleep.

MIXED AND TRANSFORMATIONAL HEADACHE PATTERNS

A commonly encountered headache in clinical practice is the mixed or transformed headache. As the names imply, this headache shares features of both migraine and the tension-type headache and often evolves from an episodic-headache pattern (usually migraine). Typically, there is a baseline headache on which is superimposed periods of more migraine-like activity. Depending on the phase of headache activity during which the patient is evaluated, clinical symptomatology can span the spectrum of migraine and tension headache.

Transformational and mixed headache disorders are frequently associated with medication misuse, depression, sleep disturbances, and anxiety disorders (19, pp. 138–145; 24).

DRUG-ASSOCIATED HEADACHE DISORDERS

Perhaps one of the most difficult headache disorders encountered in clinical practice is the medication-associated chronic daily headache. Physicians and patients alike are often tempted to increase drugs that are at least partially effective against headache, or to add more drugs to already existing treatment plans. This can be an imprudent practice since research has suggested that these drugs may in fact perpetuate the headache cycle when used on a daily or near-daily basis (25). The types of drugs most frequently implicated in drug-rebound headaches are the over-the-counter analgesics, caffeine, prescription analgesics, anxiolytics and ergotamines (26). The exact magnitude of this problem is unknown, but it is probably significant given the vast quantities of analgesic medication consumed in the United States.

Analgesic- and ergotamine-induced headaches are characterized by a daily headache pattern that typically fluctuates in intensity. The baseline headache is dull in quality, bilateral, and generally not associated with significant nausea, photophobia, or phonophobia (27). However, migraine-like attacks may be superimposed on this headache pattern. As patients self-medicate, the period of symptomatic relief shortens and a habituation cycle becomes perpetuated. Withdrawal of the offending agent typically results in a severe rebound headache. Diagnosis is confirmed after withdrawal of the offending drug produces improvement in the daily headache pattern.

CLUSTER HEADACHE

Cluster headache is a devastating headache that is far less prevalent than migraine, afflicting an estimated 0.1% of the population (28). It afflicts men approximately five times more frequently than women, and does not appear to have a clear familial association (29). Typically, cluster begins in the second and third decade of life. Those with cluster headaches have a high predilection for tobacco use compared with the migraine or non-headache population (30,31).

Cluster headaches are characterized by periods of sudden excruciating pain lasting 15 minutes to 3 hours, although most are between 30 and 45 minutes (19, p. 81). *Cluster* refers to the fact that these headaches occur at least once a day for periods of 3 to 16 weeks, then resolve for periods of months to years. There may be seasonal periodicity in some patients.

The headache is associated with ipsilateral autonomic disturbances such as conjunctival erythema, nasal congestion, lacrimation, or localized facial edema. In approximately 60% of cases, there is a partial Horner's syndrome with pupillary constriction and ptosis (32).

Cluster pain usually affects the periorbital area, temple, or frontal area, although it can be localized to the jaw, nose, chin, and teeth (13,33). Gastrointestinal symptoms commonly seen in migraine are absent in cluster headache. During a cluster attack, an individual often appears restless and agitated. They frequently pace and are unable to find a comfortable position.

Cluster headaches often occur shortly after falling asleep, resulting in patients' fearing sleep. Vasodilators, particularly alcohol, can precipitate cluster attacks (13, pp. 121–122). Cluster can be *episodic*, with discrete periods of cluster activity, or *chronic*, in which the cluster period lasts more than one year with no period of relief lasting more than 14 days (2, pp. 35–37).

CHRONIC PAROXYSMAL HEMICRANIA

Chronic paroxysmal hemicrania (CPH) is a rare headache disorder that shares many clinical features with cluster (2, pp. 37–38). This syndrome is characterized by multiple short, excruciating periorbital headaches that occur on a daily basis. Each attack is of short duration, averaging 1–2 minutes but they may last up to 45 minutes. They recur on average 14 times per day, but periods of activity may vary. (Diagnostic criteria require a frequency above five attacks a day more than half the time.) This syndrome is characterized by ipsilateral autonomic dysfunctions similar to those noted with cluster. It occurs more frequently in females, and the headache is responsive to indomethacin (34). Recently, episodic paroxysmal hemicrania has been described (35).

HEADACHES OF SHORT DURATION

Headaches of short duration are a heterogeneous group of headache disorders that are typically benign, although in some instances may herald underlying organic disease (2, pp. 39–41). They are characterized by brief, often intense periods of headache pain.

The *idiopathic stabbing headache*, sometimes nicknamed "jabs and jolts" syndrome or the "icepick headache," is a common short-duration headache. Approximately 40% of migraineurs note these headaches either in conjunction with migraine attacks or between attacks (35). These headaches occur predominately in the distribution of the first branch of the trigeminal nerve and last for only a fraction of a second. They can occur as a single stab or in a brief series of stabs. They are considered to be benign.

Headaches arising from cold stimulus, or "ice cream headaches," are common in both the headache and non-headache population. These headaches can occur as the result of either external application or ingestion of something cold. The pain is generally felt in the middle of the forehead between the eyes and resolves when the cold stimulus is removed. In migraineurs, the pain may be referred to the usual site of migraine pain.

Benign cough headache and *benign exertional headache* are similar in mechanism and may herald organic disease in about 10% of cases (35). Exertional headaches are more common in younger adults and cough headaches are more common in older adults.

Headache associated with sexual activity, or coital headache, may also be a sign of underlying pathology, although most are not. They are more common in men and may occur during sexual arousal or orgasm. A third variant is related to low CNS pressure, presumably due to a meningeal tear (35), and is associated with assuming an upright posture.

CHRONIC DAILY HEADACHE DISORDERS

Chronic daily or near-daily headaches are not easily classified in the IHS system. They have usually been classified under chronic tension headache. However, it is frequently noted that chronic daily headaches evolve from episodic migraine and that these headaches retain many features of migraine. Thus, it may be inappropriate to classify them as chronic tension headache.

Migraine and tension headache have long been considered distinct clinical entities, but some clinicians and researchers believe that migraine and tension headache represent different points on a spectrum rather than distinct clinical entities.

A practical classification for primary care physicians of chronic daily or near-daily headache is shown below.

1. Transformed migraine
   A. With medication overuse
   B. Without medication overuse

(The initial headache was episodic migraine that over time evolved into daily or near-daily headache. These headaches often retain many clinical features of the underlying migraine headache.)

2. Chronic tension-type headache
   A. With medication overuse
   B. Without medication overuse

(The initial primary headache pattern was episodic tension headache that over time has evolved into daily or near-daily headache. These headaches retain many clinical features of tension headache.)

3. New daily persistent headache
   A. With medication overuse
   B. Without medication overuse

(These headaches begin as chronic daily or near-daily headaches without an obvious evolution from an episodic headache disorder.)

This classification system has not yet been incorporated into the IHS guidelines. However, it is a practical clinical guide to chronic daily headaches and offers therapeutic considerations.

CONCLUSION

The diagnosis of headache can at times be simple, and yet its subtlety can perplex even the experienced headache specialist. The most fundamental tool to ensure accurate diagnosis is the patient's history. Therefore, compassion and understanding of the fear, suffering, and disability that headache can produce are paramount in establishing a therapeutic relationship. With an accurate diagnosis and a strong physician–patient relationship, headache is a malady that can be successfully managed.

REFERENCES

1. Which Headache? A Guide to the Diagnosis and Management of Headache. Worthing, England: Professional Postgraduate Services Europe Ltd., 1991.
2. Headache Classification Committee of the International Headache Society. Classification and diagnostic criteria for headache disorders, cranial neuralgias, and facial pain. Cephalalgia 1988; 8:(suppl 7):1–96.
3. Russell MB, Holm-Thomsen O. Migraine in primary care: Diagnosis of migraine, treatment with subcutaneous sumatriptan. Presented at 9th Migraine Trust International Symposium, Sept. 7–10, 1992.
4. Saddier P, Michel P, Jacquier-Garcia M, Tison S, Vivares C, Milan JJ, et al. Migraine and headache: physicians' diagnostic skills and prescriptions in current medical practice. Presented at 9th Migraine Trust International Symposium, Sept. 7–10, 1992.

5. Klassen AC, Berman M. Medical care for headache—a consumer survey. Cephalalgia 1991; 11(suppl 11):105.
6. Blau JN. Migraine: clinical, therapeutic, conceptual, and research aspects. London: Chapman and Hall, 1987:4–7.
7. Stewart WF, Lipton RB, Celentano DD, Reed ML. Prevalence of migraine headache in the United States: relation to age, income, race, and other socio-demographic factors. JAMA 1992; 267:64–69.
8. Maytal J, Lipton RB, Solomon S, Shinnar S. Childhood onset cluster headaches. Headache 1992; 32:275–279.
9. Silberstein SD. Evaluation and emergency treatment of headache. Headache 1992; 32:396–407.
10. Silberstein SD, Silberstein MM. New concepts in the pathogenesis of headache. Pain Management 1990; 297–303.
11. Dailies DJ. Wolf's Headache and Other Head Pain. 3rd ed. New York: Oxford University Press, 1972.
12. Travel J, Simon D. Myofascial Pain and Dysfunction: The Trigger Point Manual. Baltimore: Williams and Wilkins, 1983:165–329.
13. Kudrow L. Cluster headaches. In: Blau JN, ed. Migraine: Clinical and Research Aspects. Baltimore: Johns Hopkins University Press, 1987:113–133.
14. Celentano DD, Stewart WF, Lipton RB, Reed ML. Medication use and disability among migraineurs: a national probability sample survey. Headache 1992; 32:223–228.
15. Mathew NT, Stubis E, Nigam MP. Transformation of episodic migraine into daily headache: analysis of factors. Headache 1982; 22:66–68.
16. Mathew NT, Reuveni U, Perez F. Transformed or evolutive migraine. Headache 1987; 27:102–106.
17. Henry JB. Clinical Diagnosis and Management by Laboratory Methods. 17th ed. Philadelphia: W.B. Saunders, 1984.
18. Brust JCM. In: Rowland LP, ed. Merritt's Textbook of Neurology. 7th ed. Philadelphia: Lea & Febiger, 1984.
19. Diamond S, Dailies DJ. The Practicing Physician's Approach to Headache. 5th ed. Baltimore: Williams and Wilkins, 1992.
20. Selby G. Investigating migraine: when, why and how. In: Blau JN, ed. Migraine: Clinical and Research Aspects. Baltimore: Johns Hopkins University Press, 1987:81–83.
21. Smith R. Management of chronic headache. Can Fam Physician 1989; 35: 1835–1839.
22. Celentano DD, Stewart WF, Lipton RB, Reed ML. Medication use and disability from severe headache: a national probability sample. Cephalalgia 1991; 11(suppl 11):105.
23. Blau JN. Adult migraine: the patient observed. In: Blau JN, ed. Migraine: Clinical and Research Aspects. Baltimore: Johns Hopkins University Press, 1987:3–17.
24. Mathew NT, Stubis E, Nigam MP. Transformation of episodic migraine into daily headache: analysis of factors. Headache 1982; 22:66–68.

25. Kudrow L. Paradoxical effects of frequent analgesic use. Adv Neurol 1982; 33:335–341.
26. Mathew N. Reuvenie UR. Drug induced refractory headache: clinical features and management. Headache 1987; 27:305.
27. Rapoport AM. Analgesic rebound headache. Headache 1988; 28:662–665.
28. Ekbom K, Ahlborg B, Schele R. Prevalence of migraine and cluster headache in Swedish men of 18. Headache 1978; 18:9–19.
29. Lance JW. Mechanism and Management of Headache. 4th ed. London: Butterworth Scientific 1982:22–23, 211–220.
30. Graham JR. Cluster headache. Headache 1972; 11:175–185.
31. Kudrow L. Physical and personality characteristics in cluster headache. Headache 1974; 13:197–201.
32. Kudrow L. Cluster Headache: Mechanism and Management. London: Oxford University Press, 1980:10–20.
33. Manzoni GC, Terzano MG, Bono G, Micieli G, Martucci N, Nappi G. Cluster headache—clinical findings in 180 patients. Cephalalgia 1983; 3:21–30.
34. Antonaci F, Sjaastad O. Chronic paroxysmal hemicrania (CPH): A review of the clinical manifestations. Headache 1989; 29:648–656.
35. Solomon S. Headaches of short duration. In: Update on Headache: A Comprehensive Course in Mechanisms and Management. AASH 1992:192–200.

7

Perspectives on Headache Management
Concepts and Commentary

Roger K. Cady

Shealy Institute for Comprehensive Health Care
Springfield, Missouri

INTRODUCTION

Plato, commenting on comprehensive treatment of headache, offered a prescription of pain reliever in exchange for a patient's consent to have his soul treated first: "for in order to treat the eyes you have to treat the head, and for this you have to treat the whole body, and in order to treat the body you have to treat the soul" (1). Neglect of this principle explains the frequent failure of Greek physicians. While most physicians today would agree that patients are best understood in their human context, it is often difficult to integrate this concept into daily practice.

Perhaps reflecting this, surveys among the headache population suggest significant dissatisfaction about medical care. In one study (2), nearly three-fourths of migraineurs expressed discontent, citing as sources of their dissatisfaction physician bias, lack of compassion and understanding, and inadequate explanation of their disorder. Other studies suggest that physicians' appraisal of therapeutic interactions may differ from that of the patients. Of 158 migraineurs participating in a clinical trial (3), only 11% described their usual headache therapy as very good and only 6% felt the number of doses of medication prescribed to treat a migraine attack was adequate.

Migraine is a disorder frequently misunderstood by friends, family, coworkers, employers, and the health-care system. Bias abounds; society tends to view headache as a source of humor and those suffering with them as being weak and ineffective in managing their lives. These factors often deter sufferers from seeking medical care.

Without confirmatory diagnostic tests, the relationship between physician and migraineur becomes the most important component of successful diagnosis and management. However, effective management demands that physicians reach beyond traditional standards of successful therapy and comprehend the web of medical, psychological, and social interactions confronting the headache patient.

The current treatment paradigm for headache needs to be expanded. Traditionally, physicians have viewed their role in headache with ambiguity. On the one hand, a diagnosis needs to rule out "serious disease"; on the other, an acute attack demands a remedy. There are long-term management needs to be addressed as well. This chapter extrapolates from epidemiological and clinical factors in headache to suggest a model for comprehensive management.

MIGRAINE AS A PUBLIC-HEALTH ISSUE

Early identification and aggressive management of many chronic disorders, such as hypertension, hyperlipidemia, and diabetes, have been credited with decreasing morbidity and improving quality of life. In order for a particular disease to warrant this intensive approach, it must fulfill several criteria, including:

1. Significant prevalence within the population
2. Evidence that a significant portion of the population with this condition is currently undiagnosed and undertreated
3. Acknowledged consequences of inadequate identification and treatment of the disorder
4. Availability of effective therapy
5. Evidence that instituting this therapy changes the outcome of the underlying disorder in a positive manner

The best studied of the headache disorders is migraine. Evidence that it fulfills all these criteria is accumulating but remains incomplete. However, available information does warrant consideration of a comprehensive management model for primary care of migraine.

MANAGEMENT

Recent epidemiological data (4,5) describe migraine as a highly prevalent, underdiagnosed, and undertreated disease that causes decades of disability for many sufferers. It is, in many respects, a chronic disease. Management models successfully applied to other chronic disease states suggest that early identification and adequate treatment can diminish long-term morbidity. Migraine lends itself to such a management model, which can be divided into five basic components: 1) education, 2) acute treatment strategies, 3) prophylactic strategies, 4) nonpharmacological therapies, and 5) long-term follow-up.

Education

As with all chronic disorders, education of the patient is the cornerstone of successful management. Education should emphasize the biological basis for migraine and invite the patient to be a participant in management of the disorder. Several areas of migraine education are important to address.

Headache Threshold

Many believe that the barrier that protects the integrity of the central nervous system from various stressors is genetically vulnerable in migraineurs (6). Migraine occurs when stressors accumulate beyond a critical level, over the threshold. In other words, there is an interrelationship between environment, the genetically determined stressor threshold, and the occurrence of migraine.

The concept of migraine "triggers" has been emphasized in the past but many now view triggers as risk factors that accumulate to create an environment in which migraine is likely to occur. It is important to educate patients about precipitating factors, including those that might not be obvious, such as dietary substances. Encouraging the development of a migraine-protective environment that includes daily stress management, physical exercise, regular sleep, and consistent mealtimes is also helpful.

Use of Medication

A migraineur in the midst of an acute attack may overutilize available medication, resulting in disruptive side effects. Others, fearing or anticipating an attack, may take acute treatment medications, a habit that can lead to medication misuse and migraine transformation (see Chapter 5).

Still others may see medication as the last resort and view intervention as a sign of failure. Often there is confusion about prophylactic versus acute treatment medications. Once these issues are explained, the informed headache sufferer may use medication not only more responsibly but also more effectively.

Coping Strategies

Fear and anticipatory anxiety are often prominent features in the migraine population. Some migraineurs withdraw and avoid activities that are potentially stressful and capable of provoking a migraine. Others deny the migraine and ignore the process until debilitating symptoms force them into retreat. In contrast, others passively accept migraine as a way of life or a family curse.

Migraine is a process of the body that often forces the person to withdraw from external stimulation and seek rest and solitude. As the headache sufferer recognizes this process, working with the physiological messages may help him achieve relief. Examples include getting sufficient rest, buffering oneself from stressful situations, and, often, early appropriate pharmacological intervention.

At times, education needs to include family and/or employers. Such interventions may stop the fear/anxiety spiral that precipitates further headache activity.

Acute Treatment Strategies

Migraineurs most often encounter the medical system seeking medication for relief from acute headache attacks. Even though there are many effective medications available, none is effective for everyone. In addition, although migraine is not curable, it is a manageable disease. Understanding this distinction is the key to realistic expectations, for physicians as well as patients.

The goals of acute therapy are fourfold: 1) to ameliorate migraine pain and associated symptoms, 2) to minimize disability and restore the patient to normal function as quickly as possible, 3) to provide therapy that is predictable and effective over extended periods of time, and 4) to ensure that these benefits are achieved safely.

Studies show that a majority of migraineurs rely on nonprescription therapy (5). In a sample population of migraineurs, 60% of women and 70% of men relied on over-the-counter medications for acute attacks of migraine (7). Many patients, once identified and prescribed headache medication, will discontinue it on their own because of side effects, ineffectiveness, or unreasonable expectations of results.

Medical utilization by migraineurs is significantly higher than that of the non-migraine population, offering physicians frequent opportunities to diagnose migraine (see Chapter 3). These encounters are often for reasons other than headache, suggesting a need for physicians to actively solicit information leading to a headache diagnosis. Then, in determining the course of treatment, the physician must take into account the patient's therapeutic needs. For example, a person who is awakened in the early morning by severe migraine-related nausea is unlikely to absorb oral medication.

For patients, the desperation generated by intense head pain may render unimportant the fact that utilization of narcotics, phenothiazines, and other medications can prolong migraine disability. This leads to medication misuse. The headache sufferer needs guidance on when and how to use acute treatment medication before reaching this extreme condition. Therapy is available that disrupts the process of migraine rather than merely controlling symptoms. As a result, migraine-related disability can be minimized.

Prophylactic Medication

Migraineurs with frequent or disabling attacks may be helped by prophylactic medication. There are no clear guidelines governing the indications for prophylaxis; in general, however, it is warranted when migraine occurs more than twice a month, is disabling, and is not readily controlled with acute therapy (see Chapter 11).

Before prophylaxis is initiated, the physician and patient should review possible precipitating factors of headache as well as lifestyle changes that might prevent future attacks. The physician should also explain the importance of regulating acute treatment medication. The goals of the therapy are outlined, and the potential risks and benefits of the proposed medications are clarified.

It can take weeks or months of monitoring and adjustment before a prophylactic regimen demonstrates success. The physician may ask the patient to keep a diary to help them both evaluate prophylaxis. Prophylactic medication can usually be withdrawn after a period of 6 to 12 months without increasing headache activity. This is particularly true if lifestyle factors have been modified and effective acute therapy instituted.

Resistance to prophylactic medication has been noted to develop over time (8), and overreliance on acute treatment drugs can interfere with prophylactic therapies (9). If resistance is suspected, the initial drug should be discontinued and another prophylactic medication prescribed. This avoids the polypharmacy characteristic of the headache population. Multiple-drug prophylaxis is generally indicated only after several attempts with single therapy have failed.

Prophylaxis represents a long-term expense for the patient: The average cost of a prophylactic regimen can easily exceed $1000 per year. The frequency of adverse effects, such as weight gain, is another of the aspects of long-term prophylaxis that should be discussed carefully with the patient.

Not all prophylactic regimens require prescription medication. These include herbal products (e.g., feverfew), fish oil (omega-3 fatty acids), magnesium, and a daily aspirin tablet. If a patient wants to explore these options and there are no contraindications, physician encouragement will help the patient step closer toward personal responsibility for health.

Nonpharmacological Therapy

Nonpharmacological interventions for headache can be divided into two categories: 1) those that relieve headache and 2) those that enhance a headache-protective environment. These therapies can be active and patient-directed or passive and provider-directed. After an initial training period, self-directed therapies are usually more effective.

Examples of nonpharmacological headache treatment include modalities such as transcutaneous and/or transcranial electric stimulation, acupuncture, and osteopathic manipulative therapy. These modalities may prove helpful in selected patients.

Examples of nonpharmacological therapy that enhances a headache-protective environment include relaxation therapy, biofeedback, patient and/or family counseling, and exercise. Good nutrition, adequate sleep, massage, physical therapy, and osteopathic manipulative therapy could also fall into this category.

Long-Term Medical Needs

Migraine is a chronic disease. Like many other chronic disorders, such as hypertension or hyperlipidemia, establishing a long-term therapeutic relationship with the patient is essential to optimal care. Historically, migraineurs have not been engaged in chronic disease dynamics. However, there are good reasons to consider this model of health care, including the opportunity to educate the patient, monitor acute treatment or prophylactic medications, and screen for other associated disorders.

MIGRAINE AS A CLINICAL MARKER FOR OTHER DISEASE: THE SEROTONIN CONNECTION

Serotonin (5-HT) has been proposed as a central neurochemical in migraine pathophysiology (10,11). Recent research has proposed that serotonin interacts with a number of different serotonin receptor classes and subclasses (12). This array of serotonin receptors modulates a wide variety of diverse neurophysiological mechanisms including pain, vascular activity, mood, sexual behavior, sleep, and appetite (13,14). This may explain serotonin's involvement in a wide variety of clinical disorders and leads to speculation about migraine's relationship to other serotonergic disorders.

Migraine is associated with several other disorders of serotonin metabolism, including depression, irritable bowel syndrome, anxiety disorders, fibromyalgia, and sleep disturbance (see Chapter 13). Identifying and adequately treating migraine in early life may provide the opportunity to minimize the impact of these related disorders.

BIOPSYCHOSOCIAL MODEL

Many chronic disorders are best managed in what has been defined as the biopsychosocial model, which expands the traditional disease model by recognizing that, over time, chronic disease encompasses more than nociceptive mechanisms. After all, uncontrolled headache affects a patient's life even during headache-free periods. This is reflected in the downward socioeconomic stratification of the headache population as well as quality-of-life changes attributable to headache. Recognition of the "bigger picture" validates the importance of adequate headache management. Physicians who measure the success of therapy beyond traditional treatment parameters provide a service and an understanding that are valuable and appreciated by patients.

Beyond the biochemical/nociceptive mechanisms of headache, there are the consequences of living with a chronic disorder. As part of the natural history of migraine, there may ensue a more generalized neurochemical disruption that, over time, will be manifested in more frequent headaches and other serotonin-related clinical syndromes. Viewing migraine as a clinical marker of this "at-risk" population underscores the value of early diagnosis, treatment, and long-term follow-up. Recurrent uncontrolled attacks of migraine can lead to poor self-esteem, disruption of family life, decreased performance at work, and more frequent medical encounters. All these factors are part of the bigger picture of migraine, and effective management of migraine should be designed to address as many of them as possible.

CONCLUSION

Headache may be a specific disease state, a symptom of other underlying diseases, or part of a broader clinical complex. It can challenge the diagnostic and management skills of health-care providers, yet, properly managed, it can be a rewarding disease to treat. Assisting sufferers to effectively manage headache can improve their quality of life and allow them to enjoy greater productivity. A comprehensive management style can help physicians to achieve this goal.

REFERENCES

1. Quoted in Ref. 6, p 661.
2. Klassen AC, Berman M. Medical care for headaches—a consumer survey. Cephalalgia 1991; 11(suppl 11):85–86.
3. Cady RK, Dexter J, Sargent JD, Markley H, Osterhaus JT, Webster CJ. Efficacy of sumatriptan in repeated episodes of migraine. Neurology 1993; 43:1363–1368.
4. Stewart WF, Lipton RB, Celentano DD, Reed ML. Prevalence of migraine headache in the United States. JAMA 1992; 267:64–69.
5. Celentano DD, Stewart WF, Lipton RB, Reed ML. Medication use and disability from severe headache: a national probability sample. Cephalalgia 1991; 11(suppl 11):105.
6. Lance JW. A concept of migraine and the search for the ideal headache drug. Headache 1990; 30(suppl 1):17–23.
7. Celentano DD, Stewart WF, Lipton RB, Reed ML. Medication use and disability from severe headache: a national probability sample. Cephalalgia 1991; 11(suppl 11):85–86.
8. Raskin NH, Schwartz RK. Interval therapy of migraine: long-term results. Headache 1980; 20:336–340.
9. Rapaport AM, Weeks RE, Sheftell FD, Baskin SM, Verdi J. Analgesic rebound headache: theoretical and practical implications. Cephalalgia 1985; 5(suppl 3):448–449.
10. Lance JW, Lambet GA, Goadsby PJ, Zagami AS. 5-Hydroxytryptamine and its putative aetiological involvement in migraine. Cephalalgia 1989; 9(suppl 9):7–13.
11. Humphrey PPA, Feniuk W, Perren MJ, Beresford IJM, Skingle M, Walley ET. Serotonin and migraine. Ann NY Acad Sci 1990; 600:587–598.
12. Peroutka SJ. The pharmacology of current anti-migraine drugs. Headache 1990; 30(suppl 1):5–11.

13. Fuller RW, Wong DT. Serotonin uptake and serotonin reuptake inhibition. Ann NY Acad Sci 1990; 600:68–80.

14. Csernansky JG, Poscher M, Faull KF. Serotonin in schizophrenia. In: Coccaro EF, Murphy DL, eds. Serotonin in Major Psychiatric Disorders. Washington, DC: American Psychiatric Press, 1990.

8

Drug Treatment of Acute Migraine

Seymour Solomon and Richard B. Lipton

*Albert Einstein College of Medicine
and Montefiore Medical Center
Bronx, New York*

INTRODUCTION

The ideal therapy for an attack of migraine would quickly, permanently, and invariably abort the headache and associated features without side effects (1). The therapy would allow a prompt return to normal activity without residual symptoms of migraine or medication use. Although there are no perfect remedies, highly effective therapeutic strategies can be found for most patients.

There are several modes of drug administration and several medications designed to achieve therapeutic goals. In treating an individual patient, the response of that patient is paramount; efficacy and toxicity data generated for groups of patients are less important. Some people who do not respond to first-line medication inexplicably respond to second- or third-line drugs. In addition, it is sometimes necessary to use combinations of these agents. Finally, it must be emphasized that all medications may be overused or abused. Drugs designed for an occasional acute headache, if taken daily, may evoke and perpetuate daily headaches (2,3).

We will first review the pharmacology of the antimigraine drugs, then consider their use at different stages of the acute attack: onset, midstage, incapacitating, and intractable (status migrainosus). Finally, we will discuss other factors to be considered in prioritizing treatment.

PHARMACOLOGICAL ACTION OF ANTIMIGRAINE MEDICATIONS

Because the pathophysiology of migraine is not fully understood, the mechanisms of action for drugs used to abort attacks is, in part, speculative. Migraine attacks occur in individuals with innate susceptibility to migraine. In migraine sufferers, a lower threshold permits factors in the environment or the internal milieu to readily trigger an attack. The triggering impulses reach brain stem neurons (probably in the raphe nuclei and locus ceruleus), which in turn may then set off the cascade of events called migraine (4). The aura of migraine is probably due to spreading depression of cortical neuronal activity (5). The pain of migraine is probably caused by perivascular neurogenic inflammation; neurotransmitters released from the periarterial trigeminal nerve endings cause inflammation and vasodilation (6). Many of the drugs effective for acute treatment act at the trigemionovascular junction, inhibiting release of neurotransmitters, presumably through agonist activity at presynaptic serotonergic autoreceptors of the 5HT1 type (see Chapter 9). Other acute agents may act in the brain stem on serotonergic or opioid receptors (e.g., narcotics), or on centers that mediate nausea and vomiting (e.g., phenothiazines). We now discuss the pharmacology of agents used in the treatment of acute attacks. The new antimigraine drug sumatriptan is discussed in Chapter 10.

Ergotamine Tartrate

There is considerable variability in the absorption of ergotamine following oral, sublingual, or rectal administration. Rectal administration produces peak concentrations approximately 20 times greater than those produced by oral or sublingual administration (7). Clearance of ergotamine and its metabolites is mainly through biliary secretion. The mean elimination half-life of the drug is approximately 2 hours, but the biological half-life is significantly greater (8,9) due to the activity of persistent metabolites (10). In addition, ergotamine may dissociate slowly from the serotonin receptors that mediate drug action (11); the significance of this is discussed in Chapter 10.

In cranial blood vessels, vasoconstriction evoked by ergotamine occurs in the external rather than the internal carotid arterial tree (12,13). Ergotamine acts as a vasoconstrictor if the tonus of the vessel is low, as is the case with the dilated external carotid arterial bed during migraine headache, but may also act as a vasodilator if the tonus is high (14). Cranial vasodilation in migraine is associated with mediators of periarterial inflammation. Ergotamine's vasoconstricting action may be related to its ability to block the release of peptides from periarterial trigeminal nerve endings. This action blocks experimentally induced neurogenic inflammation in the dura mater of laboratory animals (15). In addition, some of ergotamine's beneficial action may be due to the depression of serotonergic neurones of the brain stem raphe nuclei, which may mediate pain transmission and regulate cranial circulation (16).

The most common side effects of ergotamine are nausea, vomiting, and epigastric discomfort; diarrhea and restlessness may also occur (17). More serious adverse effects include paresthesias, cramps, and weakness of the extremities, angina or other precordial distress, transient alterations in cardiac rate, and, rarely, localized edema and pruritus. Ergotamine has occasionally produced several problems, including gangrene and myocardial and cerebral infarction (18). The risk may be increased if ergotamine is given with other antimigraine vasoconstricting agents, e.g., methysergide (18). When severe peripheral ischemia occurs, parenteral infusion of nitroprusside or papaverine usually reverses the process (19).

Excessive use of ergotamine on a daily or almost-daily basis may cause rebound headache, a self-sustaining cycle of frequent headache perpetuated by medication overuse (20). Prophylactic therapy is often ineffective until the cycle of rebound headache and ergotamine overuse is discontinued. To prevent this physical dependence, ergotamine tartrate should not be taken more than 2 days a week. A nonsteroidal anti-inflammatory analgesic and a preventive agent (often a tricyclic antidepressant/ centrally acting analgesic) are substituted for the ergotamine in withdrawing patients from this drug. Hospitalization is sometimes required for this purpose.

Ergotamine is contraindicated in people who have peripheral vascular disease and other systemic vascular disease, including severe hypertension (17). Because of its gastrointestinal effects, ergotamine is contraindicated in people who have gastric or duodenal ulcer. It should not be used in patients who have renal or hepatic disease or in the presence of infection. Ergotamine tartrate and most other agents used for acute migraine are contraindicated during pregnancy.

Dihydroergotamine

Dihydroergotamine (DHE) is administered parenterally because it undergoes extensive first-pass metabolism in the liver when administered by the oral route (9,21). The elimination half-life of DHE is approximately 30 minutes, but with its metabolites the half-life is approximately 1 day. The peak plasma concentration occurs at 30 minutes with intramuscular administration and 45 minutes via the subcutaneous or intranasal routes (22,23). Intranasal DHE will soon be available in the United States.

The mechanism of action of DHE is similar to that of ergotamine tartrate. It has high affinity for 5HT-1D and 5HT-1A receptors and alpha 1- and 2-adrenergic receptors, but also for other serotonergic, adrenergic, and dopaminergic receptors (24). Although it was thought that DHE did not cross the blood–brain barrier, labeled DHE has been found in brain stem serotonergic centers in experimental animals (25). DHE has several advantages over ergotamine tartrate. It is more venoconstrictive than arterial constrictive, thereby decreasing the potential for serious adverse effects (26,27). After intramuscular administration of DHE, nausea is less prominent than with ergotamine tartrate. However, after intravenous administration, nausea is prominent enough to merit coadministration of an antiemetic.

The side effects of DHE are similar to but much less prominent than those of ergotamine tartrate. Diarrhea is the most common adverse reaction; muscle aches and abdominal cramps sometime occur. The contraindications for DHE are also similar to those cited for ergotamine tartrate, but DHE has a greater margin of safety and there is little risk of rebound (28). Nevertheless, when DHE is used in individuals at risk for coronary artery disease it is wise to monitor the electrocardiogram after initial parenteral administrations.

Open trials suggest that intramuscular DHE is effective in terminating migraine during an attack in patients presenting to the doctor's office. Intravenous DHE is similarly effective in patient presenting to emergency departments and in terminating status migrainosus (28–30). A course of intravenous DHE over a period of a few days will usually break the cycle of chronic daily headaches that may have evolved from migraine (28).

Isometheptene

Isometheptene is a sympathomimetic agent that may relieve migraine pain through its vasoconstrictive actions (31,32). It is not available alone but rather in a combination with other agents [e.g., dichloralphenazone and acetaminophen (Midrin)] (33). This combination tablet is an effective, acute treatment for some migraine sufferers and may produce less nausea than ergotamine (31–33). Reactions range from insomnia to drowsiness, sensations of dizziness and generalized weakness, paresthesias, and palpitations. The precautions cited for the ergot preparations apply to isometheptene. Isometheptene is used the same way and for the same situations as ergotamine tartrate.

Nonsteroidal Anti-Inflammatory Drugs (NSAIDs)

Simple aspirin can abort mild attacks of migraine for some sufferers (34); patients satisfactorily treated with aspirin generally do not consult doctors. In specialized headache clinics, naproxen is probably the most commonly used NSAID in treating acute migraine (35,36). Naproxen is well absorbed following oral administration. Peak plasma concentrations occur 1 hour after administration of naproxen sodium (the salt) and 2 hours after naproxen (the acid). Plasma concentrations are higher after the salt than after the acid when a standard dose is administered (37,38). Approximately 60% of the dose is eliminated by the kidneys within 12 to 15 hours (39). The analgesic action becomes apparent within 1 hour and persists for approximately 8 hours.

The NSAIDs are effective in treating migraine at least in part because of their nociceptive action; they block cyclooxygenase and thus inhibit the biosynthesis of the prostanoids that modulate the excitability of neuro-receptors (40). Many of these agents have central activity independent of prostaglandin inhibition as well as peripheral analgesic action (41,42). In addition to their analgesic action, the anti-inflammatory activity of these drugs may be a factor in countering the periarterial inflammatory reaction associated with a migraine headache.

The most common adverse reactions of the NSAIDs are related to their effect on the gastrointestinal tract: nausea, heartburn, and abdominal discomfort are common; gastritis or ulceration may occur. In addition, they may evoke vague dizziness, drowsiness, and pruritus (40). Repeated use may be associated with peripheral edema and weight gain. Renal failure may be precipitated in patients with impaired kidney function (43).

NSAIDs should not be used in patients who have active peptic ulcers and should be used with care in people with a history of ulcer disease. Caution should also be exercised in patients who have impaired renal function or congestive heart failure. Serious hepatotoxicity is rare. Like aspirin, the NSAIDs inhibit platelet aggregation and may induce bleeding. Naproxen is highly bound to plasma protein and may displace other albumin-bound drugs from their binding sites (40). Therefore, patients receiving oral anticoagulants or hydantoins should be closely observed for interactions.

The NSAIDs, in high oral dosage, are used instead of or with ergotamine or isometheptene to abort acute migraine in its early stage. Particularly when the vasoconstrictors are contraindicated, the NSAIDs are the drugs of choice. If nausea and vomiting prevent oral administration, then indomethacin can be administered as a rectal suppository, or ketorolac may be given parenterally. The parenteral action is rapid and particularly useful for treatment in mid-attack.

Other Analgesics

Other peripherally and centrally acting analgesics and narcotics can abort migraine. Many of these agents have sedative effects that may ameliorate some of the associated symptoms, but the mechanism for terminating all features of the attack is unknown. Their beneficial effects probably relate to their action on serotonergic and other biochemical systems in the brain stem and hypothalamus.

Analgesics (aspirin or acetaminophen) are often combined with caffeine in over-the-counter preparations (e.g., Anacin or Excedrin), and prescription formulations typically add a barbiturate (e.g., butalbital in Fiorinal, Fioricet, Esgic); finally, codeine may also be added (44). Caffeine enhances absorption and has some analgesic action in itself (45,46). The barbiturate-evoked sedation may help ameliorate the attack. These combinations are more effective than their individual ingredients used alone (44). They are most effective when used at the onset of the attack. Caution is necessary with these agents, as medication overuse and rebound may develop.

Narcotics may also be used for the acute treatment of migraine. Simple analgesics combined with codeine are effective in some patients. Narcotics more potent than codeine, e.g., meperidine, have been used parenterally to abort migraine at the height of an attack (47). Phenothiazines, which per se have antimigraine action, are commonly used with the opioid (48,49). Recently, butorphanol, a partial opioid agonist, has been marketed as a nasal spray for the acute treatment of migraine (50).

Phenothiazines

Two phenothiazines have received widespread use in acute migraine: chlorpromazine (Thorazine) and prochlorperazine (Compazine). Chlorpromazine (as the prototype phenothiazine) is metabolized in the intestinal wall and liver, decreasing its bioavailability to approximately 33%

(51). The onset of action occurs within 20–30 minutes, and peak plasma concentration occurs in 2 to 4 hours. After intramuscular administration, the plasma concentrations are up to 10 times greater than after oral administration (52). The elimination plasma half-life is approximately 30 hours, but months later some metabolites still persist in the urine (51). These agents have also been used intravenously in the acute treatment of migraine.

The phenothiazines are recognized as having antiemetic and tranquilizing properties. Both factors are useful in treating the associated symptoms of migraine. These agents also abort the pain as well as the associated symptoms of the attack (48,49). The effectiveness in stopping the pain of migraine is probably related to their strong antiadrenergic activity and perhaps to their slight antiserotonergic and antihistaminic action (51). The phenothiazines are potent antagonists of dopamine transmission, accounting in part for their psychotropic benefits and extrapyramidal side effect (53).

There are many side effects of phenothiazine use; only those associated with treatment for acute migraine need to be considered here (51). The most common behavioral effect is sedation, but paradoxically insomnia may occur as well as confusion and impairment of psychomotor activity. Orthostatic hypotension is another common adverse effect. Anxiety, tremor, and laryngeal and pharyngeal spasm may occur, as well as excessive sweating, pallor, and fever. Akathisia may appear almost immediately after acute administration. The adverse effects of Parkinsonism do not occur after an initial dose, but may occur as early as after a few days of daily therapy. Acute dystonic reactions occasionally occur but usually respond promptly to treatment. The neuroleptic malignant syndrome and tardive dyskinesia are rare. Anticholinergic symptoms (dryness of the mouth, tachycardia, blurred vision, urinary retention, and constipation) may also occur. Rare reactions are agranulocytosis and cholestatic jaundice.

Phenothiazines should be administered with caution in those who are receiving other sedative medication and in people who have cardiovascular, liver, or renal disease (51). Their depressant effect may further impair respiration in patients who have chronic respiratory disorders. Because of anticholinergic activity, caution is warranted in patients with glaucoma. These agents may lower the convulsive threshold and diminish the effect of oral anticoagulants.

The phenothiazines are most often used in mid-attack for incapacitating migraine or status migrainosus (48,49). They counteract withdrawal symptoms in patients being weaned from excessively used acute headache medications.

PRIORITIZING THERAPY

The Use of Medications at Different Stages of Migraine

Most often, with the treatments described in this chapter, medication is or should be taken by the patient at the onset of a migraine attack. Sometimes administration may be deferred until the attack is full-blown. A small minority of attacks are treated in the middle of a severe bout in the doctor's office or emergency department. Rarely, hospitalization is required for status migrainosus.

Treatment of Migraine at Onset

Using conventional therapy, the greatest success is attained by intervention at the earliest stage. But sometimes migraine cannot be treated early for several reasons. Severe headaches may awaken the patient from sleep. Sometimes people with two headache types have difficulty determining at onset whether a particular headache will become a full-blown migraine attack. Mild, interval headaches may subside spontaneously or with over-the-counter analgesics. Many patients are reluctant to initiate antimigraine therapy until they are sure the attack is truly migrainous, often hoping against hope that the headache will "go away." Patients with frequent headaches must delay treatment to avoid medication overuse. The physician's instruction may create a bind; early treatment of every headache may lead to medication overuse. On the other hand, treatment may be less effective or ineffective for a full-blown attack. In patients with frequent headaches, the risks of rebound headache must be balanced against greater efficacy with early treatment. As a general rule, unless the headaches are frequent, with associated danger of excessive repeated use of medications, patients should be advised to begin treatment at the first inkling of migraine even if there is uncertainty about its validity. The strategy of early drug administration has some drawbacks. It may lead headache sufferers to overestimate therapeutic efficacy; spontaneous remission may be mistaken for therapeutic success.

An antinauseant such as metoclopramide is usually recommended just before use of the antimigraine drug (see "Symptom Profiles: Treatment of Nausea and Other Associated Features" later in this chapter) (55). The antinauseant not only counters the nausea and vomiting usually accompanying the headache, but also enhances gastric motility and helps to prevent the nausea often evoked by many of the agents used to abort migraine (56).

The standard prescription for acute treatment for the past half century has been ergotamine tartrate. Because this agent effects the external rather than the internal carotid arterial tree, it may be taken at the onset of a brief aura (57). However, if the aura is severe or prolonged, agents with vasoconstricting properties should not be used. Ergotamine tartrate is often combined with caffeine. The most commonly used form is an oral tablet that consists of ergotamine tartrate 1 mg and caffeine 100 mg. Two tablets are to be taken at onset and, if necessary, one tablet every $1/2$ hour to a maximum of six tablets per attack. (Variations in these as well as other dosages should be made according to the patient's response and tolerance.) The most effective mode of administration of ergotamine tartrate is the rectal suppository (having the same constituents as the oral preparation but double the amount of ergotamine) (7,58). It is best to start with one-quarter of the suppository, repeating that dose every $1/2$ hour if necessary. If that initial dose is ineffective, one-half, three-quarters, or the whole suppository should be tried for subsequent attacks. Ergotamine tartrate (2 mg) without caffeine may also be administered as a sublingual tablet. In some countries dihydroergotamine is available as a nasal spray (59). These modes of administration, avoiding first-pass liver metabolism, may result in more rapid blood levels and are useful for those patients who do not tolerate caffeine.

Isometheptene has actions that parallel those of ergotamine. It can be purchased only in combination with other medications [e.g., isometheptene mucate 65 mg, acetaminophen 324 mg, and dichloralphenazone 100 mg (Midrin)] and is taken by mouth (33). It is generally considered somewhat less potent than ergotamine tartrate but is also associated with a more favorable side-effect profile. The dosing schedule is the same as that for oral ergotamine tartrate.

High dosage of NSAIDs may abort an acute attack of migraine. Naproxen, indomethacin, meclofenamate, ibuprofen, piroxicam, diclofenac, and ketoproten taken by mouth are agents that have been effective in anecdotal and scientific studies (36,38,60–64). A typical dose of naproxen is 750 mg at onset of migraine and, if necessary, 500 mg 2 hours later. Indomethacin is also available by rectal suppository in the United States, and other NSAIDs are available as suppositories in other countries.

Many combinations of medications are often useful in aborting migraine. Aspirin or acetaminophen are combined: with caffeine (Anacin or Excedrin), with caffeine and a barbiturate [butalbital (Fiorinal, Fioricet, Esgic)], with caffeine and orphenadrine (Norgesic), with other agents (e.g., muscle relaxants, antihistamines), or with narcotics (codeine, its analogs, or propoxyphene). These combinations are more effective than the individual ingredients administered separately; there appears to be adjuvant action (44). If aspirin irritates the stomach, the acetaminophen combinations are preferred.

A more subtle danger is habituation and rebound headache. Many headache patients seen in headache clinics relate a history of increasingly frequent use of analgesics with progressive increase in the frequency and duration of headache, leading to chronic daily headaches/chronic tension-type headaches (2). These daily headaches appear to be due to a rebound phenomenon. As the blood level of the medication drops (between doses), the next headache is triggered. Agents designed to treat an attack of episodic headaches must not be used daily—preferably no more than 2 days per week (3).

As a rule, narcotic medications are best avoided in the treatment of benign pain syndromes. But this dictum is not absolute. Codeine, its analogs, or propoxyphene in combination with aspirin, acetaminophen, or caffeine (e.g., Percodan, Darvocet, Fiorinal #3) is sometimes necessary to abort an attack of migraine. The use of narcotics is perfectly legitimate if infrequent headaches are successfully treated and normal function is restored. However, the frequency of use must be monitored to prevent addiction or rebound headaches.

Treatment of Migraine in the Midst of an Attack

When people often find themselves in the midst of a severe migraine attack, the migraine is more difficult to treat successfully. Part of the difficulty in treating established attacks stems from failure to absorb oral agents, and alternative routes of administration should then be used. All the agents described above may be effective in established attacks. But if they fail it will be necessary to use higher dosages or combinations of drugs, or both. For example, an ergotamine or an isometheptene preparation may be used with an NSAID or a codeine compound. If the nausea is severe or vomiting has occurred, a phenothiazine and ergotamine should be given by rectal suppository. A sedative to induce sleep would be more appropriate at this stage than at the onset of attack. Patients may be taught to inject DHE intramuscularly (1.0 mg) if they find themselves in this predicament. Administration of butorphanol by nasal spray may be appropriate at this stage of migraine (50). It is effective in stopping an attack but is often associated with side effects (dizziness, nausea/vomiting, drowsiness, confusion), requiring bed rest or preventing return to normal activities (65).

Treatment of Incapacitating Migraine

Sometimes the pain and associated symptoms of a migraine attack are severe, intolerable, and totally disabling. In this setting, parenteral therapy is usually required. Patients may treat themselves at home but more often come to the doctor's office or to an emergency department to be treated. DHE 0.5 mg intravenously (I.V.) (over 2–3 minutes) given with 10 mg of metoclopramide has become a standard treatment. Patients may self-administer intramuscular DHE, 0.5 to 1 mg at home. I.V. administration of a phenothiazine (e.g., chlorpromazine 25 mg or prochlorphenazine 10 mg) may be used alone or instead of metoclopramide with DHE. Parenteral phenothiazines in themselves have a high success rate in aborting migraine (66,67). Unfortunately, akathisia often occurs with intravenous metoclopramide as well as the other phenothiazines; acute dystonic reactions are rare and may be treated with benztropine (Cogentin) 2 mg I.V. The NSAID ketorolac (30 to 60 mg intramuscularly) is effective for about half of patients, but experience with this agent is limited (68).

Narcotics (e.g., meperidine 100 mg) are still the most widely used parenteral treatments in emergency rooms. Although narcotic addiction is not an important consideration with occasional use, narcotics are not highly effective. Both DHE and prochlorperazine have been shown to be more effective than meperidine in emergency room–based studies (69). In addition, narcotics may produce drowsiness, hampering the patient's return to normal function and prolonging the emergency room stay.

As discussed in Chapter 10, sumatriptan may be used by subcutaneous injection at home or in the doctor's office or emergency room as an acute treatment for migraine.

The emergency department (ED) is not a good place to treat the severe migraine attack. A patient with severe pain, photophobia, and phonophobia is often kept waiting, sometimes for hours, in a brightly lit, noisy environment while doctors treat life-threatening conditions. Moreover, the ED doctor may fear the patient is seeking narcotics and subtly communicate this concern to the patient. Even optimal ED treatment is very expensive and (for migraine) inefficient. The patient's physician should develop a treatment plan that will keep the patient out of the ED.

Treatment of Intractable Migraine: Status Migrainosus

On rare occasions, all the above remedies fail and prolonged incapacitation occurs. Status migrainosus is the term applied to a migraine attack of more than 3 days' duration. Hospitalization is often warranted under these circumstances. Nausea and vomiting may have caused dehydration, requiring I.V. fluid and electrolyte replacement. Loss of sleep may have caused exhaustion or agitation; a sedative or anxiolytic may be warranted.

For the status migrainosus patient, a regimen of I.V. DHE and metoclopramide has become standard (28). Start with 10 mg of metoclopramide, then 0.5 mg of DHE injected I.V. over 2 to 3 minutes. If the headache persists, the DHE dose is repeated in 1 hour. The subsequent doses of DHE are adjusted depending on the patient's response; if at a dose of 0.5 mg nausea persists, but not headache, the dose of DHE may be lowered to 0.3 mg. If headache persists without nausea, the dose may be raised to 0.75 mg. If nausea persists, additional metoclopramide may be advisable. DHE with or without metoclopramide is generally administered every 8 hours for 1 to 3 days to break the cycle of pain.

When headache persists in spite of the above regimen, phenothiazines other than metoclopramide are administered parenterally (66). Prochlorperazine 10 mg or chlorpromazine 25 mg is given intravenously; doses may be titrated upward until the patient is moderately drowsy, pain-free, or both. Because these agents (especially chlorpromazine) may cause orthostatic hypotension, patients should remain in bed for at least 1 hour after administration. Additional parenteral pain relief medication may be warranted. The narcotics meperidine, butorphanol, morphine, or hydromorphone may be used, again altering dosage by judging relative degrees of pain or drowsiness but also paying attention to potential respiratory depression (70). Because of the latter we now use ketorolac before narcotics (69).

Parenteral steroid therapy is warranted in patients who do not respond to DHE or have a contraindication to it. We use an initial dose of 10 mg of dexamethasone, followed by 4 mg every 6 hours until the attack breaks (71). In addition to the common side effects of fluid retention and upper gastrointestinal ulceration, aseptic neurosis of the head of the femur and mental-status changes are rare and unpredictable complications.

Other Factors To Be Considered in Prioritizing Therapy

In addition to the stage of migraine, one must also consider the features of the attack, the properties of the medication, and the value judgments of the patient.

Symptom Profiles: Treatment of Nausea and Other Associated Features

One of the major features of migraine is nausea, with or without vomiting. Unfortunately, this symptom may be aggravated by many of the acute treatments discussed above. Moreover, gastric stasis occurs with the attack and inhibits the absorption of antimigraine agents taken by mouth (56). To counter these conditions it is often advisable to prescribe an antiemetic— e.g., metoclopramide (10 mg), prochlorperazine (5 to 25 mg), or trimethobenzamide (250 mg)—to be taken by mouth or by rectal suppository about

10 minutes before taking antimigraine medication (54,55). As noted above, the phenothiazines also have antimigraine action in themselves (48). Sumatriptan has the advantage of terminating nausea as well as headache (see Chapter 10). The treatment of nausea, often overlooked, may mean the difference between therapeutic success and failure.

Anxiety is sometimes a troubling symptom during an attack of migraine. When present, it may be treated with a benzodiazepine. Migraineurs prefer to lie down, rest, and, if possible, sleep during an attack; many awaken free of headache. Administering a sedative to evoke sleep may be helpful. Some patients consider the disability caused by sleep preferable to disabling pain. However, it is ideal to abort the headache with medication that restores normal function.

The severity and frequency of attacks and the response to therapy will be factors in choosing medication. If the pain is mild, over-the-counter medication may be adequate. If the attack is disabling and results in missed work or school, the cost-effectiveness of parenteral medication is evident. High-frequency attacks (two or more per week) may lead to overuse of preparations containing ergotamine, barbiturate, or caffeine, and the evolution of chronic daily headaches. Under these circumstances, prophylactic measures are almost mandatory and acute treatments unlikely to cause rebound headache should be selected.

Properties of Antimigraine Agents

Rapidity of action of a drug is an important feature, especially for treating attacks that are quickly disabling. Parenteral therapy works rapidly but is more difficult to administer than other modes of administration. Similarly, rectal suppositories (ergotamine tartrate) and nasal sprays may rapidly produce high blood levels but are less convenient than the oral preparations. In choosing an agent, the doctor must help the patient trade off convenience and rapidity of action to optimize the patient's satisfaction with therapy.

The relative effectiveness of various acute treatments has not been well studied. Oral sumatriptan is more effective than metoclopramide and aspirin or ergotamine tartrate in a large series (72). Similarly, in one study (73), naproxen had some advantages over ergotamine. But, in choosing from among effective treatments, it is important to determine what works best for a particular patient.

The side effects of drugs are important considerations. The NSAIDs are contraindicated in patients with a peptic ulcer, and the ergot alkaloids should not be used in patients with cardiovascular disease or Raynaud's syndrome.

Value Judgments of the Patient

The feelings of patients with regard to their ailment and its treatment are important considerations. Some patients fear severe and disabling attacks of migraine, even if they are rare. They will accept side effects of medications, such as the drowsiness evoked by a narcotic, as long as the pain is relieved. Others find such side effects unacceptable and would rather put up with some degree of headache. To some patients, an injectable agent or suppository is anathema while others welcome the more rapid, complete relief these modes of administration may offer. The route of administration depends on acceptability to the patient as well as convenience, suitability, and effectiveness.

Finally, the cost of medication is a consideration. On one hand, no one would prescribe a costly medication if aspirin successfully aborts the attack. On the other hand, an expensive medication is cost-effective if it quickly aborts an attack that would have prevented the patient from going to work or would otherwise have been treated in an emergency department. Fortunately, the physician and patient can take heart in the knowledge that a migraine attack is self-limiting.

REFERENCES

1. Steiner TJ, Rose FC. Problems encountered in the assessment of treatment of headache and migraine. In: Hopkins A, ed. Headache: Problems in Diagnosis and Management. Philadelphia: W.B. Saunders, 1988:307–348.
2. Mathew NT, Stubits E, Nigam MP. Transformation of episodic migraine into daily headache: analysis of factors. Headache 1982; 22:66–68.
3. Saper JR. Changing perspectives on chronic headache. Clin J Pain 1986:19–28.
4. Lance JW, Lambert GA, Goadsby PJ, Duckworth JW. Brainstem influences on the cephalic circulation: experimental data from cat and monkey of relevance to the mechanism of migraine. Headache 1983; 23:258–265.
5. Lauritzen M, Olesen J. Regional cerebral blood flow during migraine attacks by Xenon-133 inhalation and emission tomography. Brain 1984; 107:447–461.
6. Moskowitz MA. The visceral organ brain: implications for the pathophysiology of vascular head pain. Neurology 1991; 41:182–186.
7. Sanders SW, Haering N, Mosberg H, Jaeger H. Pharmacokinetics of ergotamine in healthy volunteers following oral and rectal dosing. Eur J Clin Pharmacol 1986; 30:331–334.
8. Rosenthaler J, Munzer H. 9-10-Dihydroergotamine production of antibodies and radio-immunoassay. Experientia 1976; 32:234–235.
9. Aellig WH, Nuesch E. Comparative pharmacokinetic investigations with tritium-labelled ergot alkaloids after oral and intravenous administration in man. Int J Clin Pharmacol 1977; 15:106–112.

10. Tfelt-Hansen P, Paalzow L. Intramuscular ergotamine: plasma levels and dynamic activity. Clin Pharmacol Ther 1985; 37:29–35.

11. Fozard JR. The pharmacological basis of migraine treatment. In: Blau JN, ed. Migraine: Clinical and Research Aspects. Baltimore: Johns Hopkins University Press, 1987:165–184.

12. Lance JW, Spira PJ, Mylecharane EJ, Lord GDA, Duckworth JW. Evaluation of drugs applicable to treatment of migraine in the cranial circulation of the monkey. Res Clin Stud Headache 1978; 6:13–18.

13. Edmeads J. Cerebral blood flow in migraine. Headache 1977; 17:148–152.

14. Aellig WH, Berde B. Studies of the effect of natural and synthetic polypeptide type of ergot compounds on a peripheral vascular bed. Br J Pharmacol 1963; 36:561–570.

15. Saito K, Markowitz S, Moskowitz MA. Ergot alkaloids block neurogenic extravasation in dura mater, proposed action in vascular headaches. Ann Neurol 1988; 24:732–737.

16. Perrin VL. Clinical pharmacokinetics of ergotamine in migraine and cluster headache. Clin Pharmacokinet 1985; 10:334–352.

17. Rall TW. Oxytocin, prostaglandins, ergot alkaloids, and other drugs; tocolytic agents. In: Gilman AG, Rall TW, Nies AS, Taylor P, eds. Goodman and Gilman's The Pharmacologic Basis of Therapeutics. 8th ed. New York: Pergamon Press, 1990:933–953.

18. Galer BS, Lipton RB, Newman LC, Solomon S. Myocardial ischemia related to ergot alkaloids: a case report and literature review. Headache 1991; 31: 446–450.

19. Carliner NH, Denune DP, Finch CS Jr, Goldberg LI. Sodium nitroprusside treatment of ergotamine-induced peripheral ischemia. JAMA 1974; 227: 308–309.

20. Saper JR, Jones JM. Ergotamine tartrate dependency: features and possible mechanism. Clin Neuropharmacol 1986; 9:244–256.

21. Little PJ, Jennings GL, Skews H, Bobik A. Bioavailability of dihydroergotamine in man. Br J Clin Pharmacol 1982; 13:785–790.

22. Lindblad B, Abisch E, Bergqvist D. The pharmacokinetics of subcutaneous dihydroergotamine with and without a Dextran infusion. Eur J Clin Pharmacol 1983; 24:813–818.

23. Tfelt-Hansen P, Holm JW, Fahr A, Rosenthaler J. Bioavailability of dihydroergotamine as a nasal spray. In: Lance JW, ed. Recent Trends in the Management of Migraine. Aulendorf: Editio Cantor, 1987:23–25.

24. McCarthy BG, Peroutka SJ. Comparative neuropharmacology of dihydroergotamine and sumatriptan (GR 43175). Headache 1989; 29:420–422.

25. Goadsby PJ, Gunlach AL. Localization of 3H-dihydroergotamine-binding sites in the cat central nervous system: relevance to migraine. Ann Neurol 1991; 29:91–94.

26. deMetz JE, van Zwieten PA. Differential effects of dihydroergotamine on the circulatory actions of arterial and venous dilators in the rat. J Cardiovasc Pharmacol 1981; 3:217–227.

27. Anderson AR, Tfelt-Hansen P, Lassen NA. The effect of ergotamine and dihydroergotamine on cerebral blood flow in man. Stroke 1987; 18:120–123.
28. Raskin NH. Repetitive intravenous dihydroergotamine as therapy for intractable migraine. Neurology 1986; 36:995–997.
29. Raskin NH. Treatment of status migrainosus: the American experience. Headache 1990; 30(suppl 2):550–553.
30. Callaham M, Raskin NH. Controlled study of dihydroergotamine in the treatment of acute migraine headache. Headache 1986; 26:168–171.
31. Yrill GM, Swinburn WR, Liversedge LA. A double-blind crossover trial of isometheptene mucate compound and ergotamine in migraine. Br J Clin Pract 1972; 26:76–79.
32. United States Pharmacopeial Drug Information for the Health Care Professional. Vol. 1B. Isometheptene, dichloralphenazone and acetaminophen. Rockville, Md.: United States Pharmacopeial Convention, 1992: 1655–1658.
33. Diamond S. Treatment of migraine with isometheptene, acetaminophen, and dichloralphenazone combination: a double-blind, crossover trial. Headache 1976; 15:282–287.
34. Ross-Lee L, Eadie MJ, Tyrer JH. Aspirin treatment of migraine attacks: clinical observations. Cephalalgia 1982; 2:71–76.
35. Nestvold K, Kloster R, Partinen M, Sulkava R. Treatment of acute migraine attack: naproxen and placebo compared. Cephalalgia 1985; 5:115–119.
36. Johnson ES, Ratcliffe DM, Wilkinson M. Naproxen sodium in the treatment of migraine. Cephalalgia 1985; 5:5–10.
37. Moyer S. Pharmacokinetics of naproxen sodium. Cephalalgia 1986; 6(suppl 4): 77–80.
38. Nestvold K. Naproxen and naproxen sodium in acute migraine. Cephalalgia 1986; 6(suppl 4):81–84.
39. Verbeeck RK, Blackburn JL, Loewen GR. Clinical pharmacokinetics of nonsteroidal anti-inflammatory drugs. Clin Pharmacokinet 1983; 8:297–331.
40. Insel PA. Analgesic-antipyretics and anti-inflammatory agents: drugs employed in the treatment of rheumatoid arthritis and gout. In: Gilman AG, Rall TW, Nies AS, Taylor P, eds. Goodman and Gilman's The Pharmacological Basis of Therapeutics. 8th ed. New York: Pergamon Press, 1990:638–681.
41. Berge OG. Regulation of pain sensitivity, influence of prostaglandins. Cephalalgia 1986; 6(suppl 4):21–23.
42. Abramson S, Korchak H, Ludewig R, et al. Modes of action of aspirin-like drugs. Proc Natl Acad Sci 1985; 82:7227–7331.
43. Fox DA, Jick H. Nonsteroidal anti-inflammatory drugs and renal disease. JAMA 1984; 251:1299–1300.
44. Friedman AP, Boyles WF, Elkind AH, et al. Fiorinal with codeine in the treatment of tension headache—the contribution of components to the combination drug. Clin Ther 1988; 10:303–315.
45. Laska EM, Sunshine A, Mueller F, Elvers WB, Siegel C, Rubin A. Caffeine as an analgesic adjuvant. JAMA 1984; 251:1711–1718.

46. Ward N, Whitney C, Avery D, Dunner D. The analgesic effects of caffeine in headache. Pain 1991; 44:151–155.

47. Mathew NT. The abortive treatment of migraine. In: Gallagher RM, ed. Drug Therapy for Headache. New York: Marcel Dekker, 1991:100.

48. Iverson KV. Parenteral chlorpromazine treatment of migraine. Ann Emerg Med 1983; 12:756–758.

49. Lane PL, Ross R. Intravenous chlorpromazine—preliminary results in acute migraine. Headache 1985; 25:302–304.

50. Elenbaas RM, Iacono CU, Koellner KJ, et al. Dose effectiveness and safety of butorphanol in acute migraine headache. Pharmacotherapy 1991; 11:56–63.

51. Baldessarini RJ. Drugs and the treatment of psychiatric disorders. In: Gilman AG, Rall TW, Nies AS, Taylor P, eds. Goodman and Gilman's The Pharmacologic Basis of Therapeutics. 8th ed. New York: Pergamon Press, 1990: 386–404.

52. Dahl SG, Strandford RE. Pharmacokinetics of chlorpromazine after single and chronic dosage. Clin Pharmacol Ther 1977; 21:437–438.

53. Iverson S. Psychopharmacology: Recent Advances and Future Prospects. New York: Oxford University Press, 1985:204–215.

54. Albibi R, McCallum RW. Metoclopramide: pharmacology and clinical application. Ann Intern Med 1983; 98:86–95.

55. Hakkarainen H, Allonen H. Ergotamine vs metoclopramide vs their combination in acute migraine attacks. Headache 1982; 22:10–12.

56. Carstairs LS. Headache and gastric emptying time. Proc R Soc Med 1958; 51:790–791.

57. Saxena PR, De Vlaam-Schluter GM. Role of some biogenic substances in migraine and relevant mechanism in antimigraine action of ergotamine— studies in an experimental model for migraine. Headache 1974; 13:142–163.

58. Wilkinson M. Treatment of the acute migraine attack—current status. Cephalalgia 1983; 3:61–67.

59. Rohr L, Dufresne JJ. Dihydroergotamine nasal spray for the treatment of migraine attacks: a comparative double-blind crossover study with placebo. Cephalalgia 1985; 5(suppl 3):142–143.

60. Pradalier A, Clapin A, Dry J. Treatment review: nonsteroidal anti-inflammatory drugs in the treatment and long term prevention of migraine attacks. Headache 1988; 28:550–557.

61. Treves TA, Streiffler M, Korczyn AD. Naproxen sodium versus ergotamine tartrate in the treatment of acute migraine attacks. Headache 1992; 32:280–282.

62. Havanka-Kanniainen H. Treatment of acute migraine attack: ibuprofen and placebo compared. Headache 1989; 29:507–509.

63. Peatfield RC, Petty RG, Rose FC. Double blind comparison of mefenamic acid and acetaminophen (paracetamol) in migraine. Cephalalgia 1983; 3: 129–134.

64. Massiou H, Serrurier D, Lasserre O, Bousser MG. Effectiveness of oral diclofenac in the acute treatment of common migraine attacks: a double-blind study versus placebo. Cephalalgia 1991; 11:59–63.

65. Hoffert MJ, Couch JR, Diamond S, Elkind AH, Goldstein J, Kohlerman NJ, Saper JR, Solomon S. Transnasal butorphanol in the treatment of acute migraine. Headache. Submitted.
66. McEwen JI, O'Connor HM, Dinsdale HB. Treatment of migraine with intramuscular chlorpromazine. Ann Emerg Med 1987; 16:758–763.
67. Jones J, Sklar D, Dougherty J, White W. Randomized double-blind trial of intravenous prochlorperazine for the treatment of acute headache. JAMA 1989; 261:1174–1176.
68. Klapper JA, Stanton JS. Ketorolac versus DHE and metoclopramide in the treatment of migraine headaches. Headache 1991; 31:523–524.
69. Duarte C, Dunaway F, Turner L, Aldag J, Frederick R. Ketorolac versus meperidine and hydroxyzine in the treatment of acute migraine headache: a randomized, prospective, double-blind trial. Ann Emerg Med 1992; 21: 1116–1121.
70. Belgrade MJ, Ling LJ, Schleevogt MB, Ettinger MG, Ruiz E. Comparison of single dose meperidine, butorphanol and dihydroergotamine in the treatment of vascular headache. Neurology 1989; 39:590–592.
71. Gallagher RM. Emergency treatment of intractable migraine. Headache 1986; 26:74–75.
72. The Multinational Oral Sumatriptan and Cafergot Comparative Study Group. A randomized, double-blind comparison of sumatriptan and Cafergot in the acute treatment of migraine. Eur Neurol 1991; 31:314–322.
73. Sargent JD, Baumel B, Peters K, et al. Aborting a migraine attack: naproxen sodium v ergotamine plus caffeine. Headache 1988; 28:263–266.

9

Serotonin, Receptors, and Migraine

Anthony W. Fox

Cypros Pharmaceutical Corporation
Carlsbad, California

INTRODUCTION

The treatment of migraine, and its modern developments, depend on fundamental concepts of receptor research. A historical approach is used in this chapter to show how the various serotonin (5-hydroxytryptamine [5-HT]) receptors have been identified. The receptors govern the actions of ergot-type drugs, both their wanted and unwanted effects. Only one type of 5-HT receptor is actually relevant in the effective acute therapy of migraine. Precise understanding of this receptor led to the discovery of sumatriptan and other drugs with similar pharmacology, which are much more receptor-selective than ergot-type drugs.

SEROTONIN, ENTERAMINE, AND 5-HYDROXYTRYPTAMINE

Two lines of research led to the discovery of endogenous 5-HT. First, Rapport et al. (1) isolated a vasoconstrictor substance from the supernatant of clotted blood (serum); they gave this unidentified substance the descriptive name serotonin. Second, a substance from the gastrointestinal tract with similar properties was found; it was an amine and so was called enteramine. In 1952, Erspamer isolated and chemically characterized the mystery substance, showing it to be 5-HT.

The principal interest in 5-HT was initially in connection with studies of the control of blood pressure. Serotonin was considered something of an irritating artefact: if blood clotted in the vessels of experimental animals, then serotonin confounded precise measurements of the effects of the autonomic nervous system on vascular homeostasis. The serotonin came from platelets, and was released during the clotting process. Somewhat later, the ubiquitous presence of 5-HT along the gastrointestinal tract was recognized, and later still its presence in the central nervous system (CNS) and its possible role as a neurotransmitter. Many thought that this was simply a reflection of the similar, endodermal origins of the gastrointestinal mucosa and the CNS. In the 1960s, only the eccentric were interested in 5-HT, regarding it as an enigma, and the substance was a "hormone without a cause."

MIGRAINE

Until the 1960s a purely pragmatic approach to migraine therapy was taken. Many physicians were frustrated by the narrow range of therapies that they could offer, and their patients' frequent relapses. Early therapies included ergot-type drugs, opioids, and nonopioid analgesics. Antiemetics were in their infancy.

Clinically, migraine research began with the publication of case reports, together with the seminal publications by Wolff and others. Prospective clinical trials of therapies started in earnest only about 30 years ago.

Serotonin became a migraine research target after Sicuteri et al. (2) made the observation that, in a subset of migraineurs, an increase in urinary excretion of 5-hydroxyindole acetic acid (5-HIAA, the metabolite of 5-HT) was associated with the onset of a migraine attack. This finding was interpreted as an excessive release of 5-HT as part of the pathogenetic mechanism of the disease. This finding was not reproduced in one study of nine patients (3) or in another study of three patients (4), but finally was confirmed (again only in a subset of patients) in a careful study by the group led by Lance (5). It was speculated that the large circulating amounts of 5-HT came from platelets.

A general theory then guided further research, that migraine was fundamentally a disorder of 5-HT metabolism. Typically, a theory is of use if it fulfills two criteria: that it 1) explains a large class of previous observations and 2) predicts the results of future experiments. As we shall see, the 5-HT general theory has been only partially useful.

EXPERIMENTS WITH SEROTONIN IN MIGRAINE

The mere infusion of 5-HT, leading to an increase in urinary excretion of 5-HIAA (imitating the finding of Sicuteri et al. described above), does not create migraine headache (4). This simple experiment, now more than 30 years old, precludes any simple relationship between circulating, free 5-HT and migraine pain. Similarly, the infusion of 5-hydroxytryptophan, the metabolic precursor of 5-HT, is also not migrainogenic (4).

The converse experiment was to attempt to treat migraine headache with an infusion of 5-HT. This somewhat counterintuitive experiment was accomplished independently by at least two groups (4,6). Although associated with a wide variety of unwanted effects (mimicking the carcinoid syndrome), an intravenous injection of 2.5–5.0 mg of 5-HT does indeed relieve the pain of migraine. Clearly, this result showed that the general theory, based on an interpretation that excessive 5-HT provokes migraine headache, could be supported only with caveats.

Studies with reserpine complicated matters further. Reserpine is a drug that depletes the body of biogenic amines, among which is counted 5-HT. This depletion is initiated by an excessive release of amines from their stores. Kimball et al. (4) demonstrated that an injection of reserpine was associated with the typical unilateral pain of migraine some 6 hours later; this time course was consistent with that for the antihypertensive effects of the drug. Here was another thread of evidence that excessive release of 5-HT could provoke migraine. However, given the nonmigrainogenic effects of injected 5-HT, the relationship between serotonin release and a migraine headache could not be simple.

In summary, these experiments showed that a) 5-HT is widely distributed in the human body, b) intravenous 5-HT can treat the headache of acute migraine at the cost of diverse adverse effects, c) there is some evidence relating endogenous 5-HT concentration changes with migraine, but d) there is no clear, direct relationship between 5-HT release or metabolism and the disease.

The general theory that migraine was fundamentally a disorder of serotonin metabolism has therefore only partly fulfilled the two criteria for a useful theory. Only some observations have been explained by it.

Attempts to define more precisely what that metabolic disorder might be have given conflicting results. There is still no general theory that directly relates the onset of migraine attacks to alterations in 5-HT release.

RECEPTOR CHARACTERIZATION

Nonetheless, even though it only partly fulfills the two criteria, the general theory has been absolutely crucial for progress in migraine research. The general theory has led to a more restricted theory, and the restricted theory has led to practical benefits for patients with migraine.

Simply stated, the restricted theory is that experimental activation of the right type of 5-HT receptor can effectively treat migraine. Experimental evidence demonstrates that the restricted theory not only fulfills the two criteria for a useful theory, but also has led to the development of sumatriptan and other agonists that activate only 5-HT1 receptors. These selective agonists have great promise for medical use.

In order to discuss the restricted theory, we must consider the methods that are available for the examination of receptors. Receptors—essentially a special class of proteins—may be characterized in three ways: radioligand binding studies, functional pharmacology, and cloning to identify the absolute, primary chemical structure of the receptor. So far, migraine research has exploited the first two techniques, although the third holds great promise for the future.

Radioligand Binding Studies

Radioligand binding studies measure the ability of drug molecules to attach themselves to receptors. The principal measure of interest in these studies is the equilibrium dissociation constant (the Kd or Ki). The Ki is measured in terms of the concentration of drug needed to occupy 50% of the receptors at equilibrium, and drugs can be screened against a variety of receptors (for example, see Table 1 in Chapter 10). The lower the Ki concentration, the better the fit between drug and receptor. If the concentration is less than 1 micromolar, then this would be a good rule of thumb for an excellent fit between drug and receptor.

In addition, receptor binding studies can measure the time course of binding and dissociation of drug from receptor (7). It is important to understand how long a drug stays on the receptor once bound because this can alter the duration of action of the drug. Very often, drug action lasts longer than the period of time during which the drug can be detected in the circulation; one reason may be that the drug remains on its receptors long after plasma clearance (long-acting opioids such as buprenorphine are good examples of this).

Although helpful in identifying different binding sites and measuring how well drugs bind to receptors, radioligand binding studies are an incomplete way to study drug–receptor interactions. For example, we need to know, whether the drug, once bound, is an antagonist or an agonist (or something in between—a partial agonist). A receptor comprises not only a binding site but also a transduction mechanism. The transduction mechanism is usually a group of enzymes that control second-messenger formation, and ultimately some sort of response on the part of the cell. Radioligand binding studies tell us little about whether the receptor is of physiological or medical significance. To explore events after a drug has bound with a receptor, we must use functional pharmacology.

Functional Pharmacology Studies

Functional pharmacology studies involve measuring responses of people, organisms, tissues, cells, or enzymes after they have been exposed to drugs. In functional pharmacology studies, we indirectly infer the properties of receptors from dose-response curves.

A common problem (and one that is very relevant to migraine research) is determining whether two receptor types are the same or different. A common strategy is to compare the responses of two tissues to a range of drugs. If the drugs appear to have the same rank order of potency in the two tissues, then it can be inferred that the two tissues contain the same type of receptor. Conversely, if the rank order of potency of a variety of antagonists is different in two tissues, then this is clear evidence that the tissues contain different receptor types.

Identifying an unknown receptor type is another common pharmacological problem, and again one that has arisen in migraine research. Typically, an unknown receptor is characterized using a range of drugs with known properties. The spectrum of activity of the range of drugs is then compared to previously recorded spectra: either the unknown receptor matches a previously identified one or it is declared to be novel. The one danger here is that sometimes new drugs identify new receptors, and vice versa—new receptors sometimes tell us new things about old drugs. A circular logic can thus be engaged, which, without external reference, can defy interpretation as a whole.

Second-messenger production can also be used to classify receptors, and obviously can be studied only in functional studies (8). If there is a shortage of selective drugs that could distinguish two closely related receptors, then they can sometimes be identified by the way in which they produce different second messengers. For example, the vasopressin-1 and -2 receptors bind agonists such as antidiuretic hormone very similarly. However, their second messengers are different: vasopressin-1 receptors produce inositol phosphates, while vasopressin-2 receptors make cyclic AMP. In serotonin research, we are just starting to learn about the different second messengers produced by all the various receptor types and subtypes.

Functional pharmacology at at least the cellular level always tells us more about the physiological importance of the receptor under study than a radioligand binding study. Similarly, we can learn whether drugs are agonists or antagonists. On the negative side, functional studies are always more costly and time-consuming than radioligand binding studies.

STRUCTURAL STUDIES: MOLECULAR BIOLOGY

It is now possible to make large quantities of pure receptor protein and to document the order of amino acids along the length of the receptor. Molecular biology allows us to identify receptors from their primary, chemical structures.

Most 5-HT receptors are of the serpentine type—a long chain of amino acids that passes in and out of the cell wall, like a thread in a tapestry, or like the common representation of the Loch Ness monster (Figure 1). There are three loops and a loose end projecting outside the cell wall, and another three loops and a loose end passing down into the cell. The arrangement of the outside loops and the outside loose end, together with the physicochemical properties of the amino-acid chains themselves, govern which, and how well, drugs will bind to the receptor. The amino acids in the chain define not only the shape of the pocket into which the drug fits but also the electrochemical properties needed for a drug to bind.

Primary receptor structure is of great current scientific interest. However, so far, advances in migraine research have not depended on a knowledge of molecular biology, at this most submicroscopic level. The future may be different.

5-HYDROXYTRYPTAMINE RECEPTORS

In 1957, with very limited functional pharmacology methods available to them, Gaddum and Picarelli (9) were able to distinguish two types of 5-HT receptor, which they called D and M. The diverse properties of 5-HT in humans were shown to be much more complicated than could be

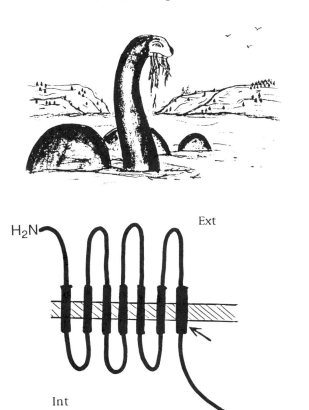

H₂N

Ext

Int

CO₂H

Figure 1 Receptors for 5-HT belong to the serpentine class, and resemble the Loch Ness Monster (upper panel). The primary structure of the receptor (lower panel) is a polypeptide chain, with the N-terminal end outside the cell (Ext), and the carboxyl end in the cytoplasm (Int). The receptor is anchored to the cell membrane (cross-hatched) by seven lipophilic regions in the polypeptide (shown as dilatations of the polypeptide chain, one of which is arrowed). Variations in the head end, three external loops, three internal loops, and/or the tail differentiates members of the class (e.g., the various 5-HT receptors, alpha-adrenergic receptors, etc.). The receptor may adopt a three-dimensional structure, arranging its loops in a circle; this creates an attractive pocket for the ligand between the three external loops and the head. Nessie is shown making a left-hand turn, and thus she is imitating the three-dimensional structure of a receptor. (Upper panel: illustration by Patricia Miesner.)

explained by this simple classification. But it was a start at identifying the 5-HT receptors, and all the more impressive given the technical limitations of that time.

With more sophisticated techniques, it was recognized that there were at least three 5-HT receptor types, labeled 5-HT1, 5-HT2, and 5-HT3 (10). The latter two types probably correspond to the older D and M classification.

Today it is recognized that these three 5-HT receptor types are actually families or classes of receptor. For example, there are at least five members of the 5-HT1 class (called 5-HT1A, 5-HT1B, etc.). In addition, a new class has been discovered and labeled 5-HT4 (11). Altogether, at least 11 different 5-HT receptors have now been identified.

RECEPTORS FOR THE TREATMENT OF MIGRAINE

Fortunately, out of this multitude of 5-HT receptors, we can concentrate on just one with regard to the acute treatment of migraine. This receptor has been studied both in animals and man. It is a member of the 5-HT1 class of receptors.

There is no doubt that migraine is a disease that expresses itself in the cranial arteries; this is true regardless of whether one believes more in the vascular or neurogenic hypotheses for the etiology of migraine. The receptor that can be used to normalize these arteries is termed "5-HT1-like" in humans, but if not the same is very similar to the 5-HT1D receptor that has been studied in detail in animals (some laboratories use the terms 5-HT1-like and 5-HT1D interchangeably, to the irritation of the purists!). This receptor exists in cranial arteries of animals (12), the human basilar artery (13), and the arteries supplying the human dura mater (14).

Activation of the 5-HT1-like receptor (i.e., the binding of a receptor to an agonist) causes smooth muscle contraction and constriction of the cranial artery. Most human cranial arteries probably also contain populations of 5-HT2 receptors (15). Small populations of 5-HT1-like receptors probably exist in the human coronary artery, although these contract the artery weakly in comparison to 5-HT2 receptors which are also present (17,18). 5-HT1-like receptors have not been found in any other human artery to date, although 5-HT2 receptors may be ubiquitous in the human cardiovascular system.

The restricted theory was developed from this knowledge of the distribution of 5-HT receptors in the human vasculature (5-HT1-like predominant in the cranial vasculature, 5-HT2 predominant elsewhere). The restricted theory was that if 5-HT1-like receptors could be activated, then this would presumably reverse the process that causes migraine symptoms. Furthermore, it could be anticipated that if a selective agonist for only the 5-HT1-like receptor could be found, this drug would probably not have more generalized effects throughout the body. This restricted theory could be tested with appropriate pharmacological innovation, regardless of whether endogenous 5-HT had any role in the genesis of migraine attacks. No matter what the cause of acute migraine, activation of 5-HT1-like receptors could be the way to treat it.

THERAPEUTIC AGENTS AND 5-HT1-LIKE RECEPTORS

Before all this receptor research, the only disease-specific drugs for acute attacks of migraine were of the ergot type. Drugs such as methysergide and propranolol found prophylactic use, but were not of value for treating the acute attacks.

The pharmacology and clinical pharmacology of dihydroergotamine and ergotamine are described in Chapters 8 and 10. These two drugs comprise almost all the acute ergot-type therapies. There is no doubt that these agents are effective antimigraine medications in large numbers of patients, and that they are associated with a wide variety of adverse events.

These acute, ergot-type drugs clearly bind and activate the 5-HT1-like receptor; this is presumably the mechanism for their beneficial therapeutic effects. The Kd for the binding is in the submicromolar range; the ergot drugs fit the 5-HT1-like receptor well. However, the ergot-type drugs also bind well to a variety of other receptors (19); they are nonselective and bind to dopamine and adrenergic receptors (see Table 1 in Chapter 10).

Why should ergot-type drugs be so receptor-nonspecific? The ergot molecules are relatively large in comparison to 5-HT. It may be assumed that the information a molecule contains depends on some part of its three-dimensional structure. One or more aspects of the molecule must fit the receptor; the analogy of a lock and key has often been used. It could be imagined that a large molecule is able to orient itself in a number of ways, each presenting a differently shaped aspect of the molecule (with different electrochemical properties, too). Different aspects of large molecules could therefore offer a wide variety of parts, capable of binding with a wide variety of receptors. A smaller molecule has fewer different aspects, and can offer fewer shapes and electrochemical options to a variety of receptors. Large molecules may therefore be compared to a collection of keys welded together that can open various locks, whereas a small molecule may be viewed as a unique key.

The functional pharmacology when arteries are exposed to ergot-type drugs appears to add further complexity. In human arteries, in the submicromolar range, ergotamine is capable of both contracting arteries and, under some conditions, blocking the ability of 5-HT itself to contract arteries (20). It may be that this is due to some partial agonist activity in some tissues, or that there are complex interactions among all the various types of receptor that may be bound by the drug.

Ergot-type drugs, then, interact potently with 5-HT1-like receptors. However, these are not selective agents. Ergot-type drugs can have effects at many types of receptor in diverse parts of the human cardiovascular system.

The discovery of ergot-type drugs occurred well before all this understanding of their receptor pharmacology. Research into the therapy of migraine was stimulated by the new understanding and by experience of the limitations of the older drugs. The objective was then to find agents that activate only the 5-HT1-like receptor, and not all the other types. The restricted theory suggested that this would confer effects beneficial for the therapy of acute migraine.

Several agents are now known that are selective for 5-HT1-like receptors. Sumatriptan, GR85548, L705126, and BW311C are four examples. Sumatriptan was discovered after a search through 850 other compounds, and has recently been introduced into medical practice. The three other compounds are in clinical trials for the acute treatment of migraine. If the measure of the worth of any theory is that an advance in medical practice results, then the restricted theory has proved itself.

REFERENCES

1. Rapport, MM, Green AA, Page IH. Serum vasoconstrictor (serotonin). IV. Isolation and characterisation. J Biol Chem 1948; 176:1243–1251.
2. Sicuteri F, Testi A, Anselmi B. Biochemical investigations in headache: increase in the hydroxyindole acetic acid excretion during migraine attacks. Int Arch Allergy 1961; 19:55–58.
3. Curzon G, Theaker P, Phillips B. Excretion of 5-hydroxyindole acetic acid (5-HIAA) in migraine. J Neurol Neurosurg Psychiat 1966; 29:85–90.
4. Kimball RW, Friedman AP, Vallejo E. Effect of serotonin in migraine patients. Neurology 1960; 10:107–111.
5. Curran DA, Hinterberger H, Lance JW. Total plasma serotonin, 5-hydroxyindoleacetic acid and p-hydroxy-m-methoxymandelic acid excretion in normal and migrainous subjects. Brain 1965; 88:997–1010.

6. Lance JW, Anthony M, Hinterberger H. The control of cranial arteries by humoral mechanisms and its relation to the migraine syndrome. Headache 1967; 7:93–102.

7. Minneman KP, Fox AW, Abel PW. Occupancy of alpha-1 adrenergic receptors and contraction of rat vas deferens. Mol Pharmacol 1983; 23:359–368.

8. Hoyer D, Boddeke H, Schoeffter P. Second messengers in the definition of 5-HT receptors. In: Fozard JR, Saxena PR, eds. Serotonin: Molecular Biology, Receptors and Functional Effects. Berlin: Birkhauser Verlag, 1991:117–132.

9. Gaddum JH, Picarelli ZP. Two types of tryptamine receptor. Br J Pharmacol Chemother 1957; 12:323–328.

10. Bradley PB, Engel G, Feniuk W, Fozard JR, Humphrey PPA, Middlemiss DN, Mylecharane EJ, Richardson BP, Saxena PR. Proposals for the classification and nomenclature of functional receptors for 5-hydroxytryptamine. Neuropharmacology 1986; 25:563–576.

11. Clarke DE, Craig DA, Fozard JR. The 5-HT4 receptor: naughty but nice. Trends Pharmacol Sci 1989; 10:385–386.

12. Connor HE, Feniuk W, Humphrey PPA. Characterisation of 5-HT receptors mediating contraction of canine and primate basilar artery by use of GR43175, a selective 5-HT1-like receptor agonist. Br J Pharmacol 1989; 96:379–387.

13. Parsons AA, Whalley ET, Feniuk W, Connor HE, Humphrey PPA. 5-HT1-like receptors mediate 5-hydroxytryptamine-induced contraction of the human basilar artery. Br J Pharmacol 1989; 96:434–449.

14. Humphrey PPA, Feniuk W, Motevalian M, Parsons AA, Whalley ET. The vasoconstrictor action of sumatriptan on human isolated dura mater. In Fozard JR, Saxena PR, eds. Serotonin: Molecular biology, Receptors and Functional Effects. Berlin-Birkhauser Verlag, 1991:421–429.

15. Edvinsson L, Jansen I. Characterization of 5-HT receptors mediating contraction of human cerebral, meningeal and temporal arteries: target for GR43175 in acute treatment of migraine. Cephalalgia 1989; 9(suppl 10):39–40.

16. Connor HE, Feniuk W, Humphrey PPA. 5-hydroxytryptamine contracts coronary arteries predominantly via 5-HT2 receptor activation. Eur J Pharmacol 1989; 161:91–94.

17. Chester AH, Martin GR, Bodelsson M, Arneklo-Nobin B, Tadjkarimi A, Tornebrandt K, Yacoub MH. 5-Hydroxytryptamine receptor profile in healthy and diseased human epicardial coronary arteries. Cardiovasc Res 1990; 24: 932–937.

18. MacIntyre PD, Bhargava B, Hogg KJ, Gemmill JD, Hillis WS. The effect of i.v. sumatriptan, a selective 5-HT1 receptor agonist, on central hemodynamics and the coronary circulation. Br J Clin Pharmacol 1992; 34:541–546.

19. McCarthy BG, Peroutka SJ. Comparative neuropharmacology of dihydroergotamine and sumatriptan (GR43175). Headache 1989; 29:420–422.

20. Oestergard JR, Mikkelsen E, Vodby B. Effects of 5-hydroxytryptamine and ergotamine on human superficial temporal artery. Cephalalgia 1981; 1:223–228.

10

Selective Serotonin-Receptor Medications
Dihydroergotamine and Sumatriptan

Egilius L. H. Spierings

*Brigham and Women's Hospital
and Harvard Medical School
Boston, Massachusetts*

INTRODUCTION

Dihydroergotamine (DHE) and sumatriptan are two antimigraine medications available for parenteral administration. DHE is a hydrogenated derivative of another antimigraine medication, ergotamine (which is used orally or rectally). Sumatriptan, on the other hand, is an analog of the endogenous biogenic amine 5-hydroxytryptamine, or serotonin (Figure 1).

DHE was introduced for the acute treatment of migraine in 1945 (1). It is marketed in the United States as a mesylate, under the tradename D.H.E.45. Each ampule of D.H.E.45 contains 1 mg dihydroergotamine mesylate in a 1 ml solution. The medication can be given by subcutaneous, intramuscular, or intravenous route.

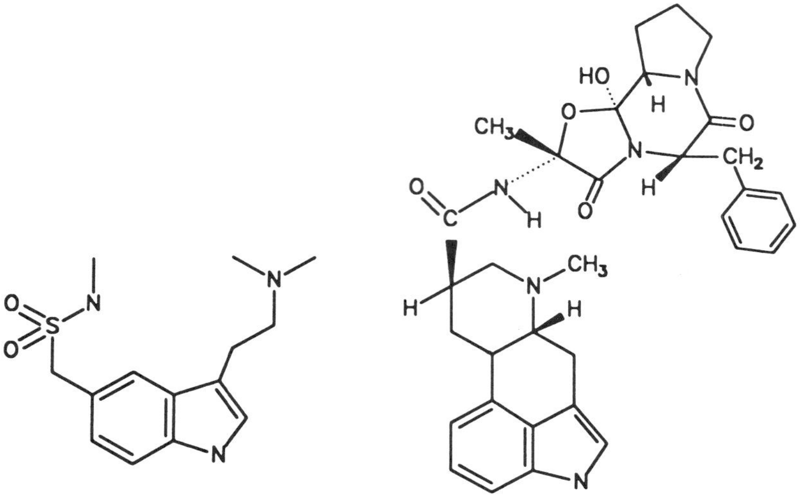

Figure 1 The structural formulae of (left) sumatriptan and (right) dihydroergotamine (see Ref. 3).

Sumatriptan was first shown to be effective for the acute treatment of migraine in 1988 (2). It is marketed in the United States and Canada as Imitrex and elsewhere as Imigran. The Imitrex or Imigran ampule contains 6 mg sumatriptan succinate in a 0.5 ml solution. Imitrex is administered subcutaneously, and is available either in vials or as prefilled syringes, which may be used with an autoinjector device.

This chapter is concerned with these two acute, parenteral migraine therapies. The experimental data (receptor, animal, and human) will be reviewed, taking a critical approach.

RECEPTOR PHARMACOLOGY

The affinities of DHE and sumatriptan for the various serotonergic and adrenergic receptors are shown in Table 1. DHE has a good affinity for all the receptors shown, except for the serotonin-3 and beta-adrenergic receptors (3). Sumatriptan, on the other hand, has affinity for only the serotonin-1A and serotonin-1D receptors.

DHE and sumatriptan have a remarkably similar affinity for the serotonin-1D receptor. They are also both agonists at this receptor site (4).

Table 1 Affinities of Dihydroergotamine
(DHE) and Sumatriptan for the Serotonergic
and Adrenergic Receptors

Receptor	Ki (nM)[a]	
	DHE	Sumatriptan
Serotonin		
-1A	1.2	100
-1C	39	>10,000
-1D	19	17
-2	78	>10,000
-3	>10,000	>10,000
Adrenergic		
Alpha-1	6.6	>10,000
Alpha-2	3.4	>10,000
Beta	960	>10,000

[a]Values shown are dissociation constants (nM); the
lower the value, the greater the affinity.
Source: Ref. 3.

It is therefore tempting to suggest that the two medications exert their
abortive antimigraine effect through stimulation of these serotonin-1D
receptors.

ANIMAL PHARMACOLOGY

DHE and sumatriptan lack a general analgesic effect (5). Therefore,
the two agents must exert their beneficial effect in migraine through an
interaction with specific migraine mechanisms. The mechanisms that are
involved in the pathogenesis of acute migraine are unknown; the various
hypotheses include extracranial arterial dilation (6), extracranial
neurogenic inflammation (7), opening of extracranial arteriovenous
anastomoses (8), and dysinhibition of central pain transmission (9). DHE
and sumatriptan are potent vasoconstrictor agents and have been shown
in animal studies to decrease carotid blood flow and to reduce extracranial
arteriovenous shunting (10,11). The two drugs have also been shown to
inhibit the development of neurogenic plasma extravasation in the rat
dura mater (12,13). The location of the neurogenic inflammation in the rat,

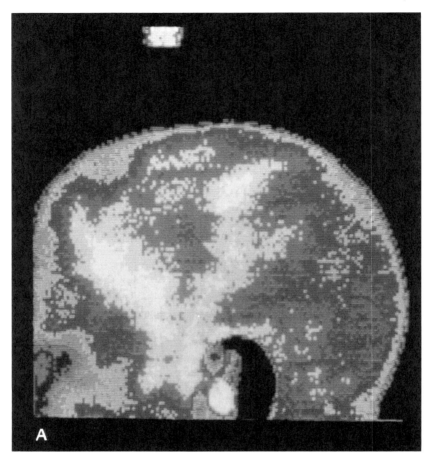

Figure 2 Thermography of the lateral skull (A) before and (B) after administration of 0.5 mg I.V. dihydroergotamine. Note the pronounced reduction in heat emission from the superficial temporal artery after administration of dihydroergotamine.

as well as difficulties extrapolating to the human migraineur, raises questions about the relevance of these studies (7).

   After intravenous administration of DHE, drug binding has been observed in the area of the raphe nuclei in the brain stem (14). These nuclei play an important role in the inhibition of transmission of pain signals in the central nervous system. Only 0.05% of a large radioactive, intravenously administered dose of sumatriptan has been found in the brain, with

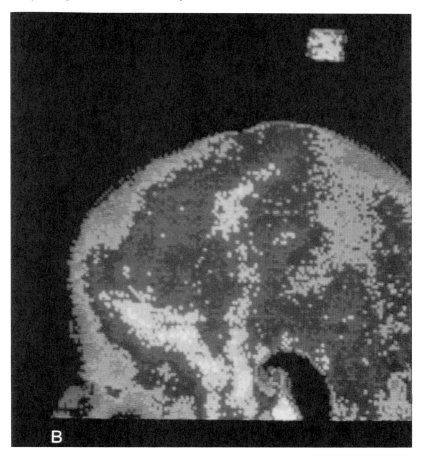

the highest levels present in the ventricles (15). It is therefore questionable whether, under ordinary conditions, sumatriptan crosses the blood–brain barrier.

HUMAN PHARMACOLOGY

DHE potently constricts the extracranial arteries in humans (e.g., the superficial temporal artery, Figure 2). DHE also increases the difference in blood oxygen gradient between extracranial arteries and veins (Figure 3, right). In experiments with cats, we determined that the arteriovenous oxygen content difference over the external circulation was a function of external carotid blood flow (Figure 4) rather than of arteriovenous

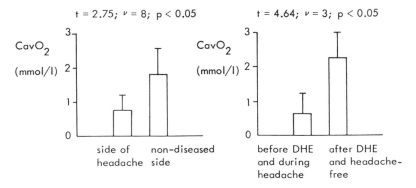

Figure 3 The arteriovenous oxygen content difference ($CavO_2$) over the extracranial circulation in man (left) during migraine and (right) before and after the administration of dihydroergotamine (see Ref. 8). Note the decreased arteriovenous oxygen content difference on the side of the headache during migraine, and the increase after administration of dihydroergotamine.

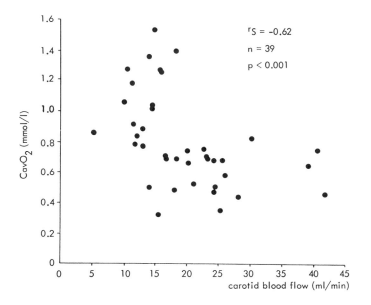

Figure 4 Scatter diagram in which the arteriovenous oxygen content difference over the extracranial circulation ($CavO_2$) is plotted against (external) carotid blood flow. Note the negative correlation between the two variables, which is significant at $p < 0.001$ (see Ref. 16).

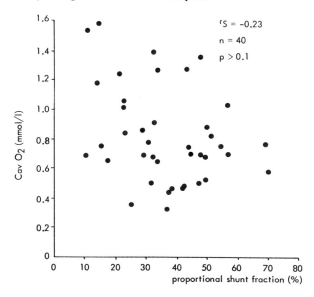

Figure 5 Scatter diagram in which the arteriovenous oxygen content difference over the extracranial circulation ($CavO_2$) is plotted against proportional shunt fraction, i.e., the proportion of (external) carotid blood flow shunted through the arteriovenous anastomoses. Note the absence of a statistically significant correlation between the two variables ($p > 0.1$) (see Ref. 16).

shunting (Figure 5) (17). While data of this type might be interpreted as evidence for arteriovenous shunting, these shunts probably do not play a role in migraine.

Sumatriptan also potently constricts the human cerebral, meningeal (dural), and superficial temporal arteries (18). The drug was most potent in constricting the meningeal artery by activating serotonin-1-like receptors. However, there is no clinical evidence for the involvement of the meningeal arteries in the pathogenesis of the migraine headache. Although the superficial temporal artery is also potently constricted by sumatriptan, the mechanism is obscure because this artery is devoid of serotonin-1 receptors (19; Figure 6).

Transcranial Doppler and high-resolution ultrasound can image middle cerebral and superficial temporal arteries noninvasively in migraine patients. Dilation of these arteries is seen during a migraine attack on the same side as the headache (20,21). The dilation of the middle cerebral artery was reversed after administration of sumatriptan, simultaneous with the relief of the headache. However, again, there is no

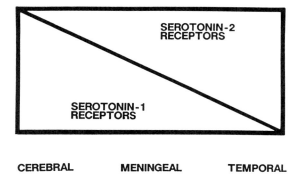

CEREBRAL   MENINGEAL   TEMPORAL

Figure 6 Relative distribution of serotonin-1 and -2 receptors on the human cerebral, meningeal, and temporal arteries. Note the absence of serotonin-1 receptors on the human superficial temporal artery (see Ref. 18).

evidence to date for the involvement of the middle cerebral artery as the anatomical source of the migraine headache. The dilation of the middle cerebral artery as observed may be an epiphenomenon of the migraine headache and may not be causally related to the generation of pain. For example, attempts to use physical means to reduce the pulsation of these arteries does not result in a reduction of the pain during migraine (22).

CLINICAL PHARMACOLOGY

Dihydroergotamine

DHE has been studied most extensively after intravenous administration. However, there were fewer than 50 patients in each study, and only one study was placebo-controlled. The majority of the DHE studies were retrospective or open-label, which decreases the reliability of the results reported.

There have been two studies of DHE administered I.V. alone, at doses of 0.5 to 2 mg (23,24). In one retrospective study, 22 of 23 patients obtained relief of their migraine. However, almost all these patients experienced nausea or increased nausea after administration of the medication. The other study, which was prospective, gave 1–2 mg DHE to 26 patients, 23% of whom obtained relief of their migraine 1 hour after treatment and 53% after 24 hours. The average decrease in headache intensity was 37% after 1 hour. Among these patients, 58% experienced adverse effects that were described as "severe gastrointestinal."

There is one study of DHE (1 mg I.V.) with metoclopramide (10 mg), again prospectively designed. Of the 21 patients who received this combination, 70% obtained relief of headache within half an hour of treatment. In terms of adverse events, dysphoria was experienced by 43%, nausea by 33%, and restlessness, an adverse effect of metoclopramide, by 19%. Two further intravenous studies have used a combination of DHE and prochlorperazine. One was prospective (26) and the other was retrospective (27). In the prospective study, 37 patients were given 5 mg prochlorperazine intravenously followed by 0.75 mg DHE or placebo. A half hour after treatment with prochlorperazine alone, before administration of DHE or placebo, the average headache intensity had decreased by 37%. Administration of DHE resulted in a further reduction in headache intensity of 11% and placebo of 16%, 1 hour after treatment. After an additional half hour, i.e., 60 minutes after the DHE or placebo, the average headache intensity in the DHE group had decreased a further 75%, while improvement had remained the same in the placebo group. Nausea, the most common adverse effect of DHE reported in this study, occurred in seven of 19 patients (37%) who had received the medication. These data suggest, on an uncontrolled basis, that prochlorperazine may have a beneficial effect in migraine. Further, on a controlled basis, there is no doubt that DHE can have a large beneficial effect that is additive to anything achieved by the antiemetic.

The second study used prochlorperazine (3.5 or 10 mg) with DHE (1 mg). Using the lower dose of the antiemetic ($n = 38$), 89% of patients obtained complete relief of headache within 4 hours of treatment, with a relapse rate of 26% within 24 hours. Sedation, an adverse effect of prochlorperazine, occurred in 38% of patients and nausea in 14%. Another 28 patients received 1 mg DHE with 10 mg prochlorperazine. Of these patients, 95% obtained complete relief of headache within 4 hours of treatment, with a relapse rate of 14% within 24 hours. Sedation as an adverse event occurred in 73% and nausea in 5%. These studies show clearly the dose-related beneficial and adverse effects of prochlorperazine, although good response rates with regard to the treatment of the migraine attack.

Both studies of DHE (1 mg) given intramuscularly are retrospective (28,29). In the first, 20 patients with migraine were treated, of whom 85% obtained complete or very marked relief of headache within 80 minutes. Five percent of these patients experienced nausea as an adverse effect of DHE. In the second study, 43 patients were treated, of whom 71% obtained complete relief within 24 hours. Most of the relief was obtained within 4 hours of treatment, and the relapse rate was 13% within 24 hours. Sedation was experienced by 25% of patients and nausea by 24% as adverse effects of DHE.

There is also a retrospective study of DHE (1 mg) given by the subcutaneous route (30). Fifty-one patients participated; 22% used an antiemetic to decrease the occurrence of gastrointestinal side effects. Seventy-six percent of the patients obtained more than 50% relief of headache with the medication, and 46% more than 90%. In terms of adverse effects, nausea was experienced by 33%, burning at the injection site by 21%, and muscle cramps by 19%.

Sumatriptan

Two major double-blind, placebo-controlled studies have been performed of subcutaneous sumatriptan (6 mg) as acute treatment for migraine (31,32). A prior dose-ranging study had found 6 mg to be the most effective dose with fewest adverse effects (33). The first study (n = 1104 patients) was conducted at 61 sites in the United States, and the second had 533 patients from Canada and several countries in Europe. The protocols were similar, as were the results, and only the larger study will be reviewed here.

Of the 1104 patients, 11% were men and 89% were women; they ranged in age from 18 to 65 years. All patients had migraine with or without aura, and experienced one to six headaches per month. Of these 1104, 734 received sumatriptan and 370 placebo. Headache intensity was graded on a four-point scale: no headache, mild headache, moderate headache, or severe headache. The headaches that were treated were all moderate (49%) or severe (51%) in intensity, and were associated with nausea in 84% of the sumatriptan group and 81% of the placebo group. Vomiting rates were low, 9% for the active treatment group and 11% for placebo. The headaches were associated with photophobia in 95% and 93%, respectively.

At 1 hour after treatment, 70% of the patients in the sumatriptan group and 22% of those who received placebo had mild or no headache. In the sumatriptan group, 49% of the patients had no headache at all; this was the case in only 9% of those in the placebo group. Most of the effect of sumatriptan on headache intensity developed within the first 40 minutes of treatment. At 1 hour after treatment, nausea was decreased from 84% to 27% in the sumatriptan group, and from 81% to 51% in the placebo group. Vomiting was decreased from 9% to less than 1% in the sumatriptan group, and from 11% to 3% for placebo. Photophobia was decreased from 94% to 43% in the sumatriptan group and from 93% to 76% in the placebo group.

Subsequently, the efficacy of sumatriptan was determined separately for the patient with and without aura. At 1 hour after treatment, 63% of the patients with aura and 72% of those without aura had no or mild headache. Of the patients with aura, 41% had no headache at all and of those without aura, 50%. The observed differences in efficacy of sumatriptan in these subgroups were not significant.

Of the 734 patients who received sumatriptan, 365 still had headache 1 hour after the injection. These 365 patients were then rerandomized, and 187 received a second injection of sumatriptan while the remaining 178 patients received placebo. The efficacy of sumatriptan was again determined 2 hours after treatment, i.e., 1 hour after the second injection. The patients who received two active injections (total dose 12 mg) were compared to those who received only one active injection (6 mg). The observed differences in efficacy between the 12 mg and 6 mg subgroups, compared to placebo, were not significant.

Rescue medications were permitted at 2 hours after treatment. At that time, 20% of the patients in the sumatriptan group and 59% of those in the placebo group took rescue medications. Of the patients in the sumatriptan group, 69% were discharged from the centers without headache, which was the case in only 22% in the placebo group. Of the patients treated with sumatriptan, 34% remained completely headache-free for 24 hours after treatment, compared to 11% after placebo.

The adverse effects observed with sumatriptan were grouped into two categories: injection-site reactions and systemic adverse events. Injection-site reactions occurred in 59% of the patients who received sumatriptan, compared to 24% after placebo. These reactions consisted of a generally brief stinging or burning sensation at the site of injection. Systemic adverse events occurred in 11–14% of the sumatriptan group, and consisted of a warm, hot, tight, or tingling sensation, generally in the upper half of the body, and lightheadedness. The occurrence of these adverse effects in the placebo-treated patients was 3–4%.

Similar results, as discussed above, were obtained when sumatriptan was administered by the patients themselves at home with the use of the autoinjector (34). In a recent double-blind, placebo-controlled study (35), sumatriptan has also been shown to maintain its efficacy when administered for up to three separate attacks.

DIHYDROERGOTAMINE VERSUS SUMATRIPTAN

Provided that DHE is given together with an antiemetic, the efficacy of the medication is similar to that of sumatriptan. When DHE is given by S.C.

injection, which is probably the way it should be administered if it is used by patients themselves at home, the antiemetic can generally be taken as an oral tablet or rectal suppository. It is important to allow at least 15 to 30 minutes between administration of the antiemetic and that of DHE. The dose of DHE is 0.5 to 1 mg, which can be repeated, if necessary, with intervals of at least 1 hour to a maximum of 2 mg per day.

In the office or emergency department, DHE can be given by intravenous or intramuscular injection. With intravenous administration of the medication, it is important to remember that DHE is a potent (arterial) vasoconstrictor and that angina and myocardial infarction have been reported with its use (36). The antiemetic should be given at least 15 minutes prior to the DHE and is best administered I.V. or I.M. Metoclopramide, a reliable antiemetic, is a good choice and can be given safely by I.V. injection because it does not have cardiovascular effects. It also does not cause drowsiness or any other adverse effects, except for restlessness, which occurs in 5 to 10% of patients. The restlessness, if it occurs, can easily be treated with a small dose of a sedative, such as diazepam, given I.V. In addition, metoclopramide, when given in a dose of 10 mg I.V., has an abortive antimigraine effect itself, which has been reported in a double-blind, placebo-controlled study to be 67% (37). Again, the dose of DHE is 0.5 to 1 mg and can be repeated, if necessary, with intervals of at least 1 hour to a maximum of 2 mg per day.

DHE is a relatively slow-acting medication, evidenced by the fact that, even with I.V. administration, the medication takes more than a half hour to develop its effect (26). With I.M. or S.C. injection, it may take as long as 4 hours for the effect to fully develop (29). However, the effect of medication seems to last longer, as indicated by a low relapse rate of 13–26% within 24 hours (27,29). In contrast, most of the effect of sumatriptan administered by S.C. injection develops within 40 minutes. However, the relapse rate is 66% within 24 hours due to the relatively short duration of action of the medication.

Sumatriptan is undoubtedly much better tolerated than DHE. Nausea occurs as an adverse event of DHE in 5 to 58% of patients, depending on the route of administration, dose of the medication, and pretreatment with an antiemetic. Another common adverse effect of DHE is muscle cramps, especially in the legs, which occur in almost 20% of patients. With sumatriptan, adverse effects of a systemic nature occur in 11–14% of patients and consist of a warm, hot, tight, or tingling sensation, generally in the upper half of the body, and lightheadedness (31). Sumatriptan does not cause nausea and in fact has been shown to reduce nausea in association with relief of the migraine headache.

Sumatriptan has recently been shown, under placebo-controlled conditions, to have a very reproducible beneficial effect; i.e., the response rates are similar for successive migraine attacks. Furthermore, in studies to be published soon, sumatriptan has been shown to be effective orally, and also may be used to treat recurrence of migraine pain after an initial response wears off. It has also been demonstrated that the efficacy and adverse effects of sumatriptan are similar, no matter at what stage of a migraine attack it is used (for a description of the various stages, see Chapter 6). There are no comparable data for DHE.

CONCLUSION

In summary, DHE and sumatriptan are probably equally effective in the acute treatment of migraine. However, sumatriptan, having fewer adverse effects, is better tolerated than DHE. The onset of action is also faster with sumatriptan although of shorter duration. Therefore, in patients with prolonged migraine headaches, DHE may still be the medication of choice.

REFERENCES

1. Horton BT, Peters GA, Blumenthal LS. A new product in the treatment of migraine: a preliminary report. Proc Staff Mtg Mayo 1945; 20:241–248.
2. Doenicke A, Brand J, Perrin VL. Possible benefit of GR43175, a novel 5-HT-1-like receptor agonist for the acute treatment of severe migraine. Lancet 1988; i:1309–1311.
3. McCarthy BG, Peroutka SJ. Comparative neuropharmacology of dihydro-ergotamine and sumatriptan (GR43175). Headache 1991; 29:420–422.
4. Deliganis AV, Peroutka SJ. 5-Hydroxytryptamine-1D receptor agonism predicts anti-migraine efficacy. Headache 1991; 31:228–231.
5. Skingle M, Birch PJ, Leighton GE, Humphrey PPA. Lack of anti-nociceptive activity of sumatriptan in rodents. Cephalalgia 1990; 10:207–212.
6. Graham JR, Wolff HG. Mechanism of migraine headache and action of ergotamine tartrate. Arch Neurol Psych 1938; 39:737–763.
7. Chapman LF, Ramos AO, Goodell H, Silverman G, Wolff HG. A humoral agent implicated in vascular headache of the migraine type. Arch Neurol 1960; 3:223–229.
8. Heyck H. Pathogenesis of migraine. Res Clin Stud Headache 1969; 2:1–28.
9. Anselmi B, Baldi E, Casaci F, Salmon S. Endogenous opioids in cerebrospinal fluid and blood in idiopathic headache sufferers. Headache 1980; 20:294–299.
10. Den Boer MO, Heiligers JPC, Saxena PR. Carotid vascular effects of ergotamine and dihydroergotamine in the pig: no exclusive mediation via 5-HT-1-like receptors. Br J Pharmacol 1991; 104:183–189.

11. Den Boer MO, Villalon CM, Heiligers JPC, Humphrey PPA. Role of 5-HT-1-like receptors in the reduction of porcine cranial arteriovenous anastomotic shunting by sumatriptan. Br J Pharmacol 1991; 102:323–330.
12. Saito K, Markowitz S, Moskowitz MA. Ergot alkaloids block neurogenic extravasation in dura mater: proposed action in vascular headache. Ann Neurol 1988; 24:732–737.
13. Buzzi MG, Moskowitz MA. The anti-migraine drug sumatriptan (GR43175) selectively blocks neurogenic plasma extravasation from blood vessels in dura mater. Br J Pharmacol 1990; 99:202–206.
14. Goadsby PJ, Gundlach AL. Localization of tritiated-dihydroergotamine binding sites in the cat central nervous system: relevance to migraine. Ann Neurol 1991; 29:91–94.
15. Humphrey PPA, Feniuk W, Marriott AS, Taner RJN, Jackson MR, Tucker ML. Preclinical studies on the anti-migraine drug sumatriptan. Eur Neurol 1991; 31:282–290.
16. Spierings ELH. The pathophysiology of the migraine attack. Alpher aan den Rijn, The Netherlands: Stafleu's Scientific Publishing, 1980.
17. Spierings ELH, Saxena PR. Anti-migraine drugs and cranial arteriovenous shunting in the cat. Neurology 1980; 30:696–701.
18. Jansen I, Edvinsson L, Mortensen A, Olesen L. Sumatriptan is a potent vasoconstrictor of human dural arteries via a 5-HT-1-like receptor. Cephalalgia 1992; 12:202–205.
19. Edvinsson L, Jansen I. Characterization of 5-HT receptors mediating contraction of human cerebral, meningeal, and temporal arteries: target for GR43175 in acute treatment of migraine. Cephalalgia 1989; 9(suppl 10):30–40.
20. Friberg L, Olesen J, Iversen HK, Sperling B. Migraine pain associated with middle cerebral artery dilation: reversal by sumatriptan. Lancet 1991; 338:13–17.
21. Iversen HK, Nielsen TH, Olesen J, Tfelt-Hansen P. Arterial responses during migraine headache. Lancet 1990; 336:837–839.
22. Schumacher GA, Wolff HG. Experimental studies on headache: A. Contrast of histamine headache with the headache of migraine and that associated with hypertension. B. Contrast of vascular mechanisms in pre-headache and in headache phenomena of migraine. Arch Neurol Psych 1941; 45:199–214.
23. Tillgren N. Treatment of headache with dihydroergotamine. Acta Med Scand 1947; 196(suppl):222–228.
24. Bell R, Montoya D, Shuaib A, Lee MA. A comparative trial of three agents in the treatment of acute migraine headache. Ann Emerg Med 1990; 19:1079–1082.
25. Belgrade MJ, Ling LJ, Schleevogt MB, Ettinger MG, Ruiz E. Comparison of a single-dose meperidine, butorphanol and dihydroergotamine in the treatment of vascular headache. Neurology 1989; 39:590–592.
26. Callaham M, Raskin N. A controlled study of dihydroergotamine in the treatment of acute migraine. Headache 1986; 26:168–171.
27. Saadah HA. Abortive headache therapy in the office with intravenous dihydroergotamine plus prochlorperazine. Headache 1992; 32:143–146.

28. Hartmann MM. Parenteral use of dihydroergotamine in migraine. Ann Allergy 1945; 3:440–442.
29. Saadah HA. Abortive headache therapy with intramuscular dihydroergotamine. Headache 1992; 32:18–20.
30. Klapper JA, Stanton J. Clinical experience with patient administered subcutaneous dihydroergotamine mesylate in refractory headaches. Headache 1992; 32:21–23.
31. Cady RK, Wendt JK, Kirchner JR, Sargent JD, Rothrock JF, Skaggs H. Treatment of acute migraine with subcutaneous sumatriptan. JAMA 1991; 265:2831–2835.
32. The Subcutaneous Sumatriptan International Study Group. Treatment of migraine attacks with sumatriptan. N Engl J Med 1991; 325:316–321.
33. The Sumatriptan International Study Group. Subcutaneous sumatriptan in the acute treatment of migraine. J Neurol 1991; 238:S66–S69.
34. The Sumatriptan Auto-Injector Study Group. Self-treatment of acute migraine with subcutaneous sumatriptan using an auto-injector device. Eur Neurol 1991; 31:323–331.
35. Cady RK, Dexter J, Sargent JD, Markley H, Osterhaus JT, Webster CJ. Efficacy of subcutaneous sumatriptan in repeated episodes of migraine. Neurology 1993; 43:1363–1368.
36. Galer BS, Lipton RB, Solomon S, Newman LC, Spierings ELH. Myocardial ischemia related to ergot alkaloids: a case report and literature review. Headache 1991; 31:446–450.
37. Tek DS, McClellan DS, Olsaker J, Allen CL, Arthur DC. A prospective, double-blind study of metoclopramide hydrochloride for the control of migraine in the emergency department. Ann Emerg Med 1990; 19:1083–1087.

11

Prophylactic Pharmacology for Migraine

Joseph D. Sargent

Menninger Clinic
Topeka, Kansas

Prophylactic therapy involves the taking of one or more medications on a daily basis over a sustained period with the goal of reducing headache frequency or severity. Such terms as *preventive* or *suppressive* have been used in conjunction with this method of treatment. The goal of prophylactic therapy is not to totally eliminate or cure headaches, but rather to ameliorate disability caused by headache activity.

Medications for the treatment of acute migraine are used on an as-needed basis whenever a headache develops and probably should not be used every day over a prolonged period of time. Many times these medications will lose their effectiveness when used every day and can lead to rebound headache (see Chapter 5).

CURRENT RATIONALE FOR ETIOLOGY OF MIGRAINE

The vascular model for the pathogenesis of migraine was proposed by Wolff in the 1930s (1,2). Simply stated, it was hypothesized that vasoconstriction of the intracranial arterial systems prior to the onset of headache sometimes led to aura. After onset of headache, the extracranial arterial system then dilated; this theory provided a rationale for the use of ergot alkaloids, with ergotamine and dihydroergotamine being the best known. The drugs in this class are vasoconstrictors that relieve headache by reversing vasodilation in the extracranial arterial system.

However, researchers began to doubt this rational because reversal of arterial vasodilation did not always relieve migraine. The neurogenic hypothesis was then devised and proposed that migraine was a primary disorder of the central nervous system rather than a condition originating in the vascular system. Sicuteri (3), who was the first researcher to suggest serotonin as a major participant in the etiology of migraine, helped to develop methysergide, the first truly effective prophylactic medication for migraine. With the emergence of sumatriptan as an effective treatment for acute migraine, interest has increased in serotonin as the key to unlocking the migraine mystery. Whether serotonin is the molecular basis for either the vascular or neurogenic hypotheses in migraine patients remains to be seen.

WHEN SHOULD PROPHYLACTIC TREATMENT BE CONSIDERED?

Not all migraine patients should be placed on prophylactic treatment. Prophylaxis should be considered for those who have two or more disabling headaches per month that last more than 24 hours. Menstrual migraine is a unique situation for female migraine sufferers because it occurs predictably once a month (4). Episodic prophylactic treatment is commonly given then to control menstrual migraine.

Prophylactic therapy is not as prevalent for children with migraine as it is for adults. The reasons are unclear, but it may be because childhood migraine responds better to acute treatment. In addition, children with migraine respond better to nonpharmacological treatment than do adults.

NONPHARMACOLOGICAL TREATMENT

My experience during many years of treating migraine headache has shown that some patients respond poorly to the whole range of available medications. In pondering how these migraine patients differ, I have concluded that many live more turbulent lives. This group of migraineurs, who would benefit most from changes in lifestyle, provides substantial evidence for the role of nondrug factors in perpetuating migraine. Areas that need careful attention in all migraine sufferers are diet, sleep, and recreation.

I approach dietary restrictions differently than some physicians. Migraine patients often suffer from other medical conditions that require dietary modifications, and I have been dismayed with the skewed diets of some migraineurs. Therefore, I encourage migraine sufferers to become familiar with the types of foods that can trigger migraine (see Table 1). By being their own detectives, they can discover what foods might trigger their migraine, thus avoiding the unnecessary elimination of foods from their diet that are not responsible for migraines. Treaters should caution migraineurs against the fairly common practice of skipping meals.

Lack of sleep is a major exacerbating factor in increased migraine activity. Since patients tend to underestimate the contribution made by a loss of sleep, some simple prophylactic precautions against it can be quite effective. Some migraineurs also find that sleeping late on weekend mornings will trigger a migraine. All migraine sufferers should determine their

Table 1 Foods That May Trigger a Migraine

Ripened cheeses (cheddar, emmentaler, gruyère, stilton, brie, and camembert)
Herring
Vinegar (except white vinegar)
Anything fermented, pickled, or marinated
Sour cream, yogurt
Nuts, peanut butter
Hot fresh breads, raised coffee cakes, and doughnuts
Pods of broad beans (lima, navy, and pea)
Any foods containing large amounts of monosodium glutamate
Onions
Canned figs
Citrus fruits (no more than one orange per day)
Bananas (no more than 1/2 banana per day)
Pizza
Pork
Excessive tea, coffee, cola beverages (no more than 4 cups per day)
Avocado
Fermented sausage (bologna, salami, pepperoni, summer sausage, and
    hot dogs)
Chicken livers
Alcoholic beverages of any type, especially wine; if alcohol is consumed, it
    should be done sparingly

---

individual sleep requirements and then obtain that amount of sleep as regularly as possible.

Recreation encompasses a broad range of activities that renew strength and refresh spirits. A period should be set aside from daily chores when recreational activities can be enjoyed at the individual's own pace. Recreation should be planned, however, because too often the best intentions end up being sacrificed to the demands of daily living. Which activities renew the strength and refresh the spirits varies with the individual patient, and can range from those requiring considerable physical exertion, such as swimming or jogging, to sedentary activities, such as reading.

A number of nonpharmacological techniques including biofeedback-assisted relaxation can be used to enhance sleep and recreation, and these are covered in Chapter 17. These techniques do not cure but are tools that migraineurs can use to gain control over the discomfort caused by their headaches.

Patients with headaches have sometimes developed profound changes in their emotional state that might benefit from psychotherapy. Although these patients may find it difficult to acknowledge their emotional distress, the physicians using patience and compassion can help them recognize this aspect of their problem and then make the referral for psychotherapy. However, premature referral can lead the patient to resist the idea of psychotherapy.

PROPHYLACTIC TREATMENT WITH MEDICATION

The choice of an initial prophylactic agent from among the many available is not a simple one. Many different classes of agents contain many individual medications from which to choose (see Table 2). The initial agent chosen should be one with which the individual physician has the greatest experience and comfort level in prescribing. If that initial choice proves ineffective, a second and even a third agent can be tried. After that, a referral to a headache center would be appropriate. The treatment of choice will have fewest adverse effects and most consistent efficacy.

If a medication proves satisfactory for the patient, then that treatment regimen is continued unless adverse effects intercede. At the end of the first year, the patient is gradually withdrawn from medication. If headache recurs, then the medication may be restarted. Two or more failed annual attempts to withdraw therapy may be needed before continuing prophylaxis indefinitely.

Prophylactic headache management truly involves the art of medicine, and how a patient is treated depends on the clinician's knowledge of and expertise in treating headaches. My initial choice would be made from the calcium channel blocker group or the beta-blocker group, because as an internist I am familiar with their use in the treatment of hypertension and cardiovascular disease. Factors such as the patient's allergies, sensitivities, and previous therapeutic experience would also influence such a decision. With any prophylactic medication, initial dosages should be low. The dosage can be increased gradually over time, depending on the response of migraine to the medication and the appearance of drug-related side effects. Sometimes a combination of medications is necessary to control a particular patient's migraine.

CALCIUM CHANNEL BLOCKERS

In 1989, Amery (5) reviewed the prophylactic treatment of migraine with calcium channel blockers. These medications, which are very heterogeneous biochemically and pharmacologically, are divided into six classes based on their pharmacological and clinical profiles. Only agents from class I, II, and VI have been tested in randomized trials for migraine. The rationale for use of class I and II agents was based on Wolff's concept of the vasoconstriction-vasodilation etiology of migraine, while the use of class VI agents was based on their prevention of focal hypoxia.

The data for verapamil—a class I agent—and nifedipine and nimodipine—class II agents from drug trials—are inconclusive as to their clinical effectiveness. The clinical efficacy of flunarizine, a class VI agent, has been well documented in studies, but this agent is not available in the United States because of its unsatisfactory side-effect profile. In 1988, Spierings (6) added a review of diltiazem, which has been investigated only in an open study. Leandri et al. (7), in a double-blind cross-over design, found nicardipine to be effective against migraine and well tolerated by a majority of patients. No data are available on isradipine, felodipine, and bepridil in the treatment of migraine. The clinical effectiveness of the agents discussed so far remains in doubt scientifically, but personal clinical experience has convinced me that they are clinically useful in migraine prophylaxis.

BETA-BLOCKERS

Beta-blockers have many side effects that are usually mild and seen only at high dosages. However, the common side effects of lethargy and a subtle dysphoric state, somewhat akin to overt clinical depression, may occur

Table 2 Prophylactic Medications for Migraine

Medications	Dosage	Some common side effects
I. Calcium Channel Blockers		
A. Verapamil	Up to 480 mg/day	Constipation, dizziness, nausea, hypotension, headache, peripheral edema
B. Diltiazem	Up to 240 to 360 mg/day	Peripheral edema, headache, nausea, dizziness, skin eruption, weakness
C. Nifedipine	Up to 120 mg/day	Peripheral edema, dizziness, nausea, headache and flushing, weakness, transient hypotension
D. Nimodipine	30–60 mg q. 4 hrs	Hypotension, headache, nausea, bradycardia, abnormal liver function tests, edema
E. Nicardipine	20–40 mg t.i.d.	Peripheral edema, dizziness, headache, asthenia, flushing, increased angina
F. Israpine (Dynacirc)	2.5 mg b.i.d. up to 10 mg/day	Headache, dizziness, edema, palpitations, fatigue, flushing
G. Felodipine (Plendil)	5 mg once/day up to 20 mg once/day	Peripheral edema, headache, flushing, dizziness, URI, asthenia
H. Bepridil (Vascor)	200–400 mg once/day	Dizziness, GI symptoms, ventricular arrhythmias, syncope
II. Beta-blockers		
A. Nonselective		
1. Propranolol	Up to 640 mg/day	Bradycardia, hypotension, light-headedness, bronchospasm, lassitude, mental depression, nausea
2. Timolol	20–30 mg/day	Bradycardia, fatigue, dizziness, dyspnea, headache
3. Nadolol	Up to 240 or 320 mg once/day	Bradycardia, peripheral vascular insufficiency, congestive heart failure, hypotension, cardiac arrhythmia, dizziness, fatigue
B. B-1 selective		
1. Metoprolol	100–400 mg once/day or in divided doses	Tiredness, dizziness, depression, shortness of breath and bradycardia, diarrhea, pruritis or rash
2. Atenolol	50–100 mg once/day	Bradycardia, dizziness, nausea, diarrhea, vertigo, lethargy

Table 2 (Continued)

Medications	Dosage	Some common side effects
III. Tricyclic antidepressants		
A. Amitryptyline	Up to 150 mg/day	Anticholinergic effects (dry
B. Nortriptyline	Up to 150 mg/day	mouth, constipation, urinary
C. Doxepin	Up to 150 mg/day	retention, visual blurring),
D. Imipramine	Up to 150 mg/day	photosensitization
E. Desipramine	Up to 200 mg/day	
IV. Nonsteroidal anti-inflammatory drugs (NSAIDs)		
A. Naproxen (Naprosyn)	250–500 mg b.i.d.	Constipation, heartburn, abdominal pain, nausea, headache, dizziness, drowsiness, pruritus and skin eruption, tinnitus, edema
B. Ibuprofen	Up to 3200 mg/day	Nausea, epigastric pain, heartburn, dizziness, rash
C. Flurbiprofen (Ansaid)	200–300 mg/day	Dyspepsia, diarrhrea, abdominal pain, nausea, headache, edema
D. Sulindac (Clinoril)	Up to 400 mg/day	Dyspepsia, nausea, diarrhea, constipation, dizziness, headache
E. Diflunisal (Dolobid)	250–500 mg b.i.d.	Nausea, dyspepsia, GI pain, diarrhea, rash, headache
F. Piroxicam (Feldene)	10–20 mg once/day	Epigastric distress, nausea, decreased hemoglobin
G. Indomethacin (Indocin)	50–150 mg/day	Nausea, dyspepsia, dizziness, headache
H. Etodolac (Lodine)	Up to 1200 mg/day	Abdominal pain, diarrhea, flatulence, nausea, dizziness, asthenia
I. Meclofenamate (Meclomen)	Up to 400 mg/day	Diarrhea, nausea, vomiting, abdominal pain, rash, headache, dizziness
J. Fenoprofen (Nalfon)	200 mg q. 4–6 hrs	Dyspepsia, nausea, constipation, headache, somnolence, pruritus, rash
K. Ketoprofen (Orudis)	150–300 mg/day	Dyspepsia, flatulence, nausea, abdominal pain, diarrhea, constipation, headache, insomnia, elevated blood ureanitrogen

Table 2   (Continued)

Medications	Dosage	Some common side effects
L. Tolmetin sodium (Tolectin)	Up to 1800 mg/day	Nausea, dyspepsia, GI distress, abdominal pain, diarrhea, flatulence, vomiting, headache, asthenia, elevated blood pressure, edema, weight gain or loss
M. Diclofenac sodium (Voltaren)	25–75 mg t.i.d.	Abdominal pain, headache, diarrhea, indigestion, nausea, constipation
V. Alpha2-adreno-ceptor agonist		
A. Guanfacine (Tenex)	1–3 mg/day	Dry mouth, somnolence, weakness, dizziness, constipation, impotence
B. Clonidine (Catapres)	0.2–0.6 mg/day	Dry mouth, drowsiness, dizziness, constipation, nausea and vomiting, nervousness and agitation
VI. Ergot preparations		
A. Ergotamine in Bellergal-S	1 tablet b.i.d.	Tingling and other paresthesias of extremities, blurred vision, palpitations, dry mouth, decreased sweating, decreased GI motility (not all side effects attributable to ergotamine since Bellergal-S also contains phenobarbital and alkaloid of belladonna)
B. Methysergide (Sansert)	4–8 mg/day	Fibrotic complications, nausea and vomiting, diarrhea, insomnia, drowsiness, peripheral edema, weight gain, myalgia
C. Ergonovine	0.2 mg b.i.d. or t.i.d.	Nausea, nervousness, aching of legs
VII. Monoamine oxidase inhibitors		
A. Phenelzine (Nardil)	Up to 60 mg/day	Dizziness, headache, sleep disturbances, constipation, dry mouth, weight gain, sexual disturbances

Table 2 (Continued)

Medications	Dosage	Some common side effects
B. Isocarboxazid (Marplan)	10–30 mg/day	Orthostatic hypotension, cardiac arrhythmias, dizziness and vertigo, constipation, headache, jitteriness
VIII. Other agents		
A. Cyproheptadine (Periactin)	8–16 mg/day	Sedation, dizziness, dryness of mouth, nausea, bowel disturbance, urinary retention
B. Phenytoin (Dilantin)	100 mg t.i.d. or q.i.d.	Nystagmus, ataxia, slurred speech, dizziness, insomnia
C. Valproate (Depakote)	15–60 mg/kg/day	Nausea, vomiting, indigestion, minor elevations of transaminases, sedation, photosensitivity

even at low dosages in some patients, which limits the usefulness of this class of drug. These two side effects may be more common with propranolol than with more beta-selective, less lipid-soluble beta-blockers (8,9). In my personal experience, this class of agents can be quite effective in controlling migraine provided that the patient understands what side effects to expect.

TRICYCLIC ANTIDEPRESSANTS

Of the five tricyclic antidepressants listed in Table 2, only amitriptyline has been well studied and found to be clinically effective (10–12). My own experience has been limited primarily to amitriptyline, which I have found to be particularly useful with a calcium channel blocker or a beta-blocker, and its sedative effects can be put to good use in the sleep-deprived patient. Its major limitations are its anticholinergic effects, which cause dry mouth and constipation. The other agents have been used in connection with migraine, but there are no studies available to document their efficacy. An agent from this class has not usually been one of my first choices for migraine prophylaxis but has been very useful in chronic daily headache as an agent of first choice.

NONSTEROIDAL ANTI-INFLAMMATORY DRUGS

The list of nonsteroidal anti-inflammatory agents (NSAIDs) is quite long, but most of them have not been studied to determine their efficacy in migraine prophylaxis. Diamond and Freitag (13), in an article on the use of NSAIDs in headache, reviewed studies that showed naproxen sodium to be helpful in controlling migraine. They concluded that NSAIDs should not replace other effective medications for migraine, but that they do provide an alternative for use alone or in combinations with other agents. Diamond and colleagues (14) also demonstrated that fenoprofen was a safe and effective agent in migraine prophylaxis. In a review of 12 controlled studies, Pradalier et al. (15) concluded that NSAIDs revealed no clear difference in efficacy from other prophylactic agents in comparative trials.

ALPHA₂-ADRENOCEPTOR AGONISTS

In spite of favorable results from double-blind controlled studies, Raskin (16) saw no improvement in any patient on the alpha$_2$-adrenoceptor agonist clonidine. As a result, he regarded it of little to no value in migraine prophylaxis. No data are available regarding the efficacy of guanfacine in migraine. In my clinical practice, I have used guanfacine for migraine prophylaxis with moderate success as a sole agent or in combination with other drugs.

ERGOT PREPARATIONS

The ergot preparations include ergotamines, methysergide, and ergonovine. Ergotamine in a combination product with phenobarbital and belladonna alkaloids (Bellergal-S) has been used for prevention of migraine. One of its indications in the *Physicians' Desk Reference* is as an interval treatment of recurrent throbbing headache, but in my experience it has not been particularly helpful. It should be noted that the use of ergotamine can be associated with rebound headache, and migraine transformation (see Chapter 5).

Methysergide was the first prophylactic agent to be proven effective in migraine. At first it appeared to be the answer to preventing migraine, but its side-effect profile keeps it from being the drug of first choice. In particular, the fibrotic complications have limited its use and have led to the recommendation that a patient needs a break, the so-called "drug holiday," from methysergide every 4–6 months. Raskin's book (16, pp. 164–171) on headache provides a thorough discussion of this drug.

The use of ergonovine was first introduced to me by Raskin in this textbook (16, pp. 172–174). It has proven to be a very helpful agent in migraine prophylaxis, but is not readily available because no major pharmaceutical company markets it. Methylergonovine is also available (and is a principal human metabolite of methysergide).

MONOAMINE OXIDASE INHIBITORS

The monoamine oxidase inhibitors, particularly phenelzine, have usually been used when other agents have failed, but these drugs have many undesirable side effects. A major disadvantage is that a strict tyramine-free diet must be observed to avoid a hypertensive crisis. On the whole, this group of medications has a narrow niche of usefulness in migraine treatment.

OTHER AGENTS

Cyproheptadine has both antihistamine and antiserotoninergic properties; it reduces release of serotonin outside the central nervous system. It has been used as a prophylactic agent for childhood migraine, and has been used much less in suppression of adult migraine. A suggestion has been made to combine cyproheptadine with methysergide when neither drug is effective.

Phenytoin has been used in migraine prophylaxis based on the supposed similarity between migraine and epilepsy. Anecdotally, this drug has been touted as an effective agent in migraine prophylaxis, but this claim has never been proven scientifically.

Valproate is the latest addition to the long list of medications thought to be effective in controlling migraine. Hering and Kuritsky (17) have obtained statistically significant results in the use of valproate for this purpose. The mechanism by which it works has not been clarified.

PROPHYLAXIS IN MENSTRUAL MIGRAINE

The medication mainstay for menstrual migraine is the class of NSAIDs. Gallagher (18) has also shown ergonovine to be helpful when taken at the time of the menses. Hormonal manipulation has also been tried with good results (19,20).

PROPHYLAXIS IN CHILDHOOD MIGRAINE

Cyproheptadine has been reported to be quite helpful for children, which my clinical experience confirms. Although propranolol has also proven effective, it is usually avoided in prophylactic therapy because of concern about possible long-term effects in children.

CONCLUSION

Prophylactic treatment should embrace a philosophy combining pharmacological and nonpharmacological therapies. When a prophylactic regimen is found, it should be continued for at least one year before changing it, to allow enough time to test it against the natural fluctuation in migraine. After that, changes in the prophylactic regimen can be made with reasonable assurance as to the extent that prophylactic treatment had an impact on the headache problem. Physicians should choose, as the initial agent, the one with which they are most familiar. If the initial choice proves unsuccessful, which is frequently the case, other agents should then be tried alone or in combination. The successful prophylactic treatment of headache truly depends heavily on the clinical skill of the treater, the cooperation of the patient, and the patience of both.

REFERENCES

1. Graham JR, Wolff HG. Mechanism of migraine headache and action of ergotamine tartrate. Arch Neurol Psychiatry 1938; 39:737–763.
2. Schumacher GA, Wolff HG. Experimental studies on headache. Arch Neurol Psychiatry 1941; 45:199–214.
3. Sicuteri F. Vasoneuractive substances in migraine. Headache 1966; 6:109.
4. Somerville BW. The role of estradiol withdrawal in the etiology of menstrual migraine. Neurology 1972; 22:824–828.
5. Amery WK. Prophylactic and curative treatment of migraine with calcium antagonists. Drug Des Deliv 1989; 4:197–203.
6. Spierings EL. Clinical and experimental evidence for a role of calcium entry blockers in the treatment of migraine. Ann NY Acad Sci 1988; 522:676–689.
7. Leandri M, Rigardo S, Schizzi R, Parodi CI. Migraine treatment with nicardipine. Cephalalgia 1990; 10:111–116.
8. Tfelt-Hansen P. Efficacy of beta-blockers in migraine: A critical review. Cephalalgia 1986; 6(suppl 5):15–24.
9. Beckett BE. Contemporary management of migraine. Part 2. Am Pharm 1990; NS30(4):42–45.

10. Couch JR, Ziegler DK, Hassanein R. Amitriptyline in the prophylaxis of migraine: Effectiveness and relationship of anti-migraine and anti-depressant side effects. Neurology 1976; 26:121–127.
11. Couch JR, Ziegler DK, Hassanein RS. Amitriptyline in migraine prophylaxis. Arch Neurol 1979; 36:695–699.
12. Ziegler DK, Hurwitz A, Hassanein RS, Kodanaz HA, Preskorn SH, Mason J. Migraine prophylaxis: A comparison of propranolol and amitriptyline. Arch Neurol 1987; 44:486–489.
13. Diamond S, Freitag FG. Do non-steroidal anti-inflammatory agents have a role in the treatment of migraine headaches? Drugs 1989; 37:755–760.
14. Diamond S, Solomon GD, Freitag FG, Mehta ND. Fenoprofen in the prophylaxis of migraine: A double-blind, placebo controlled study. Headache 1987; 27:246–249.
15. Pradalier A, Clapin A, Dry J. Treatment review: Non-steroidal anti-inflammatory drugs in the treatment and long-term prevention of migraine attacks. Headache 1988; 28:550–557.
16. Raskin RH. Migraine: Treatment. In: Raskin NH, ed. Headache. 2nd ed. New York: Churchill Livingstone, 1988:135–214.
17. Hering R, Kuritsky A. Sodium valproate in the prophylactic treatment of migraine: A double-blind study versus placebo. Cephalalgia 1992; 12:81–84.
18. Gallagher RM. Menstrual migraine and intermittent ergonovine therapy. Headache 1989; 29:366–367.
19. Lichten EM, Bennett RS, Whitty AJ, Daoud Y. Efficacy of danazol in the control of hormonal migraine. J Reprod Med 1991; 36:419–424.
20. O'Dea JPK, Davis EH. Tamoxifen in the treatment of menstrual migraine. Neurology 1990; 40:1470–1471.

12

Cluster Headache and Variant Syndromes

Lee Kudrow and David Kudrow

California Medical Clinic for Headache
Encino, California

Migrainous neuralgia (1), histamine cephalgia (2), and ciliary neuralgia (3) are the early terms given to the entity that is universally known today as cluster headache. Its name derives from the curious observation that attacks occur in clusters (4). Descriptions of cluster headache appear in the literature as early as 1840 (5), but the characteristic periodicity of the disorder was first described by K. A. Ekbom in 1947 (6).

Cluster headache generally occurs in two forms: *episodic cluster headache* and *chronic cluster headache*. Episodic cluster headache, the more common of the two forms, composes approximately 80% of a cluster headache population, whereas chronic cluster headache composes almost the remaining 20% (7). Episodic cluster headache is defined by a period of attack susceptibility that lasts 1–3 months followed by a remission period (headache-free interval) of generally 6 months to years in duration. Chronic cluster headache is characterized by the absence of any remission period for at least 12 months. Attack frequency may exceed that of episodic cluster headache and patients may be less responsive to prophylactic drug therapy, but these parameters vary from patient to patient. Chronic cluster headache that occurs without a preceding history of episodic cluster headache is considered primary chronic cluster headache. Secondary cluster headache defines the population of patients who have converted from the episodic pattern (8).

Chronic paroxysmal hemicrania (CPH) is considered a cluster headache variant. This disorder was first described by Sjaastad and Dale in 1974 (9), and more recently an episodic variety was described by Kudrow et al. (10). The paroxysmal hemicranias and cluster headache share certain features such as headache location, intensity, pain quality, and autonomic symptomatology. Paroxysmal hemicrania differs from cluster headache in that the frequency of attacks is 2–10 times greater, attack duration is shorter, and in paroxysmal hemicrania there is an absolute and complete response to prophylactic therapy with indomethacin.

EPIDEMIOLOGY

The mean age of onset of cluster headache is approximately 27–30 years of age (7,11,12). This is 10 years later than the mean age of onset of migraine.

Cluster headache is predominantly a male disorder. The male-to-female ratio is 4.5:1 to 6:1 (7,11–14). However, among African-Americans the male-to-female ratio is approximately 3:1, showing a relative over-representation of black women with cluster headache (7). This finding was first described by Lovshin in 1961 (14).

The incidence of cluster headache in the general population is not known. Based on prevalence rates in 18-year-old Swedish men (15) and population differences within headache clinics, the estimated incidence is approximately 1% (16).

DIAGNOSTIC FEATURES

Attack Characteristics

Within a 24-hour period, the attack frequency ranges from one to 10, with a mean of two attacks. They occur only once daily in 50% of patients, twice daily in 33% of patients, and more frequently in the remainder (17,18).

Attack duration may range from 10 minutes to 3 hours, with the mean attack duration being 45 minutes (19). Fifty to 75% of patients have nocturnal attacks (4,12,17,18). These attacks awaken the patient 90 minutes after sleep onset and are associated with the first REM period of the night. The temporal relationship between REM phase and cluster attack onset was first described by Dexter and Riley (20) and subsequently corroborated by Kudrow et al. (21).

Cluster headache pain intensity is most often described as excruciating. The character of the pain is boring with a sharp and burning quality, at times throbbing, but always penetrating. The pain is always unilateral with an occulotemporal, occulofrontal, or temporofacial distribution. It is not unusual that patients describe radiation of pain to the teeth on one side. This may obscure and delay the diagnosis, and lead to unnecessary dental procedures.

The patient's behavior during the attack is important. Many patients will pace the floor or sit in a chair leaning forward with their head in their hands and rock to and fro. The inability to lie still during an attack is constant and in fact pathognomonic of cluster headache pain. The dramatic nature of this disorder is demonstrated by the behavior of some cluster headache sufferers who, regardless of how stoic they are, cry out in desperation or smash their fists or heads against the wall during an attack. Despite the frequency and severity of attacks, and the certain anticipation of coming attacks, suicide, although contemplated by some patients, is rarely carried out. In fact, in our own population of 1200 cluster headache patients, suicide occurred in only one case and that was during a remission.

Several autonomic symptoms accompany the cluster headache attack in 72 to 84% of patients, including ipsilateral lacrimation, rhinorrhea, nasal stuffiness, and conjunctival suffusion (7). Ipsilateral ptosis and miosis (partial Horner's syndrome) have been observed during the attack in 60 to 70% of patients (7,11).

The Cluster Period

It is only during the cluster period that cluster attacks occur, whether they are spontaneous or provoked. The cluster period is therefore characterized by attack susceptibility. The period may last 2 to 4 months but the mean duration is 2 months (7,11).

Cluster period occurrence may be related to seasonal photoperiod changes. In one study (22), 900 cluster period onsets were recorded from 400 patients over a 10-year interval. The occurrence of cluster periods was found to increase during intervals of both longer and shorter photoperiods. In fact, the frequency of cluster periods peaked approximately 2 weeks following both the longest and shortest days of the year (January and June). Conversely, cluster period frequency decreased dramatically within 2 weeks of Daylight Savings and Standard Time changes. Thus, the chronobiological nature of cluster headache seems hardly disputable.

Cluster headaches may be provoked in patients during an active cluster period. Horton et al. (23) noted that attacks could be provoked by the administration of small amounts of alcohol and by subcutaneous administration of histamine. Sublingual nitroglycerin 1 mg was shown to provoke cluster headache attacks in 100% of 10 patients with cluster headache (24).

The Remission

In contrast to cluster periods, remission periods are intervals during which headaches do not occur spontaneously or by provocation. According to Ekbom (11), the average duration of remission is less than 2 years. Of 428 patients studied at the California Medical Clinic for Headache, 47.7% experienced remissions of 7 to 12 months, 19.2% had remissions of 1 to 6 months, and 14.3% had remissions of 1 to 2 years. The remainder experienced remission for more than 2 years. Remission periods may range from 1 month to 20 years (7).

DIFFERENTIAL DIAGNOSIS

Because of its unique periodicity, pain characteristics, and associated symptoms, few conditions can be mistaken for cluster headache. Other conditions, however, may share similar features.

As compared with migraine, cluster attacks are shorter in duration, occur several times per day, and are generally not associated with nausea and vomiting. There is certainly not a tendency to lie still during the cluster headache attack, in contradistinction to the migraine headache.

Pheochromocytoma (25) may produce headaches of relatively short duration and they may occur on a daily basis. The headache of pheochromocytoma, however, is generally bilateral and occipital and it is less intense. Other features of this disorder include sweating, pallor, tachycardia, and elevated blood pressure.

Temporal arteritis is generally seen in older patients. The location of the headache is usually unilateral and temporal. The intensity is not as severe as in cluster headache. The character of the headache is described as persistent and nonthrobbing. Important associated features include jaw claudication (26,27), malaise, elevated erythrocyte sedimentation rate, and the presence of a tender and tortuous, nonpulsatile temporal artery, and in some patients there may be an accompanying polymyalgia.

Trigeminal neuralgia occurs at a frequency of several times per day, like cluster headache, but the duration of headache is seconds to minutes. It is usually located in the distribution of second or third division of the trigeminal nerve, and it is usually unilateral. The pain is described as severe, burning, or lancinating. There may be a trigger zone either cutaneously or inside the mouth, which, when stimulated, may set off a paroxysm (28).

Raeder's syndrome (29), or the pericarotid syndrome (30), is a unilateral, persistent, severe pain that may be characterized as burning and either throbbing or nonthrobbing. It is generally located in the supraorbital region and may be associated with a partial Horner's syndrome.

As stated previously, chronic paroxysmal hemicrania (CPH) is a variant of cluster headache. It was first described by Sjaastad and Dale in 1974 (9). This disorder is uncommon. In 1983, Sjaastad reported having been informed of 80 cases worldwide (31). Treatment of this disorder is quite different from that of cluster headache; thus, its identification is critical. CPH may be confused with cluster headache in that it is unilateral, severe, and occulofrontal or temporal, and the pain is boring in character. Similarly, it occurs several times per day but usually much more frequently than cluster headache. The mean attack frequency in CPH is 14 per day. Attacks are shorter than cluster attacks, lasting 3 to 45 minutes, with a mean duration of 13 minutes (32).

Episodic paroxysmal hemicrania, described by Kudrow et al. (10), is similar to CPH in attack profile but its periodicity is different. Attacks occur during specific intervals of susceptibility as in episodic cluster headache, separated by long remissions. The patients described experienced cycles as long as 20 years.

The etiology and pathogenesis of the paroxysmal hemicranias are unknown. Ipsilateral intraoccular pressure, indentation pulse amplitudes, and corneal temperatures were increased on the ipsilateral side during attacks. These characteristics are similar to but more pronounced than those of cluster headache (33,34). Also, autonomic dysfunction has been found in both headache types (35,36).

Nocturnal paroxysmal hemicrania attacks are less likely to occur than cluster headaches. These headaches are unique in that they respond completely and absolutely to prophylactic treatment with indomethacin (31).

PATHOPHYSIOLOGY

Vascular Changes

During the cluster headache attack there is extracranial vasodilatation (2) and increased cerebral blood flow (19,37,38). An increase in regional cerebral blood flow has been described in the central, basal, and right parietotemporal regions (19). These findings were interpreted as being related to pain rather than being primary pathogenetic phenomena.

Impairment of autoregulatory responses has been suggested in cluster headache (37,38). There is an exaggerated vascular response to oxygen and a diminished response to carbon dioxide. Again, it is unclear whether these characteristics are primarily associated with the cluster headache syndrome or are epiphenomena related to pain activity (19).

Ekbom and Greitz (39) described the angiographic appearance of a segmental luminal narrowing on the ipsilateral internal carotid artery (ICA) during a cluster attack. These investigators interpreted this finding as being representative of luminal narrowing due to vasodilatation of the artery within a restrictive bony canal. According to this mechanism, compression of the sympathetic plexus surrounding the ICA may explain the partial Horner's syndrome.

Further evidence exists of ICA changes during cluster headache. Pulse synchronous indentation pulse waves and pulse synchronous changes in eye tension, as measured by dynamic tonometry, were found to be increased ipsilaterally (33,34). This suggests that during the cluster attack there is ophthalmic artery dilatation.

Biochemical Changes

Tryptophan, the platelet 5-HT precursor, was found to be increased in the CSF during cluster attacks (40). Similarly, whole-blood 5-HT was also shown to be elevated during the attack (41). Subsequent to these studies, it was shown that, following cluster headache attacks, the maximum rate of platelet derived 5-HT uptake was significantly decreased (42,43). Platelet-derived MAO was also found to be reduced in patients with cluster headache, but this was interpreted as being due to cigarette smoking rather than cluster headache (44–46).

The role of histamine in the pathogenesis of cluster headache is uncertain. Past studies showed increased levels of histamine in urine and blood in patients during the cluster attack (47,48). Administration of H_1 and H_2 blockers did not affect the frequency or intensity of cluster headaches (49).

Appenzeller et al. (50) and others (51) showed in electron microscopy studies that biopsies taken from temporal skin in patients with cluster headache had elevated mast cell counts and degranulation, with deposition of the mast cells around cutaneous nerves. Thus, Appenzeller et al. (50) suggested that the release of histamine by antidromal sensory nerves may be responsible for vasodilatation and the pain of cluster headaches. These results, however, could not be duplicated by others (52,53).

Cyclic Hormonal Changes

Hypothalamic dysfunction has been suggested by many investigators based on studies examining cyclic neuroendocrine derangement and chronobiological changes. Plasma testosterone levels were found to be lower in males during the active cluster period than in cluster patients during the remission (54,55). This was corroborated by others (56–59), and explanations for the phenomenon included possible hypothalamic-pituitary axis dysfunction (54,55) disordered REM states (59), and stress and secondary effects of pain (57,58). Altered circadian secretions of testosterone (56), prolactin (60,61), melatonin (62,63), cortisol (64,65,66), and β-endorphin (67) in cluster patients further contributed support for a chronobiological derangement. One study also showed a loss of circadian rhythmicity for blood pressure and body temperature (68).

Autonomic Changes

The anatomy of cluster headache is probably quite complex. Some researches have indicated that the cluster headache attack results from stimulation of the parasympathetic nuclei of the hypothalamus (69–71). The route of parasympathetic activity was described to be via the superficial petrosal nerve and sphenopalatine ganglion. Accordingly, surgical sectioning of portions of the seventh cranial nerve, including the nervous intermedius (70) or superficial petrosal nerve (67,72), did result in partial or complete relief of attacks in small numbers of patients.

A less invasive approach to the examination of the autonomic nervous system in cluster headache patients was described in a study by Fanciullacci et al. (73) in which topical 2% tyramine was used to measure pupillary responses. They showed that tyramine produced a poor mydriatic response on the symptomatic side during cluster headache attacks, interval periods, and remission. From these results they concluded that these patients had permanent dysfunction of ipsilateral sympathetic neurons. Other investigators (35,36) have shown increased facial sweating on the ipsilateral side caused by sympathetic dysfunction.

PATHOGENESIS

The cluster period is an altered physiological state during which there is occurrence of, and susceptibility to, the cluster attack. As stated previously, it is characterized by its cyclic nature, impaired autoregulatory activity, and altered neuroendocrine function. It is probably the result of abnormal hypothalamic function (7,41,74,75).

Cluster headache attacks occur in association with states in which there is hypoxemia. Such conditions include high altitude, REM sleep, and the use of some vasodilators. Oxygen inhalation aborts cluster headaches with remarkable reliability and rapidity (76). In 1983, Kudrow (77) hypothesized that cluster headache patients, during the attack-susceptible period, have a disordered physiological response to hypoxemia, probably due to chemoreceptor dysfunction. It was proposed that cluster headache patients should demonstrate a blunted chemoreceptor response to hypoxemia. This idea was recently tested in a study involving active and remission cluster headache patients as well as normal controls (78). Ten patients in active cluster periods were monitored for oxygen saturation before and after administration of sublingual nitroglycerin. The same procedure was carried out in the remission patients and controls. Following administration of nitroglycerin, all subjects showed a significant oxygen desaturation. In the remission and control groups, the oxygen saturation returned to baseline after approximately 30 minutes. In the active cluster group, the oxygen saturation continued to decrease for an additional 20 minutes, resulting in attacks in 10 of 10 patients. These results are interpreted as supporting the hypothesis that active cluster patients have an abnormal chemoreceptor response to hypoxemia (77).

Polysomnographic studies on a small group of cluster headache patients showed that there was an association between attack onset and REM period–related oxygen desaturation (21).

Moskowitz (72) introduced a trigeminovascular theory on the etiology of head pain which has been elaborated elsewhere. Siccuteri et al. (79–81) suggested that cluster headache pain results from release of substance P from trigeminal nerves. Antidromic stimulation results in release of substance P, which then causes a nociceptive response. Earlier, an antidromal mechanism mediated by histamine was postulated by Appenzeller et al. (59). As indicated earlier, more distal pathways in the production of cluster headache pain have implicated the seventh cranial nerve (69–71).

TREATMENT

Patient Education

As in all other medical disorders, patient education, prophylaxis, and symptomatic treatment are the cornerstones of successful management of cluster headache. An integral part of the management of cluster headache is informing the patient about the mechanism of the disorder in understandable terms, and assuring him that attacks can be prevented and rapidly aborted. This should alleviate some of the attendant anticipatory anxiety that plagues the patient during the cluster period. Expectations, however, should be realistic and the patient should be informed that while prophylactic and abortive medications are highly effective, they do not attenuate or prevent the cluster period.

The natural history of the disorder is such that one-third of the patients will have permanent remissions, one-third will have periods of remission alternating with cluster periods, unchanged, and one-third will improve to the extent that they have only minor attacks or they don't require medication (82).

By the time most patients present to a physician, they have already made an association between attack onset and ingestion of alcohol. Nevertheless, a warning regarding alcohol use during the cluster period will reinforce abstinent behavior. Similarly, patients should be counseled against prolonged exposure to other volatile substances that might precipitate the attack, such as solvents or gasoline.

Reduced atmospheric oxygen tensions may cause a relative hypoxemia in cluster patients. Thus, patients should be informed about the possibility of attacks occurring at high altitude. This is most apt to occur at an altitude of 5000 feet or greater (in airplane travel, cabin pressures may be equivalent to 7000–8000 feet). In such cases the patient may use ergotamine, 2 mg, 1 hour prior to air travel to prevent an attack. To abort an attack during flight, oxygen inhalation at 7 liters per minute will offer complete relief. Cluster headache attacks that are expected to occur during periods at high altitude can be prevented by the oral administration of acetoazolamide, 25 mg, twice daily for 4 days, beginning 2 days before altitude is reached.

Prophylaxis

Episodic Cluster Headache

Attacks occurring during nighttime sleeping hours generally occur 90 minutes after sleep onset, corresponding to the first REM period.

Administration of ergotamine, 2 mg, 2 hours prior to the expected onset of the attack, will usually prevent these nocturnal attacks. Frequent doses of ergotamine are contraindicated in migraine because it tends to cause a well-known rebound phenomenon. Nightly doses of ergotamine in the cluster headache population, however, do not produce rebound, and in our experience clinical ergotism is unlikely at this dosage. Ergotamine is contraindicated in the presence of peripheral vascular disease, cardiovascular disease, and cerebrovascular disease. Additionally it is contraindicated in pregnancy, liver and renal disease, and serious infection, and during postsurgical periods.

In patients who experience attacks at any time of the day or night, prophylaxis with agents such as verapamil, methysergide, lithium, or prednisone may be indicated. In our clinic, for patients under the age of 30 who have had one or two cluster periods, methysergide, 4 mg, three to four times daily is the treatment of choice. Methysergide appears to be most effective in the early course of the disease and becomes less effective with time. This medication has an approximate 65% efficacy rate in prophylaxis against cluster headache (83,84). Complications associated with this medication are well known and have been reviewed elsewhere (85).

In patients beyond the age of 30, our treatment of choice is verapamil, 80 mg, given four times daily spaced evenly throughout waking hours. Gabel and Spierings (86) have shown that its efficacy is approximately 70% in episodic and chronic cluster headache prophylaxis. Our unpublished data and others (87) corroborate this finding. Furthermore, an additional 15% of patients can be captured successfully when treated with 1–2 mg ergotamine tartrate, given 1 hour before bedtime. The mechanism of action of this verapamil in cluster headache is still uncertain. Calcium channels are widely distributed throughout the neuronal and vascular systems. The most troublesome side effect of this medication, which precludes its use in the occasional patient, is constipation. This problem appears to be more frequent with the longer-acting, sustained-release preparation. Also, 5–8% of patients may experience girdle pain and myalgia.

Lithium, 300 mg twice daily, in addition to verapamil and ergotamine, will capture the 5–10% of episodic cluster patients who are otherwise resistant to verapamil and ergotamine alone. Ekbom (88) first reported the use of lithium as a sole prophylactic agent in 1978. Lithium alone, 300 mg b.i.d., was reported to show 70–80% efficacy as a prophylactic medication in cluster headache (89–91). The use of lithium, however, is accompanied by contraindications such as the use of diuretics or severe sodium-restricted diets. The lithium ion competes with intracellular sodium and can lead to toxicity.

Despite the usual success of using verapamil and ergotamine—or even triple therapy with the addition of lithium—there may still be a small number of patients who continue to be resistant. In these patients who are under the age of 40, treatment with corticosteroids may be indicated. In our clinic, we use prednisone beginning at a total daily dose of 40 mg per day, divided, and the medication is tapered over a period of 3 weeks. With this regimen, about 80% of patients with episodic and 40% of those with chronic cluster headache should experience medication remission (84,92). However, attacks may break through when the total daily dose falls to 15 mg. Contraindications, side effects, and complications of prednisone therapy are ubiquitous and have been reported elsewhere. We have been made aware of two cases of ruptured intestinal diverticulae in patients with cluster headache over the age of 40 who were treated with prednisone. Diverticulosis, then, should be added to the list of contraindications to the use of prednisone. Of course, long-term corticosteroid use should be avoided due to the potential development of hypoadrenalism.

Chronic Cluster Headache

In a large population of chronic and subchronic (remissions lasting less than 5 months) cluster headache patients, approximately 50% were treatment-resistant (93). MMPI studies on these patients revealed that they had elevated scales for depression or hysteria and were prone to addiction (93). In patients with these traits, therapy should be initiated with verapamil, ergotamine, and lithium: triple therapy. The use of narcotic analgesics should be prohibited. Continued resistance to therapy despite this combination of medications may warrant a course of histamine desensitization, in which efficacy, either alone or in combination with prophylaxis, has been reported (94).

In the absence of a treatment-resistant history, neurosis, drug abuse, and evidence of addiction proneness, treatment is the same as that for episodic cluster headache. Lithium carbonate, 300 mg b.i.d. alone or with the addition of ergotamine 1–2 mg at bedtime, is as effective as verapamil and ergotamine.

Hering and Kuritsky (95), in an open-labeled study using sodium valproate 600–2000 mg per day, showed success in 11 of 15 patients. The medication was well tolerated in all patients except for mild nausea in three, and there was no correlation between efficacy and plasma levels. The authors suggest that sodium valproate, a GABA mimetic, inhibits interneurons in the suprachiasmatic nucleus of the hypothalamus. Their assumption lends further support to the theory that there is a chrono-biological role in cluster headache.

Bright-light phototherapy has been used successfully in treating a variety of disorders that have in common a chronobiological nature (96–98). At the California Medical Clinic for Headache, we have employed bright-light therapy in an attempt to reset circadian pacemakers. It is expected that in this way one can shift sleep–wake cycles and perhaps interrupt the hypothalamic-dependent periodicity associated with cluster headache. To date, results have been encouraging in four of eight patients (unpublished data).

Ultimately, in the event that adequate prophylaxis cannot be achieved using optimal medicinal therapy, then surgical therapy should be con-sidered. The treatment of choice in this case appears to be radiofrequency trigeminal gangliolysis. Significant success rates have been reported by Mathew and Hurt (99) in treatment of chronic cluster headache and by K. Campbell (personal communication) at the Mayo clinic.

Symptomatic Treatment of Cluster Headache

Effective symptomatic treatment is needed when patients experience "breakthrough" attacks despite adequate prophylaxis, when the use of prophylaxis is contraindicated due to concurrent medical illness, or when preventive medications are refused.

Oxygen inhalation proves to be the safest and fastest method to abort cluster headache attacks (76). In our experience, 70% of attacks can be aborted within 10 minutes and 90% within 15 minutes. The method of oxygen inhalation is of utmost importance in achieving success. The fol-lowing points should be remembered.

1. Oxygen inhalation should be started at the earliest sign of attack.
2. The oxygen tank regulator should be set such that a continuous flow of 100% oxygen is maintained at a rate of 7 liters per minute. A high level of oxygen saturation must be sustained for several minutes to achieve relief of an attack (78).
3. The method of delivery should be by facial mask, nonbreather type, held over the mouth and nose. Nasal cannulae are not adequate as there may be significant nasal congestion during an attack.
4. The patient must assume a sitting position, leaning forward, elbows on knees and face parallel to the ground to allow adequate cavernous sinus drainage. Supine or near-supine positioning will increase cavernous sinus congestion and aggravate the attack.

There are few contraindications to short-term oxygen use, and its value in aborting cluster attacks has been well established (76,100,101).

Sublingual and inhaler ergotamine preparations are also of benefit in aborting the cluster headache attack. Indeed, these preparations are more convenient to use than oxygen inhalation. The subcutaneous preparation is placed under the tongue at attack onset and left unswallowed for several minutes to maintain absorption. One may repeat this after 10 minutes if necessary. The inhaler may be used at the onset of attack and it can be repeated three times at 5-minute intervals, as needed.

Parenteral administration of DHE-45, 1 mg, may be used in an emergency room or office setting. It is generally given as an I.M. injection intragluteally.

Intranasal administration of local anesthetics such as cocaine HCL 5% (102) or lidocaine 4% (103) may also be used. The head is tilted back and turned toward the ipsilateral side. The effects of these agents are limited by the patient's intranasal anatomy, proper administration, and tolerance.

Treatment of the Paroxysmal Hemicranias

The absolute and complete response to indomethacin, which is used as a prophylactic agent in CPH, is practically diagnostic for this disorder. In our experience, indomethacin, 75–100 mg per day in divided doses, provides successful management of the paroxysmal hemicranias. Maintenance therapy may suffice even at doses as low as 25 mg per day.

Childhood-onset CPH has been reported with some frequency. However, treatment guidelines in pediatric age groups are as yet unavailable. We reported a case of a 9-year-old male (104) in whom treatment with baby aspirin 162 mg twice daily provided complete relief.

REFERENCES

1. Harris W. Ciliary (migrainous) neuralgia and its treatment. Br Med J. 1936; 1:457–460.
2. Horton BT. Histaminic cephalgia. Lancet 1952; ii:92–98.
3. Harris W. Neuritis and Neuralgia. London: Oxford University Press, 1926.
4. Kunkle EC, Pfeiffer JB Jr, Wilhoit WM, et al. Recurrent brief headache in "cluster" pattern. Trans Am Neurol Assoc. 1952; 77:240–243.
5. Romberg MH. A Manual of Nervous Diseases of Man. Sieveking EH, trans. London: Sydenham Society, 1840.
6. Ekbom KA. Ergotamine tartrate orally in Horton's "histaminic cephalgia" (also called Harris' "ciliary neuralgia"). Acta Psychiatr Scand 1947; 46(suppl): 106–113.

7. Kudrow L. Cluster Headache: Mechanism and Management. Oxford: Oxford University Press, 1980.

8. Ekbom K, de Fine Olivarius B. Chronic migrainous neuralgia—diagnostic and therapeutic aspects. Headache 1971; 11:97–101.

9. Sjaastad O, Dale I. Evidence for a new (?) treatable headache entity. Headache 1974; 14:105–108.

10. Kudrow L, Esperanca P, Vijayan N. Episodic paroxysmal hemicrania? Cephalalgia 1987; 7:197–201.

11. Ekbom K. A clinical composition of cluster headache and migraine. Acta Neurol Scand 1970; 46(suppl 41):1–44.

12. Friedman AP, Mikropoulos HE. Cluster headaches. Neurology 1958; 8:653–663.

13. Lance JW, Anthony M. Migrainous neuralgia or cluster headache. J Neurol Sci 1971; 13:401.

14. Lovshin LL. Clinical caprices of histaminic cephalgia. Headache 1961; 1:3–6.

15. Ekbom K, Ahlborg B, Schele R. Prevalence of migraine and cluster headache in Swedish men of 18. Headache 1978; 18:9–19.

16. Kudrow L. Cluster headache. In: Blau JN, ed. Migraine: Clinical, Therapeutic, Conceptual and Research Aspects. London: Chapman and Hall, 1987:113–132.

17. Ekbom K. Pattern of cluster headache with a note on the relation to angina pectoris and peptic ulcer. Acta Neurol Scand. 1970; 46:225–237.

18. Lance JW. Mechanisms and Management of Headache. 3rd ed. London: Butterworths, 1978.

19. Aebelholt-Krabbe A, Henriksen L, Olesen J. Tomagraphic determination of cerebral blood flow during attacks of cluster headache. Cephalalgia 1984; 4:17–23.

20. Dexter JD, Riley TL. Studies in nocturnal migraine. Headache 1975; 15:51–62.

21. Kudrow L, McGinty DS, Phillips ER, et al. Sleep apnea in cluster headache. Cephalalgia 1984; 4:33–38.

22. Kudrow L. The cyclic relationship of natural illumination to cluster period frequency (abstr). Cephalalgia 1987; 7(suppl 6):76–77.

23. Horton BT, MacLean AR, Craig WM. A new syndrome of vascular headache. Results in treatment with histamine: Preliminary report. Mayo Clin Proc 1939; 14:257–260.

24. Ekbom K. Nitroglycerin as a provocative agent in cluster headache. Arch Neurol 1968; 19:487–493.

25. Thomas JE, Rooke ED, Kvale WF. The neurologist's experience with pheochromocytoma: A review of 100 cases. JAMA 1966; 197:754.

26. Horton BT, Magath TB, Brown GE. An underdescribed form of arteritis of the temporal vessels. Proc Staff Meet Mayo Clin 1932; 7:700–701.

27. Huston KA, Hunder GG, Lie JT, et al. Temporal arteritis: A 25 year epidemiologic, clinical, and pathological study. Ann Intern Med 1978; 88:162–167.

28. Dalessio DJ. A reappraisal of the trigger zone of tic douloureaux. Headache 1969; 9:73–76.

29. Raeder JG. "Paratrigeminal" paralysis of oculo-pupillary sympathetic. Brain 1924; 47:149–158.
30. Vijayan N, Watson C. Pericarotid syndrome. Headache 1978; 18:244–254.
31. Sjaastad O. Chronic paroxysmal hemicrania: Clinical aspects and controversies. In: Blau JN, ed. Migraine: Clinical, Therapeutic, Conceptual and Research Aspects. London: Chapman and Hall, 1987:135–152.
32. Russell D. Chronic paroxysmal hemicrania: Severity, duration and time of occurrences of attacks. Cephalalgia 1984; 4:53–56.
33. Broch A, Horven I, Nornes H, et al. Studies of cerebral and ocular circulation in a patient with cluster headache. Headache 1970; 10:1–13.
34. Horven I, Nornes H, Sjaastad O. Different corneal indentation pulse patterns in cluster headache and migraine. Neurology 1972; 22:92–98.
35. Saunte C, Russell D, Sjaastad O. Cluster headache: On the mechanisms behind attack-related sweating. Cephalalgia 1983; 3:175–185.
36. Sjaastad O, Saunte C, Russell D, et al. Cluster headache: The sweating pattern during spontaneous attacks. Cephalalgia 1981; 1:233–244.
37. Norris JW, Hachinski VC, Cooper PW. Cerebral blood flow changes in cluster headache. Acta Neurol Scand 1976; 54:371–374.
38. Sakai F, Meyer JS. Regional cerebral hemodynamics during migraine and cluster headaches measured by the ^{133}Xe inhalation method. Headache 1987; 18:122–132.
39. Ekbom K, Greitz T. Carotid angiography in cluster headache. Acta Radiol Diagn 1970; 10:177–186.
40. Salmon S, Bonciani M, Fanciullacci M, et al. A putative 5-HT central feedback in migraine and cluster headache. In: Critchley M, Friedman AP, Gorini S, et al., eds. Advances in Neurology. Vol 33. New York: Raven Press, 1982:265–274.
41. Medina JL, Diamond S, Fareed J. The nature of cluster headache. Headache 1979; 19:309–322.
42. Swade CC, Carroll JD, Coppen A. Platelet 5-hydroxytryptamine accumulation in migrainous neuralgia. In: Rose FC, Zilkha KJ, eds. Progress in Migraine Research. Vol. 1. London: Pitman, 1981:89–92.
43. Waldenlind E, Ross SB, Saaf J, et al. Concentration and uptake of 5-hydroxytryptamine in platelets from cluster headache and migraine patients. Cephalalgia 1985; 5:45–54.
44. Glover V, Peatfield R, Zammit-Pace R, et al. Platelet monoamine oxidase activity and headache. J Neurol Neurosurg Psychiatry 1981; 44:786–790.
45. Littlewood JT, Glover V, Sandler M, et al. Migraine and cluster headache: Links between platelet monoamine oxidase activity, smoking and personality. Headache 1984; 24:30–34.
46. Waldenlind E, Saaf J, Ekbom K, et al. Kinetics and thermolability of platelet monoamine oxidase in cluster headache and migraine. Cephalalgia 1984; 4:125–134.
47. Anthony M, Lance JW. Histaminic and serotonin in cluster headache. Arch Neurol 1971; 25:225–231.

48. Sjaastad O, Sjaastad OV. Urinary histamine excretion in migraine and cluster headache. J Neurol 1977; 216:91–104.
49. Anthony M, Lord GDA, Lance JW. Controlled trials of cimetidine in migraine and cluster headache. Headache 1978; 18:261–264.
50. Appenzeller O, Becker W, Ragas A. Cluster headache: Ultrastructural aspects. Neurology 1978; 28:371.
51. Prusinski A, Liberski PO. Is the cluster headache local mastocytic diaethesis? Headache 1979; 19:102.
52. Aebelholt-Krabbe A, Rank F. Histological examination of the superficial temporal artery in patients suffering cluster headache. Cephalalgia 1985; 5(suppl 3):282–283.
53. Cuypers J, Westphal K, Bunge ST. Mast cells in cluster headache. Acta Neurol Scand 1980; 61:327–329.
54. Kudrow L. Plasma testosterone and LH levels in cluster headache. Headache 1977; 17:91–92.
55. Kudrow L. Plasma testosterone levels in cluster headache: Preliminary results. Headache 1976; 16:28–31.
56. Facchinetti F, Nappi G, Cicoli C, et al. Reduced testosterone levels in cluster headache: A stress related phenomenon. Cephalalgia 1986; 6:29–34.
57. Klimek A. Plasma testosterone levels in patients with cluster headache. Headache 1982; 22:162–164.
58. Nelson RF. Testosterone levels in cluster and non-cluster migraineurs headache patients. Headache 1978; 18:265–267.
59. Romiti A, Martelletti P, Gallo MG, et al. Low plasma testosterone levels in cluster headache. Cephalalgia 1982; 3:41–44.
60. Polleri A, Nappi G, Murialdo G, et al. Changes in the 24-hour prolactin pattern in cluster headache. Cephalalgia 1982; 2:1–7.
61. Waldenlind E, Gustafsson SA. Prolactin in cluster headache: Diurnal secretion, response to thyrotropin-releasing hormone, and relation to sex steroids and gonadotropins. Cephalalgia 1987; 7:43–54.
62. Chazot G, Claustrat B, Brun J, et al. A chronobiological study of melatonin, cortisol, growth hormone and prolactin secretion in cluster headache. Cephalalgia 1984; 4:213–220.
63. Waldenlind E, Ekbom K, Friberg Y, et al. Decreased nocturnal serum melatonin levels during active cluster headache periods. Opusc Med 1984; 29:109–112.
64. Ferrari E, Canepari C, Bossolo PA, et al. Changes of biological rhythms in primary headache syndromes. Cephalalgia 1983; 3(suppl 1):58–68.
65. Nappi G, Ferrari E, Polleri A, et al. Chronobiological study of cluster headache. Chronobiologia 1981; 2:140.
66. Waldenlind E, Gustafsson SA, Ekbom K, et al. Circadian secretion of cortisol and melatonin in cluster headache during active cluster periods and remission. J Neurol Neurosurg Psychiatry 1987; 50:207–213.
67. Nappi G, Facchinetti F, Bono G, et al. Lack of β-endorphin and β-lipotropin circadian rhythmicity in episodic cluster headache: A model for chronopathology.

In: Pfaffenrath V, Lundberg PO, Sjaastad O, eds. Updating in Headache. Berlin: Springer-Verlag, 1985.

68. Ferrari E, Martignoni E, Vailati A, et al. Chronobiological aspects of cluster headache: Effects of lithium therapy. In: Savoldi F, Nappi G, eds. Headache. Pavia: Palladio Editore, 1979:152–160.

69. Gardner WJ, Stowell A, Dutlinger R. Resection of the greater superficial petrosal nerve in the treatment of unilateral headache. J Neurosurg 1947; 4: 105–114.

70. Sachs E Jr. The role of the nervous intermedius in facial neuralgia: Report of four cases with observations on the pathways for taste, lacrimation and pain in the face. J Neurosurg 1968; 23:54–60.

71. Stowell A. Physiologic mechanisms and treatment of histaminic or petrosal neuralgia. Headache 1970; 9:187–194.

72. Moskowitz MA. The neurobiology of vascular head pain. Ann Neurol 1984; 16:157–168.

73. Fanciullacci M, Pietrini U, Gatto G, et al. Latent dysautonomic pupillary lateralization in cluster headache: A pupillometric study. Cephalalgia 1982; 2:135–144.

74. Ekbom K. Pathogenesis of cluster headache. In: Blau JN, ed. Migraine: Clinical, Therapeutic, Conceptual and Research Aspects. London: Chapman and Hall, 1987:433–448.

75. Nappi G, Savoldi F. In: Headache: Diagnostic System and Taxonomic Criteria. London: John Libbey Eurotext, 1985.

76. Kudrow L. Response of cluster headache attacks to oxygen inhalation. Headache 1981; 21:1–4.

77. Kudrow L. A possible role of the carotid body in the pathogenesis of cluster headache. Cephalalgia 1983; 3:241–247.

78. Kudrow L, Kudrow DB. Association of sustained oxyhemoglobin desaturation and onset of cluster headache attacks. Headache 1990; 30(8):474.

79. Sicuteri F, Fanciullacci M, Geppetti P, et al. Substance P mechanism in cluster headache: Evaluation in plasma and cerebrospinal fluid. Cephalalgia 1985; 5:143–149.

80. Sicuteri F, Geppetti P, Marabini S, et al. Pain relief by somatostatin in attacks of cluster headache. Pain 1984; 18:359–365.

81. Sicuteri F, Raino L, Geppetti P. Substance P and endogenous opioids: How and where they could play a role in cluster headache. Cephalalgia 1983; 3(suppl 1):143–145.

82. Kudrow L. Natural history of cluster headache. Part 1. Outcome of drop-out patients. Headache 1982; 22:203–206.

83. Friedman AP, Elkind AH. Appraisal of methysergide in treatment of vascular headaches of migraine type. JAMA 1963; 184:125–130.

84. Kudrow L. Comparative results of prednisone, methysergide and lithium therapy in cluster headache. In: Green R, ed. Current Concepts in Migraine Research. New York: Raven Press, 1978:159–163.

85. Graham JR, Suby HI, LeCompte RM, et al. Inflammatory fibrosis associated with methysergide therapy. In: Friedman AP, ed. Research and Clinical Studies in Headache. Vol. 1. Basel: Karger, 1967:123–164.

86. Gabel IJ, Spierings ELH. Prophylactic treatment of cluster headache with verapamil. Headache 1989; 29:167–168.

87. Meyer JS, Hardenberg BA. Clinical effectiveness of calcium entry blockers in prophylactic treatment of migraine and cluster headaches. Headache 1983; 23:266–277.

88. Ekbom K. Litium vid kroniska symptom av cluster headache. Opusc Med 1978; 19:148–156.

89. Ekbom K. Lithium for cluster headache: Review of the literature and preliminary results of long-term treatment. Headache 1981; 21:132–139.

90. Kudrow L. Lithium prophylaxis for chronic cluster headache. Headache 1977; 17:15–18.

91. Mathew NT. Clinical subtypes of cluster headache and response to lithium therapy. Headache 1978; 18:26–30.

92. Jammes JL. The treatment of cluster headache with prednisone. Dis Nerv Syst 1975; 36:375–376.

93. Kudrow L. Subchronic cluster headache. Headache 1987; 27:197–200.

94. Diamond S, Freitag FG, Prager J, et al. Treatment of intractable cluster. Headache 1986; 26:42–46.

95. Hering R, Kuritsky A. Sodium valproate in the treatment of cluster headache: An open clinical trial. Cephalalgia 1989; 9:195.

96. Czeisler CA, Kronauer RE, Allan JS, et al. Bright light induction of strong (Type O) resetting of the human circadian pacemaker. Science 1989; 244:1328–1333.

97. Lewy AJ, Sacks RL, Miller LS, et al. Antidepressant and circadian phase-shifting effects of light. Science 1987; 235:352–354.

98. Richardson GS, Coleman RM, Zimmerman JC, et al. Chronotherapy: Resetting the circadian clock of patients with delayed sleep phase insomnia. Sleep 1981; 4:1–21.

99. Mathew NT, Hurt W. Radiofrequency trigeminal gangliolysis in the treatment of chronic intractable cluster headache. Headache 1985; 25:166.

100. Anthony M. Treatment of attacks of cluster headache with oxygen inhalation. In: Tyrer JH, Eadie MG, eds. Clinical Experimental Neurology. Vol. 18. Sydney: Australian Association of Neurologists, 1981:195.

101. Fogan L. Treatment of cluster headache: A double-blind comparison of oxygen vs. air inhalation. Arch Neurol 1985; 42:362–363.

102. Barre F. Cocaine as an abortive agent in cluster headache. Headache 1982; 22:69–73.

103. Kittrelle JP, Grouse DS, Seybold M. Cluster headache: Local anaesthetic abortive agents. Arch Neurol 1985; 42:496–498.

104. Kudrow DB, Kudrow L. Successful aspirin prophylaxis in a child with chronic paroxysmal hemicrania. Headache 1989; 29:280–281.

13

Chronic Daily Headache and Myofascial Pain Syndromes
Pathophysiology and Treatment

Gary W. Jay

*Headache and Neurological
Rehabilitation Institute of Colorado
Denver, Colorado*

PRESENTATION

Chronic daily headache (CDH) has multiple etiologies sharing elements of at least five other types of pain syndromes. These include chronic tension-type headache, posttraumatic headache, migraine, drug-withdrawal headache, and muscle-induced pain syndromes.

Pathological changes in muscle may initiate central nervous system adaptations that modulate or perpetuate chronic headache (see Chapter 14). CDH most often presents as a tension-type headache. Tension-type headache is itself a muscle-induced pain syndrome, associated with myofascial pain syndrome (MPS) and fibromyalgia. Instead of a headache continuum spanning from migraine to chronic daily headache (acute to chronic), CDH may represent different aspects of a central nociceptive disorder with headache as the final common pathway.

MUSCLE PAIN SYNDROMES AND CHRONIC HEADACHE

There are at least three distinct muscle pain syndromes that may be concurrent with CDH: 1) localized MPS associated with trigger points, 2) fibromyalgia, which appears to be a systemic disorder that includes non-REM sleep disturbance, and 3) articular dysfunction (1) (see Chapters 14 and 15).

Myofascial Pain Syndrome

Travell and Rinzler (2) identified the contribution of musculoskeletal factors in the etiology of tension-type or chronic daily headache. They demonstrated that there are consistent patterns of referred pain from trigger points within specific muscles and defined perpetuating factors that convert acute myofascial pain into a chronic pain syndrome (3). Some headaches are specific examples of this generalized process.

MPS is a localized or regional pain problem associated with small zones of hypersensitivity within skeletal muscle called trigger points. With palpation of these points, pain is referred to adjacent or even distant areas. Trigger points in the head, neck, and upper back may elicit headache, tinnitus, vertigo, and lacrimation. These features are often noted in patients with CDH.

Trigger points may be either active (with reproducible pain upon palpation) or latent (without clinically associated complaints of pain). Although painless, latent trigger points may produce muscle dysfunction (4–7). Muscles with trigger points may show increased stiffness, fatigability, weakness, and restricted motion. As muscles shorten, pain increases if the muscle is stretched. To avoid this pain, patients often compensate by adopting unusual or poor postures (7). The resulting muscle restriction may not only perpetuate existing trigger points but aid in the development of additional ones.

Trigger points represent muscle fibers in an "energy crisis," with decreased amounts of adenosine triphosphate and other muscle metabolic chemicals. Localized vascular disturbances due to increased muscle tension result in relative tissue hypoxia (8–10). Over time, prostaglandins, bradykinin, and histamine accumulate, further sensitizing the afferent nerve endings (11). Some common referred myofascial pain patterns of the head and neck are illustrated in Figures 1–8. These can often be managed

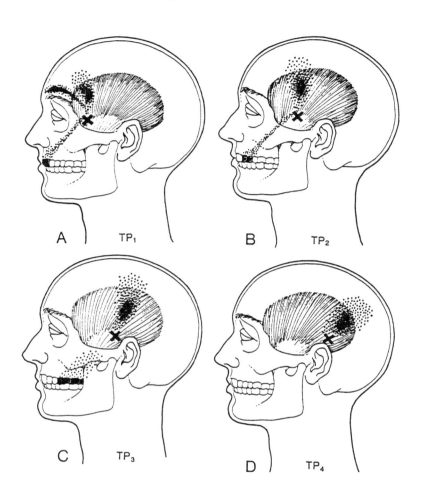

Figure 1 Referred pain patterns from trigger points (×) in the left temporalis muscle. Dark areas show essential zones; spillover zones are stippled. (A) Anterior "spokes" of pain arising from the anterior fibers—trigger point 1 region. (B and C) Middle spokes—trigger point 2 and 3 regions. (D) Posterior supra-auricular spoke—trigger point 4 region. (From Ref. 3.)

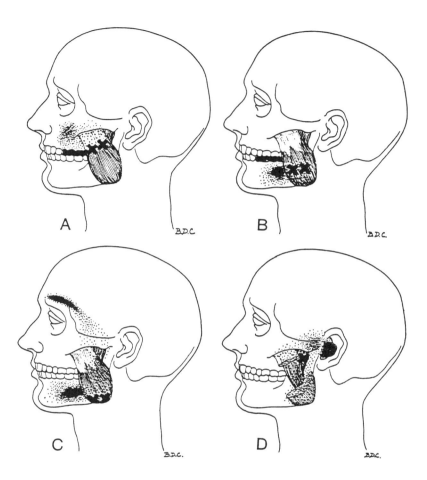

Figure 2 x's indicate trigger points in various parts of the masseter muscle. Dark areas show essential zones; spillover zones are stippled. (A) Superficial layer, upper portion. (B) Superficial layer, mid-belly. (C) Superficial layer, lower portion. (D) Deep layer, upper part—just below the temporomandibular joint. (From Ref. 3.)

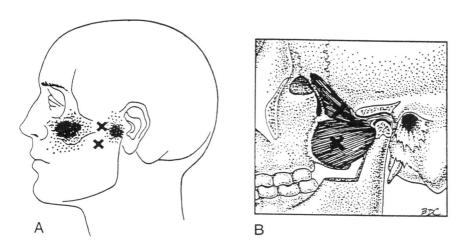

Figure 3 (A) Referred pain pattern of trigger points (×) in (B) the left lateral pterygoid muscle. Note the similarity to temporomandibular disorder. (From Ref. 3.)

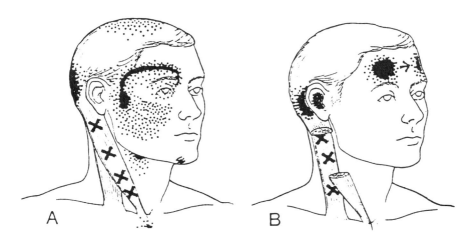

Figure 4 Referred pain patterns with location of corresponding trigger points (×) in the right sternocleidomastoid muscle. Dark areas show essential zones; spillover zones are stippled. (A) The sternal (superficial) division. (B) The clavicular (deep) division. (From Ref. 3.)

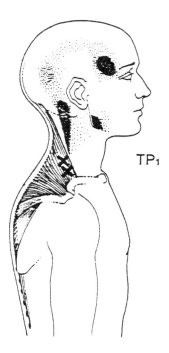

TP₁

Figure 5 Referred pain pattern and location of trigger point (×) in the upper trapezius muscle. Dark areas show essential zones; spillover zones are stippled. (From Ref. 3.)

effectively with physical therapy, spray and stretch techniques, or injection of local anesthetic.

Fibromyalgia

Fibromyalgia is a systemic disorder affecting approximately seven women for every man. The typical patient with fibromyalgia is between 30 and 50 years of age.

Diagnostically, there is at least a 3-month history of generalized symmetrical pain, and often daily headache, anxiety, depression, and irritable bowel syndrome. Similar to patients with CDH, there is an alpha-intrusion in stage IV sleep, causing "nonrestorative slumber."

The energy crisis in muscles is similar but more generalized than with MPS. From a list of clinical diagnostic criteria of 18 symmetrical tender

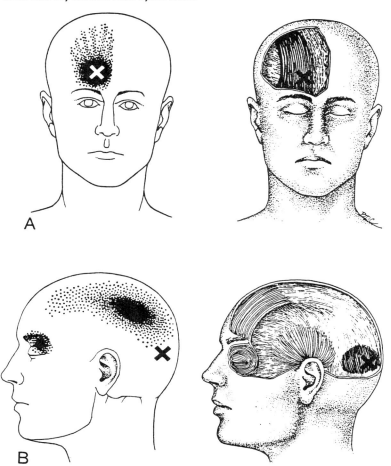

Figure 6 Pain patterns (shaded areas) referred from trigger points (×) in the occipitofrontalis muscle, commonly associated with unilateral, supraorbital, or ocular headache. (A) Right frontalis belly. (B) Left occipitalis belly.

points, at least 11 need to be found on examination to confirm the disorder (12–14). Fibromyalgia and MPS are hypothesized to be distinct disorders with the same underlying pathophysiology (15).

Oculomotor disturbances occur in patients with fibromyalgia and, to a lesser degree, in those with CDH. There is hypofunction of the sympathetic nervous system and disturbances in microcirculation resulting in the muscular energy crisis and depletion of high-energy phosphates

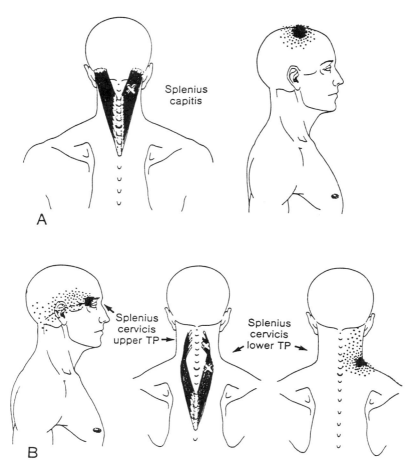

Figure 7 Trigger points (×) and referred pain patterns (shaded areas) for the right splenius capitis and splenius cervicis muscles. (A) The splenius capitis trigger point, which overlies the occipitaal triangle. (B) (Left) The upper splenius cervicis trigger point (TP) refers pain to the orbit. The dashed arrow represents the pain shooting from the inside of the head to the back of the eye. (From Ref. 3.)

(16–21). While there do not appear to be serum β-endorphin abnormalities in fibromyalgia (22), naloxone will increase pain, increase stage I sleep, and decrease stage II, III, and IV sleep (23).

Abnormalities of serotonin binding to platelets in fibromyalgia are similar to those seen in CDH (24). Epidural opiates cause analgesia,

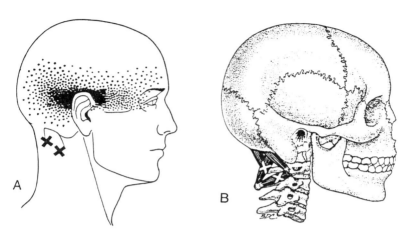

Figure 8 (A) Referred pain pattern (shaded area) of trigger points (×) in (B) the right suboccipital muscles. (From Ref. 3.)

suggesting that fibromyalgic pain may be peripheral in origin (25). In a study evaluating CDH, a continuum of severity and a progression of clinical findings were found in patients with tension-type headache, MPS, and fibromyalgia (26).

CLINICAL ASSOCIATIONS WITH CHRONIC DAILY HEADACHE

The exact role in CDH of emotional problems such as stress, anxiety, and depression is uncertain. Chronic headache has been identified as a symptom of failure to mourn (27). It is also the most common somatic component in patients who were victims of childhood sexual abuse (28). Episodic tension-type headache patients have higher levels of anxiety, depression, hostility, and suppressed anger (29).

Chronic headache patients seem to benefit simply by receiving treatment, regardless of whether their headaches improve. The patients experience a greater sense of personal control after treatment, and those with high levels of somatization expressed fewer somatic concerns in relationship to headache relief (30).

An entity described by Diamond as a "depression headache" has been characterized as a somatic manifestation of depression (31). Antidepressant medications are an effective way to treat this type of headache. Olesen (32) feels that almost any psychiatric disorder, except for psychosis, would predispose patients to tension-type headache. Anxiety may directly contribute to a psychophysiological reaction leading to tension-type headache (33), while somatization of anxiety or suppressed anger may be initiating factors (34,35).

The etiology of CDH may be neurochemical or myofascial, or both. Quite possibly, depression and CDH are due to central serotonergic dysfunction resulting from similar neurochemical changes.

Two other structural hypotheses have been evaluated: 1) cervical spondylosis, which is usually secondary to muscle contraction (32,36–38) and 2) temporomandibular joint (TMJ) dysfunction (39,40). Masticatory muscle tenderness is often seen in CDH patients (41–43). In terms of specific etiology, does intense muscle spasm of the masticatory and the occipital muscles and associated muscle regions cause secondary TMJ dysfunction? Many patients with CDH who are treated for TMJ dysfunction with tooth extractions, tooth-grinding, and various types of splints experience insignificant or transient reduction in their headache problem.

ASSOCIATED DISORDERS OF SLEEP

An important relationship exists among headache, sleep, and muscle pain syndromes. Central biogenic amines, particularly serotonin and norepinephrine, are important not only to central pain-modulation systems but also to sleep (44). Brain stem noradrenergic and serotonergic systems initiate and regulate sleep (24,45,46). At the same time, there is a high incidence of sleep disturbance in headache patients (47). Migraine is known to occur in association with REM sleep, and with excessive sleep in stages III, IV, and REM (48). Like patients with fibromyalgia, CDH patients have frequent awakenings and decreased stage IV sleep (49).

Sleep disturbances increase pain severity. CDH patients appear to have a high incidence of sleep abnormalities compared to normal, headache-free subjects. There is also an alpha non-REM pattern of stage IV sleep. Daily headache can be induced in normal patients with stage IV sleep deprivation, and is common in those suffering from rheumatoid arthritis, chronic pain syndromes including posttraumatic headache, and depression (25,50,51). Nonrestorative sleep, a hallmark of fibromyalgia, is also reported in patients with depression and posttraumatic pain syndromes (52,53).

Further study is needed to understand the interrelationships among sleep, headache, pain (including myofascial nociception), and the central neuropeptides and biogenic amines. With knowledge will come a more detailed account of pathogenesis and effective treatment of CDH patients.

SPECIFIC PATHOPHYSIOLOGY

Most CDH is of the tension-type. Muscle contraction, although traditionally heralded as the cause of tension-type headache, is probably an epiphenomenon reflecting changes in the central nervous system associated with the primary headache disorder (54–56).

The central nervous system maintains muscle tone. There is supraspinal control from the cortical, subcortical, and limbic systems. As evidenced by the spasticity developing after spinal-cord damage, the nature of these central mechanisms is largely inhibitory. Subthalamic Renshaw cells, via the inhibitory neurotransmitter gamma-aminobutyric acid (GABA), activate gamma-efferent neurons in the anterior horn cells of the spinal cord, which directly influence alphamotor neurons supplying muscle spindles. Pathological stimulation of these pathways may cause significant muscle spasm. If prolonged, the tonic muscle contraction eventually becomes associated with a sustained muscle contraction–pain cycle (31,36).

At the tissue level, it is muscle tension that may produce ischemic hypoxia via compression of small blood vessels. These conditions favor anaerobic metabolism, allowing the accumulation of pain-producing metabolites such as bradykinin, lactic acid, prostaglandins, and serotonin. These stimulate nociceptors and propagate painful muscle spasm (57–59).

A causal relationship between increased muscle tension and headache has been found (60,62), and pericranial muscle tenderness correlates directly with headache intensity (63). Differences in pressure pain thresholds are noted between chronic tension-type headache or CDH patients and normal volunteers. This finding suggests that alterations occur in central modulation of nociceptive impulses in determining muscle tension (64–66). Patients diagnosed with MPS or fibromyalgia have similar decreases in pressure pain threshold (67–69). Muscles typically involved in this process function in postural stabilization, withdrawal, and protection of the head (70).

CENTRAL NERVOUS SYSTEM PATHOPHYSIOLOGY

In the central nervous system, the endogenous opiate system (EOS) may act as a nociceptive rheostat, or "pain stat," that determines pain-modulation capacity. Factors modulating this system change an individual's pain tolerance.

Substance P, enkephalins, serotonin, various neurotransmitters, and β-endorphin may all be involved in a complex interrelationship that ultimately modulates pain. Patients with chronic neuropathic pain have low β-endorphin levels, with lower pain thresholds and lower tolerance to experimentally induced pain (71,72). Terenius (71) suggested that chronic neuropathic pain may develop into a chronic pain syndrome secondary to a deficiency in the EOS control mechanisms.

The rostral section of the analgesic system subserves the head, neck, and shoulders. It also has neuroanatomical connections with the affective areas of the brain, i.e., the limbic system. Headache and myofascial pain travel into the central nervous system through cervical roots 2 and 3 (70), passing to the trigeminal brain stem sensory complex, the major brain stem relay center for orofacial sensory information (73). Trigeminal afferents can cause release of vasoactive substances, including substance P, which induces pain and local inflammation (74).

Central modulation of pain appears to originate in the brain stem and involves at least two systems: the "descending" inhibitory analgesia system and the "ascending" pain-modulation system. The major neurotransmitters in both systems include biogenic amines, opioid peptides, and nonopioid peptides (75–77).

The "ascending" pain-modulation system, which originates in the midbrain and projects to the thalamus, may have more relevance to headache disorders (77). The serotonergic midbrain dorsal raphe nucleus projects to the medial thalamus and is associated with central pain modulation. Serotonergic projections to the forebrain involve sleep-cycle regulation, mood changes, pain perception, and hypothalamic regulation of hormone release (78).

The endogenous opiates modulate the neurovegetative triad of pain, depression, and autonomic disturbances found only in two conditions, chronic headache and morphine abstinence. Endogenous opioids are implicated as primary protagonists in idiopathic headache (79,80).

Headache is accompanied by changes in circulating endorphin and enkephalin levels (81,82). Reduced plasma concentrations of β-endorphin have been found in idiopathic headache patients, including chronic tension-type headache (82–85). Normal levels were found in one study (86).

Increased levels of β-endorphin are found at the end of a headache attack, possibly associated with the stress provoked by headache pain (87). Stress provocation is suggested by the fact that ACTH and β-endorphin are located in the same hypothalamic neurons.

An increase in plasma methionine enkephalin during headache may be related to increased serotonin levels. Both chemicals are co-stored, and they are natural antagonists.

Serotonergic uptake mechanisms in platelets are similar to those in the neurons (88). Serotonergic abnormalities in platelets reflect similar abnormalities in the central nervous system. Levels of methionine enkephalin in CDH patients are found to be decreased in platelets and increased in plasma, whereas in migraine exactly the opposite is observed (89). The existence of a diagnostic marker may therefore be hypothesized.

Substance P, an excitatory neuropeptide, is found at all levels of the neuroaxis. The levels of substance P are lower in chronic neuropathic and idiopathic headache/pain patients than in normal volunteers (90,91). After a stepwise multiple-regression statistical analysis, pain and headache were most related to levels of substance P, methionine enkephalin, and β-endorphin (92).

A primary relationship exists between the EOS and the biogenic amine systems. This is intrinsic to the pathophysiology and treatment of daily headache. A perturbation of serotonergic neurotransmission appears intrinsic to the generation of headache. Ordinary periodic headache may be the "noise" of serotonergic neurotransmission (77).

Low levels of serotonin have been found in the platelets and plasma of CDH patients, indicating an impairment of serotonergic metabolism (93,94). This suggests a central serotonergic disturbance in patients with chronic daily tension-type headache.

Platelet GABA levels in patients with chronic daily tension-type headache are significantly higher than those seen in migraine and normal controls. Increased GABA levels appear to counterbalance neuronal hyperexcitability and may be associated with emotional factors such as depression (95).

Low levels of plasma norepinephrine are found in both migraine and CDH patients in response to the cold pressor test, suggesting possible peripheral sympathetic hypofunction (96). Noradrenergic pathways may also participate in central opioid dysfunction (85). Opioid receptor mechanisms appear very susceptible to desensitization, or the development of tolerance.

In CDH or tension-type headache sufferers, opioid receptor hypersensitivity is marked, probably because of the chronically diminished secretion of neurotransmitters. This entity, which Sicuteri in 1988 named the "empty neuron syndrome" (97), may involve both autonomic and nociceptive afferent systems.

The EOS modulates monoaminergic neurons. A chronic EOS deficiency would provoke transmitter leakage, leading to neuronal exhaustion and "emptying," and compensatory effector-cell hypersensitivity.

The most important phenomena of the hypoendorphin system syndromes, including chronic headache, would appear to be the poor release of neurotransmitter and receptor hypersensitivity (79). Headache may therefore be a "pain disease" linked to the central dysmodulation of the nociceptive and antinociceptive systems, either latent or pathological in nature.

MECHANISMS OF CENTRAL DYSMODULATION

The EOS is impaired in CDH. It is uncertain whether the opioid dysfunction is based on a genetic deficiency or results from neuronal exhaustion secondary to continuous activation of the system (84,98), possibly by elements of chronic myofascial nociception. Many of the clinical phenomena of chronic daily tension-type headache may be explained by centrally related phenomena, or by chronic central stimulation from the periphery via myofascial mechanisms such as trigger points found in MPS. These factors may be reinforced or complemented by other central dysfunctions, for example, those found in associated sleep disorder that follow neurochemically.

Figure 9 (99) summarizes the pathophysiological mechanisms of chronic daily or tension-type headache.

Continuous peripheral stimulation from myofascial nociceptive input can effectively trigger a change in the central pain "rheostat" associated

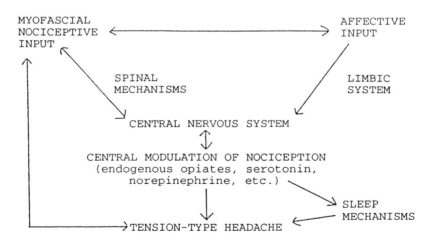

Figure 9 Pathophysiology of chronic daily or chronic tension-type headache. (From Ref. 99.)

with nociceptive input. The longer the peripheral stimulation persists, the greater the probability that the central modulating mechanisms would assume a primary rather than a secondary or reactive role in pain perception, shifting pain perception from the peripheral "muscular regions" to the central nervous system.

Such a shift may make innocuous stimuli aggravating to the pain-modulating systems. Already "dysmodulated" internal feedback mechanisms may overreact until central neurochemical mechanisms dominate via such mechanisms as neurotransmitter exhaustion, abnormal biogenic amine metabolism, and receptor hypersensitivity.

It is equally important to realize that the affective aspects of pain, including depression, fear, anxiety, and stress, can directly influence myofascial nociception. After 3 and 4 months (sooner in some patients), changes in the central nervous system's central modulation of nociception can occur. After this transition has taken place, the primary pain generator for CDH is found in the central nervous system rather than in the periphery.

The relationship between CDH, MPS, and fibromyalgia is obviously complex. There are many clinical similarities regarding the description of headache and physical findings. There are similar neurochemical abnormalities among these entities, especially relating to the serotonergic system. Significant sleep disorders have been noted in CDH sufferers and patients with fibromyalgia.

CDH or chronic tension-type headache may therefore be a disorder of perception rather than muscle, while infrequent or episodic tension-type headache is probably secondary to myofascial mechanisms.

TREATMENT

Treatment of CDH is best accomplished via an interdisciplinary rehabilitation approach.

Whatever the cause, drug detoxification is a necessary first step. Patients who take chronic daily analgesics of the simple variety (aspirin or acetaminophen), narcotics, or barbiturates must be detoxified (100). Frequent treatment failures occur with patients who continue taking chronic daily analgesics.

Chronic daily analgesic medications may prevent the appropriate functioning of the EOS. Consider the dilemma of patients with a normal thyroid who are prescribed thyroxine to increase their metabolism with the goal of losing weight. The normal thyroid gland responds to a negative feedback loop brought into play by the constant input of the exogenous thyroid medication and stops producing thyroxine naturally. Analogously, the EOS will shut down in the presence of chronic daily exogenous analgesics.

Many patients suffer vascular-rebound headaches induced by the daily or near-daily intake of vasoconstrictor medication, such as ergot derivatives and Midrin (isometheptene). During the drug detoxification period, these types of medications must be stopped. Vascular-type headache is also found to occur during or after use or abrupt withdrawal of cocaine or marijuana (101).

Clinically, an effective way to detoxify CDH patients of medication is with the repetitive intravenous DHE-45 protocol described by Raskin (78). This usually involves a 3- to 4-day period of hospitalization, during which patients receive intravenous metoclopramide and DHE-45. This is also an excellent time to start prophylactic medication.

After drug detoxification, CDH patients are best treated in an outpatient interdisciplinary headache rehabilitation program. Such programs use neuropharmacological therapy, physical therapy (102), psychotherapy, and stress management (including biofeedback-enhanced neuromuscular re-education and muscle relaxation). Hypnotherapy may also be a useful treatment modality (103). Optimal physical therapy regimes alone will not resolve myofascial difficulties if the affective, sleep, and central nervous system neurochemical dysmodulation is not concurrently and appropriately treated.

An interdisciplinary approach to treating the CDH patient enables fine-tuning of the diagnosis. Patients with CDH may have more than one etiology for their headaches. As the myofascial aspects of the problem are rectified and the patient's depression clears, an episodic migraine may be uncovered, requiring appropriate treatment. Trying to treat patients with only one aspect of this approach at a time does not address the needs of the whole patient and often results in unnecessary expense and repeated treatment failures.

Adjunctive modalities to correct central neurochemical abnormalities occurring in CDH include cortical electrical stimulation (CES). A specific 15,000 Hz bipolar CES unit produces significant increases in serotonin, β-endorphin, GABA, and ACTH in plasma and cerebrospinal fluid. Concomitant diminution of plasma cortisone and L-tryptophan occurs (104,105). Bipolar CES also potentiates neuropharmacological treatment such as the serotonergic tricyclic antidepressants (106–110).

At the Headache and Neurological Rehabilitation Institute, more than 88% of patients with CDH, including those associated with trauma and combination headache diagnoses, become headache-free. Understanding the pathophysiology and utilizing an interdisciplinary treatment model that addresses all aspects of the CDH/tension-type headache are important. The 12% of patients who do not experience total or significant diminution in their headache problem have been found to have significant premorbid psychopathology or significant secondary gain issues.

In summary, CDH patients may have many diagnoses, each of which needs to be teased out and appropriately treated. These may include chronic tension-type headache (posttraumatic in origin or otherwise), migrainous cephalalgia, analgesic-rebound headache, vascular-rebound headache, and muscle pain syndromes. The typical CDH patient has a dysmodulation of central antinociceptive systems.

The associated problems of analgesic-rebound headache and vascular-rebound headache must be dealt with before the use of prophylactic medications and an interdisciplinary headache rehabilitative approach to treatment.

Failure to treat the CDH patient with a whole-person approach (Figure 9) is responsible for multiple patient treatment failures and the expenditure of enormous amounts of money that do not generate a long-lasting response, i.e., headache remediation.

REFERENCES

1. Simons D. Muscular pain syndromes. In: Friction JR, Awad E, eds. Advances in Pain Research and Therapy. Vol. 17. New York: Raven Press, 1990:1–41.
2. Travell J, Rinzler SH. The myofascial genesis of pain. Postgrad Med 1952; 11:425–434.
3. Travell JG, Simons DG. Myofascial Pain and Dysfunction: The Trigger Point Manual. Baltimore: Williams and Wilkins, 1983.
4. Simons DG. Myofascial pain syndromes: Where are we? Where are we going? Arch Phys Med Rehabil 1988; 69:207–212.
5. Fishbain DA, Goldberg M, Meagher BR, Steele R, Rosomoff H. Male and female chronic pain patients categorized by DSM-III diagnostic criteria. Pain 1986; 26:181–197.
6. Fricton JR, Kroening R, Haley D, Siegart R. Myofascial pain syndrome of the head and neck: a review of clinical characteristics of 164 patients. Oral Surg 1985; 60:615–623.
7. Fricton JR. Myofascial pain syndrome. In: Fricton JR, Awad E, eds. Advances in Pain Research and Therapy. Vol. 17. New York: Raven Press, 1990:107–127.
8. Bengtsson A, Hendriksson KG, Larsson J. Muscle biopsy in primary fibromyalgia. Scand J Rheumatol 1986; 15:1–6.
9. Bengtsson A, Hendriksson KG, Larsson J. Reduced high-energy phosphate levels in painful muscle in patients with primary fibromyalgia. Arthritis Rheum 1986; 29:817–821.

10. Lund N, Bengtsson A, Thorborg P. Muscle tissue oxygen pressure in primary fibromyalgia. Scand J Rheumatol 1986; 15:165–173.
11. Simon DG. Myofascial pain syndromes of head, neck and low back. In: Dubner R, Gebhart GF, Bond MR, eds. Proceedings of the Vth World Congress on Pain. New York: Elsevier Science Publishing, 1988:186–200.
12. Gowers WR. Lumbago: Its lesson and analogues. Br Med J 1904; 1:117–121.
13. Wolfe F, Smyth HA, Yunus MB, et al. The American College of Rheumatology 1990 criteria for the classification of fibromyalgia: a report of the multicenter committee. Arthritis Rheum 1990; 33:160–172.
14. Campbell SM, Clark S, Tindall EA, Forehand ME, Bennett RM. Clinical characteristics of fibrositis. 1. A "blinded" controlled study of symptoms and tender points. Arthritis Rheum 1983; 26:817–824.
15. Bennett RM. Myofascial pain syndromes and the fibromyalgia syndrome: a comparative analysis. In: Fricton JR, Awad E, eds. Advances in Pain Research and Therapy. Vol. 17. New York: Raven Press, 1990:43–65.
16. Martucci N, Manna V, Porto C, Agnoli A. Migraine and the noradrenergic control of vasomotricity: a study with alpha-2 stimulant and alpha-2 blocker drugs. Headache 1985; 25:95–100.
17. Zidar J, Backman E, Bengtsson A, Henriksson KG. Quantitative EMG and muscle tension and painful muscles in fibromyalgia. Pain 1990; 40:249–254.
18. Semble EL, Wise CM. The fibrositis syndrome. Part 1. Pain Management 1988; Sept./Oct., pp. 202–214.
19. Rosenhall U, Johansson G, Orndahl G. Eye motility dysfunction in patients with chronic muscular pain and dysesthesia. Scand J Rehab Med 1987; 19:139–145.
20. Hendriksson KG, Bengtsson A. Muscle pain with special reference to primary fibromyalgia (PF). In: Dubner R, Gebhart GF, Bond MR, eds. Proceedings of the Vth World Congress on Pain. New York: Elsevier Science Publishing, 1988:232–237.
21. Vaeroy H, Zhi-Gai Q, Morkrid L, et al. Altered sympathetic nervous system response in patients with fibromyalgia (fibrositis syndrome). J Rheumatol 1989; 16:1460–1465.
22. Yunis MB, Denko CW, Masi AT. Serum β-endorphin in primary fibromyalgia syndrome: A controlled study. J Rheumatol 1986; 13:1833–1836.
23. Moldofsky H. The contribution of sleep-wake physiology to fibromyalgia. In: Fricton JR, Awad E, eds. Advances in Pain Research and Therapy. Vol. 17. New York: Raven Press, 1990:227–240.
24. Goldenberg DL. Fibromyalgia and chronic fatigue syndrome: are they the same? J Musculoskel Med 1990; 7:19–28.
25. Goldenberg DL. Diagnostic and therapeutic challenges of fibromyalgia. Hosp Prac 1989; 9:39–52.
26. Jay GW. Myofascial mechanisms in the etiology of chronic daily headache: Two syndromes, one entity? Presented at the 32nd Annual Meeting of the American Association of the Study of Headache, Los Angeles, June 1990.
27. Haiser RS, Primavera JP. Chronic headache as a symptom of failure to mourn. Headache 1992; 32:261.

28. Dawson GA, Wirtho, Turkewitz LJ, et al. Histories of childhood sexual abuse in adults with chronic headache. Headache 1992; 32:261.

29. Hatch JP, Schoenfeld LS, Boutrous NN, et al. Anger and hostility in tension-type headache. Headache 1991; 31:302–304.

30. Blanchard EB, Steffek BD, Jaccard J, Nicholson NL. Psychological changes accompanying non-pharmacological treatment of chronic headache: The effects of outcome. Headache 1991; 31:249–253.

31. Diamond S, Dalessio DJ. The Practicing Physician's Approach to Headache. 3rd ed. Baltimore: Williams and Wilkins, 1980:99–108.

32. Olesen J. Clinical characterization of tension headache. In: Olesen J, Edvinsson L, eds. Basic Mechanisms of Headache. New York: Elsevier Science Publishing, 1988:9–14.

33. Martin MJ, Rome HP, Swenson WM. Muscle contraction headache: a psychiatric review. Res Clin Stud Headache 1967; 1:184–204.

34. Gannon LR, Haynes SN, Cuevas J, Chaves R. Psychophysiological correlates of induced headaches. J Behav Med 1987; 10:411–423.

35. Ziegler DK, Hassanein R, Hassanein K. Headache syndromes suggested by factor analysis of symptom variables in a headache prone population. J Chron Dis 1972; 25:353–363.

36. Speed WG. Muscle contraction headaches. In: Saper JR, ed. Headache Disorders. Boston: John Wright, 1983:115–124.

37. Robinson CA. Cervical spondylosis and muscle contraction headaches. In: Dalessio DJ, ed. Wolff's Headache and Other Head Pain. 4th ed. New York: Oxford University Press, 1980:362–380.

38. Iansek R, Heywood J, Karnaghan J, Balla JI. Cervical spondylosis and headaches. Clin Exp Neurol 1987; 23e:175–178.

39. Forsell H. Mandibular dysfunction and headache. Proc Finnish Dent Soc 1985; 81(suppl II):591.

40. Mikail M, Rosen H. History and etiology of myofascial pain-dysfunction syndrome. J Prosthet Dent 1980; 44:438–444.

41. Langemark M, Olesen J, Poulsen DP, Bech P. Clinical characterization of patients with chronic tension headache. Headache 1988; 28:590–596.

42. Magnusson T, Carlsson GE. Comparison between two groups of patients in respect to headache and mandibular dysfunction. Swed Dent J 1978; 2:85–92.

43. Magnusson T, Carlsson GE. Recurrent headaches in relation to temporomandibular joint pain-dysfunction. Acta Odontol Scand 1978; 36:333–338.

44. Gans M. Migraine as a form of neurasthenia. J Nerv Ment Dis 1951; 113:315–331.

45. Lance JW, Lambert GA, Goadsby PJ, Duckworth B. Brainstem influences on the cephalic circulation: Experimental data from cat and monkey of relevance to the mechanisms of migraine. Headache 1983; 23:258–265.

46. Yaksh TL. Direct evidence that spinal serotonin and noradrenalin terminals mediate the spinal antinociceptive effects of morphine in the periaquaductal gray. Brain Res 1979; 160:180–185.

47. Mathew NT, Glaze D, Frost J. Sleep apnea and other sleep abnormalities in primary headache disorders. In: Rose C, ed. Migraine. Proceedings of the 5th International Migraine Symposium, London, 1984. Basel: Karger, 1985:40–49.
48. Sahota PK, Dexter JD. Sleep and headache syndromes: a clinical review. Headache 1990; 30:80–84.
49. Drake ME, Pakalnis A, Andrews JM, Bogner JE. Nocturnal sleep recording with cassette EEG in chronic headaches. Headache 1990; 30:600–603.
50. Moldofsky H, Scariabrick P, England R, et al. Musculoskeletal symptoms and non-REM sleep disturbances in patients with fibrositis syndrome and healthy subjects. Psychosom Med 1975; 37:341–351.
51. Moldofsky H, Scariabrick P. Induction of neurasthenic musculoskeletal pain syndrome by selective sleep stage deprivation. Psychosom Med 1976; 38:35–44.
52. Wittig R, Zorick FJ, Blumer D, et al. Disturbed sleep in patients complaining of chronic pain. J Nerv Ment Dis 1982; 170:429–431.
53. Saskin P, Moldovsky H, Lue FA. Sleep and post-traumatic rheumatic pain modulation disorder (fibrositis syndrome). Psychosom Med 1986; 48:319–323.
54. Riley TL. Muscle-contraction headache. Neurolog Clin 1983; 1:489–500.
55. Philips C. Tension headache: theoretical problems. Behav Res Ther 1978; 16:249–261.
56. Philips C, Hunter MS. A psychophysiological investigation of tension headache. Headache 1982; 22:173–179.
57. Dorpat TL, Holmes TH. Mechanisms of skeletal muscle pain and fatigue. Arch Neurol Psychiatry 1955; 74:628–640.
58. Perl S, Markle P, Katz LN. Factors involved in the production of skeletal muscle pain. Arch Intern Med 1934; 53:814–824.
59. Hong S, Kniffki K, Schmidt R. Pain Abstracts. Vol. 1. Second World Congress on Pain, Montreal, 1978:58.
60. Robard S. Pain associated with muscle contraction. Headache 1970; 10:105–115.
61. Marin PR, Mathews AM. Tension headaches: psychophysiological investigation and treatment. J Psychosom Res 1978; 22:389–399.
62. Sakuta M. Significance of flexed posture and neck instability as a cause of chronic muscle contraction headache. Rinsho Shinkeigato—Clinical Neurology 1990; 30(3):254–261.
63. Langemark M, Olesen J. Pericranial tenderness in tension headache. A blind, controlled study. Cephalalgia 1987; 7(4):249–255.
64. Borgeat F, Hade B, Elie R, Larouche LM. Effects of voluntary muscle tension increases in tension headache. Headache 1984; 24:199–202.
65. Langemark M, Jensen K, Jensen TS, Olesen J. Pressure pain thresholds and thermal nociceptive thresholds in chronic tension-type headache. Pain 1989; 38(2):203–210.
66. Drummond PD. Scalp tenderness and sensitivity to pain in migraine and tension headache. Headache 1987; 27:45–50.
67. Yang JC, Richlin D, Brand L, Wagner J, Clark WC. Thermal sensory decision theory indices and pain threshold in chronic pain patients and healthy volunteers. Psychosom Med 1985; 47:461–468.

68. Malow RM, Grimm L, Olsen RE. Differences in pain perception between myofascial pain dysfunction and normal subjects: a signal detection analysis. J Psychosom Res 1980; 24:303–309.
69. Quimby LG, Block SR, Gratwick G. Fibromyalgia: generalized pain intolerance and manifold symptom reporting. J Rheumatol 1988; 15:1264–1270.
70. Langemark M, Jensen K. Myofascial mechanisms of pain. In: Olesen J, Edvinsson L, eds. Basic Mechanisms of Headache. New York: Elsevier Science Publishing, 1988:321–341.
71. Terenius L. Endorphins and modulation of pain. In: Critchley M, et al. eds. Advances in Neurology. Vol. 33. New York: Raven Press, 1982:59–64.
72. von Knorring L, Almay BGL, Johnasson F, Terenius L. Pain perception and endorphin levels in cerebrospinal fluid. Pain 1978; 5:359–365.
73. Sessle BJ. Central nervous system mechanisms of muscular pain. In: Fricton JR, Awad E, eds. Advances in Pain Research and Therapy. Vol. 17. New York: Raven Press, 1990:87–105.
74. Moskowitz MA. The neurobiology of vascular head pain. Ann Neurol 1984; 16:157–168.
75. Basbaum AI, Fields HL. Endogenous pain control systems: brainstem spinal pathways and endorphin circuitry. Annu Rev Neurosci 1984; 7:309–338.
76. Andersen E, Dafny N. An ascending serotonergic pain modulation pathway from the dorsal raphe nucleus to the parafascicularis nucleus of the thalamus. Brain Res 1983; 269:57–67.
77. Raskin NH. On the origin of head pain. Headache 1988; 28:254–257.
78. Raskin NH. Headache. 2nd ed. New York: Churchill Livingstone, 1988.
79. Sicuteri F. Natural opioids in migraine. In: Critchley M, et al., eds. Advances in Neurology. Vol. 33. New York: Raven Press, 1982:65–74.
80. Sicuteri F, Spillantini MG, Fanciullacci M. "Enkephalinase" in migraine and opiate addiction. In: Rose C, ed. Migraine. Proceedings of the 5th International Migraine Symposium, London, 1984. Basel: Karger, 1985:86–94.
81. Ansalmi B, Baldi E, Casacci F, Salmon S. Endogenous opioids in cerebrospinal fluid and blood in idiopathic headache sufferers. Headache 1980; 20:294–299.
82. Mosnaim AD, Diamond S, Wolfe ME, et al. Endogenous opioid-like peptides in headache. An overview. Headache 1989; 29:368–372.
83. Genazzani AR, Nappi G, Facchinetti F, et al. Progressive impairment of CSF B-EP levels in migraine sufferers. Pain 1984; 18:127–133.
84. Facchinetti F, Genazzani AR. Opioids in cerebrospinal fluid and blood of headache sufferers. In: Olesen J, Edvinsson L, eds. Basic Mechanisms of Headache. New York: Elsevier Science Publishing, 1988:261–269.
85. Nappi G, Gacchinetti F, Legnante G, et al. Impairment of the central and peripheral opioid system in headache. Proceedings of the 4th International Symposium of the Migraine Trust, London, 1982.
86. Gawel M, Fettes I, Kuzniak S, Edmeads J. Endorphin levels in headache syndromes. In: Rose C, ed. Migraine. Proceedings of the 5th International Symposium, London, 1984. Basel: Karger 1985:66–71.

87. Bella DD, Carenzi A, Casacci F, et al. Endorphins in the pathogenesis of headache. In: Critchley M, et al., eds. Advances in Neurology. Vol. 33. New York: Raven Press, 1982:75–79.

88. Pletsher A, Affolter H, Cesuro AM, Ezne P, Muller K. Blood platelets as a model for neurons: Similarities of the 5-hydroxytryptamine system. In: Schlessberger HG, Kocheau W, Linzen B, Steinbast H, eds. Berlin: Walter de Gruyter, 1984:231–239.

89. Ferrari MD, Odink J, Frolich M, et al. Methionine-enkephalin in migraine and tension headache. Differences between classic migraine, common migraine and tension headache, and changes during attacks. Headache 1990; 30:160–164.

90. Pernow B. Substance P. Pharmacol Rev 1983; 35:85–141.

91. Almay BGL, Johansson F, von Knorring L, et al. Substance P in CSF of patients with chronic pain syndromes. Pain 1988; 33:3–9.

92. von Knorring L. Affect and pain: Neurochemical mediators and therapeutic approaches. In: Dubner R, Gebhart GF, Bond MR, eds. Proceedings of the Vth World Congress on Pain. New York: Elsevier Science Publishing, 1988:276–285.

93. Giacovazzo M, Bernoni RM, Di Sabato F, Martelletti P. Impairment of 5HT binding to lymphocytes and monocytes from tension-type headache patients. Headache 1990; 30:581–583.

94. Shimomura T, Takahashi K. Alteration of platelet serotonin in patients with chronic tension-type headache during cold pressor test. 1990; Headache 30:581–583.

95. Kowa H, Shimomura T, Takahashi K. Platelet gama-amino butyric acid levels in migraine and tension type headache. Headache 1992; 32:229–232.

96. Takeshima T, Takao Y, Urakami K, et al. Muscle contraction headache and migraine. Platelet activation and plasma norepinephrine during the cold pressor test. Cephalalgia 1989; 9:7–13.

97. Sicuteri F, Nicolodi M, Fusco BM. Abnormal sensitivity to neurotransmitter agonists, antagonists and neurotransmitter releasers. In: Olesen J, Edvinsson L, eds. Basic Mechanisms of Headache. New York: Elsevier Science Publishing, 1988:275–286.

98. Martignoni E, Facchinetti F, Rossi F, et al. Neuroendocrine evidence of deranged noradrenergic activity in chronic migraine. Psychoneuroendocrinology 1989; 14:37–363.

99. Jay GW. The pathophysiology of tension-type headache. In: Tollison CD, Kunkel RS, eds. Headache: Diagnosis and Interdisciplinary Treatment. Baltimore: Williams and Wilkins, 1993.

100. Mathew NT, Kurman R, Perez F. Drug induced refractory headache—clinical features and management. Headache 1990; 30:634–638.

101. DeMarinis M, Janiri L, Agnoli A. Headache in the use and withdrawal of opiates and other associated substances of abuse. Headache 1991; 31:159–163.

102. Jay GW, Brunson J, Branson SJ. The effectiveness of physical therapy in the treatment of chronic daily headaches. Headache 1989; 29:156–162.

103. Melis PML, Rooimans W, Spierings ELH, Hoogduin CAC. Treatment of chronic tension-type headache with hypnotherapy: A single-blind time controlled study. Headache 1991; 31:686–689.
104. Liss S, Liss B, Clossen W, Bennett A. Baseline analysis for normals with 20-minute transeramial treatment using Liss Cranial Stimulators. Private communication.
105. Clossen W. Confidential Research Report, May 1991. Private communication.
106. Clossen W. Changes in blood biochemical levels following treatment with TENS devices of differing frequency composition. Private communication, 1986.
107. Shealy CN, Cady RK, Wilkie RG, et al. Depression: A diagnostic neurochemical profile and therapy with cranial electrical stimulation (CES). J Neuro Orth Med Surg 1989; 10(4):319–321.
108. Cady RK, Shealy CN, Culver-Veeloff D, Houston R. Cerebrospinal fluid and plasma neurochemicals: response to cranial electrical stimulation. In press.
109. Hughes JR, GS, Lichstein PT, Whitlock D, Harker C. Response of plasma beta-endorphins to transcutaneous electrical nerve stimulation in healthy subjects. Phys Ther 1984; 64:1062–1066.
110. Shealy CN. Effects of transcranial neurostimulation upon mood and serotonin production: a preliminary report. Il Dolore 1979; 1:13–16.

.

14

Spinally Mediated Headache

C. Norman Shealy

Shealy Institute for Comprehensive Health Care
Springfield, Missouri

Cranial and cervical pain represent the most frequently observed clinical examples of referred pain. In 1952, Travell and Rinzler (1) delineated five cervical muscles with pain reference into the head. And, in our clinical experience, myofascial triggers of headache have been observed from every muscle in the neck and thorax, at least as low as the tenth dorsal vertebra. Furthermore, there is extensive clinical evidence of cranially referred pain from every cervical facet, intervertebral disc, and interspinous ligament. The anatomical and physiological basis for this cranial-cervical interrelationship may help us understand the often confusing differential diagnosis and assist in therapy.

ANATOMICAL CONNECTIONS

The trigeminal nerve and its interconnections offer the final common pathway for cortical awareness of cranial pain. All structures of the cranial vault, the face, and the mouth are innervated by the trigeminal nerve, which also has at least motor connections with the oculomotor, facial, and hypoglossal nerves, as well as sensory connections via the nervus intermedius. The occipital to parietal scalp is innervated by the second and third cervical nerves, which interdigitate with the frontal branches of the trigeminal nerve.

Even more critically, the spinal nucleus of the trigeminal nerve extends from the entry of the fifth nerve in the pons inferiorly, at least as caudally as the second cervical vertebra, with rich interconnections throughout the central spinal cord.

Although there are no direct anatomical connections of the trigeminal more caudally, extensive interneuronal pathways allow for potential cross-talk at least from C8 up to C1. For instance, consider the innervation of the head, neck, and arm muscles, all of which receive innervation from trigeminal and/or cervical nerves. The mechanics of muscular tension alone allow for tremendous activation of the spinal cord by any chronic muscle tension in any of these groups (Table 1).

Perhaps the most significant cord input to the trigeminal system is that from the sympathetic nervous system, which for all cranial and neck

Table 1   Muscles Feeding into the Trigeminal/Cervical Network

Tensor palati, masseter,		Spinatus	C5 and 6
temporalis, pterygoids,		Teres minor	C5
mylohyoid, digastric	Cr. V	Supraspinatus	C5 and 6
Geniohyoid and thyrohyoid	C1 and 2	Infraspinatus	C5 and 6
Rectus capitis anterior		Brachioradialis	C5 and 6
and lateralis	C1 and 2	Supinator of forearm	C5 and 6
Intrahyoids	C1-3	Teres major	C5 and 6
Longus capitis	C1-3	Serratus anterior	C5, 6, and 7
Longus colli	C2-7	Pectoralis major	C5, 6, and 7
Semispinalis cervicis		Biceps	C5, 6, and 7
and capitis	C2-7	Pronator teres	C6 and 7
Levator scapulae	C3 and 4	Spinalis cervicis	C6, 7, and 8
Sternocleidomastoid	C2 and 5,	Splenius cervicis	C6, 7, and 8
	Cr. XI	Splenius capitis	C6, 7, and 8
Trapezius	C3 and 4,	Various forearm	
	Cr. XI	muscles	C6, 7, and 8
Levator scapulae	C3 and 4	Coracobrachialis	C7
Rhomboids	C5	Triceps	C7 and 8
Subclavius	C5	Pectoralis minor	C7 and 8, T1
Deltoid	C5 and 6	Pronator quadratus	C8, T1
Subscapularis	C5 and 6	Various finger muscles	C7 and 7, T1

structures originates from T2! The fibers of the sympathetic nervous system supplying the entire head, both internally and superficially, arise from the intermediolateral cell column of the spinal cord, primarily from T1 and T2. These fibers exit the spinal cord in the motor nerves at T1 and T2, and relay through myelinated fibers to the paravertebral ganglia. All blood vessels, both veins and arteries, glands, and smooth muscle receive innervation from the sympathetic nervous system. At the level of the first thoracic ganglion is the stellate ganglion extending upward from there; the second largest, the inferior (cervical and cranial!) ganglion, lies behind the origin of the vertebral artery. The connection then goes upward to a small middle cervical ganglion in front of the inferior thyroid artery opposite the sixth cervical vertebra. The connection further extends upward to the superior cervical ganglion, which lies on the longus capitis muscle just below the base of the skull and behind the carotid sheath. Extensions from the cervical sympathetic chain continue along the carotid arteries, ultimately supplying the basilar, cerebellar, and all cerebral arteries as well as veins and even the cavernous sinus.

There are strong cross-connections through the internal carotid plexus to the trigeminal ganglion and through the deep petrosal nerve to join the greater petrosal branch of the facial nerve as well as the caroticotympanic nerve to the tympanic plexus of the middle ear. Direct fibers from the sympathetic chain pass from the superior cervical ganglion to the hypoglossal nerve to the inferior ganglion of the vagus nerve and to the glossopharyngeal nerves. The other cranial nerves receive their sympathetic fibers indirectly through the internal carotid plexus. Thus, the interconnections of the sympathetic chain originating from T1 and T2 ultimately serve the entire skin, external, and internal vascular system of the head, cranium, and brain (see Table 2 and Figures 1–4).

Obviously, the anatomy of the sympathetic chain makes it particularly susceptible to injury. The deep anterior paravertebral muscular structure, for instance, makes the sympathetic chain particularly sensitive to any kind of strain, sprain, contusion, muscle spasm, or any other form of injury. When the sympathetic supply is significantly damaged, there will be a temporary period of vasodilation followed by restoration of normal tone, but ultimately the smooth muscles (of the blood vessels) become hypersensitive to sympathicomimetic substances such as epinephrine and norepinephrine, leading to a state of facilitation—that is, they are activated by stimuli at a lower threshold than in undamaged, nonfacilitated nerves.

Although this discussion is directed at spinally mediated headache, sympathetic denervation hypersensitivity (or "facilitation") has also been reported in migraine and cluster headache (2).

Table 2 Sympathetic Control of Cranial, Cervical, and Brachial Structures

T1, T2 →	Stellate ganglion → Other cervical ganglia
	All blood vessels of brain, face, skull, neck and arms
	Cavernous sinus and all veins of same areas
	Trigeminal ganglion
	Middle ear
	Hypoglossal, vagus, and glossopharyngeal nerves
	All other cranial nerves through carotid plexus
	Skin
	Eyes
	Mouth
	Nose
	All glandular activity of these areas

SPINAL FACILITATION OF CRANIAL PAIN

Irvin Korr (3) has extensively studied the effects of spinal dysfunction on the sympathetic nervous system. The essence of his work is that strain of any kind on muscles, tendons, or joints *at any level* of the spine leads to both focal segmental hyperadrenergia and generalized hyperadrenergia or sympathicotonia under certain circumstances. Such hyperactivity of the sympathetic nervous system leads to facilitation, a state in which, as described above, the facilitated region has a lowered threshold for new stimuli, even to the point of spontaneous firing in extreme situations. In Korr's work, mostly done in the thoracic and lumbar spine, even such relatively minor strains as a 3/8" heel lift led to facilitated segments.

Both a polysynaptic and an oligosynaptic pontobulbar interneuron pathway normally suppress tension in temporalis, masseter, and trapezius muscles. These pathways are activated by stimulation of the mental nerve. In patients with all types of chronic headache this normal reflex is significantly reduced, suggesting a chronic facilitation leading to increased trapezius tension from activation of the mental nerve, perhaps by teeth-clenching. Here is an example of facilitation of the cranial nerve V system, almost certainly including its sympathetic control, centrally mediated through the T2 spinal cord and affecting the bulbar nucleus of cranial nerve XI (4).

Even in migraine headache there is significant muscle tension in cervical paraspinal muscles and trapezius muscles as is found in "tension headaches" (5). The trapezius muscles are major sites of trigger points.

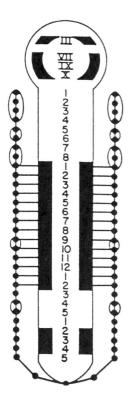

Figure 1 Paravertebral chains of sympathetic ganglia and the preganglionic fibers (leaving the spinal cord via the ventral roots and white rami between T1 and L2). Encircled pairs or groups of ganglia indicate fusions that are commonly found. (From Ref. 3.)

It appears unlikely that the altered state of tension in temporalis, masseter, and trapezius muscles is independent of accompanying hyperadrenergia seen in other areas of the body. Indeed, Korr has stated that "every neuron potentially influences, and is influenced by, almost every other neuron in the body" (6). And he noted that *all* incoming sensory information, from touch to sound to sight, influences the motor nerves. Although it is local musculoskeletal dysfunction that initiates muscle spasm and pain, it is the sustained overactivity (hyperadrenergia or sympathicotonia) that leads to the vicious cycle of ischemia, more muscle spasm, and pain (6, p. 80).

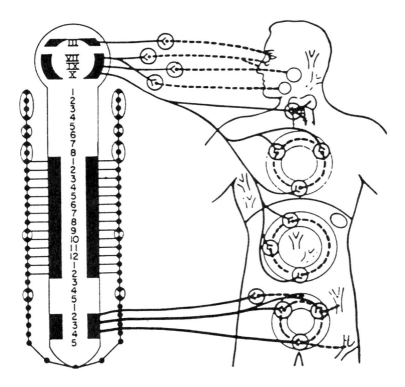

Figure 2 Visceral structures are represented within the human figure in four main groupings: those of the head and neck, thoracic, abdominal, and pelvic and genital. Only the parasympathetic innervation is shown. In this and the remaining figures solid lines represent preganglionic axons and interrupted lines represent postganglionic axons. (From Ref. 3.)

Korr noted that simple trauma led to new areas of excess sympathetic activity in dermatomes related to the site of the trauma. Of some interest is that areas Korr found responded most intensely to trauma were those of the upper posterior thorax and parascapular areas (6, p. 60)—those most prominent in myofascial pain, fibromyalgia, and cervicogenic headache. Once such segmental areas of hyperadrenergia originate, they are highly constant and reproducible in that patient for many months (6, p. 77).

Korr especially emphasized that *clinical* symptomatology was related to the tissues innervated by the facilitated sympathetic neurons, with vascular changes being the common factor (6, p. 77). Facilitation may be so

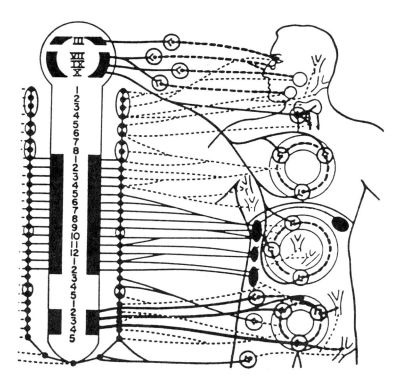

Figure 3 Sympathetic innervation of visceral structures has been added, showing dual innervation of most viscera. Note that sympathetic postganglionic innervation in head and neck and the thorax originate in paravertebral ganglia. Those of the abdomen and some pelvic organs arise in outlying ganglia (for example, celiac and mesenteric). Note also that the adrenal medulla (shown under left side of diaphragm) is innervated by sympathetic preganglionic neurons, and that blood vessels receive their innervation predominately from the sympathetic division. (From Ref. 3.)

intense that the threshold is zero, leading to spontaneous discharge without direct stimulation of receptors. He particularly noted this strong influence of the superior cervical ganglion on cortical and subcortical activity (6, p. 78).

Removal of the superior cervical ganglion leads to behavioral changes, and even in EEG voltage and in the electrical activity of the hypothalamus. Stimulation of the cervical ganglion reduces the amplitude of spontaneous electrical activity in the ipsilateral hemisphere as well as its response to

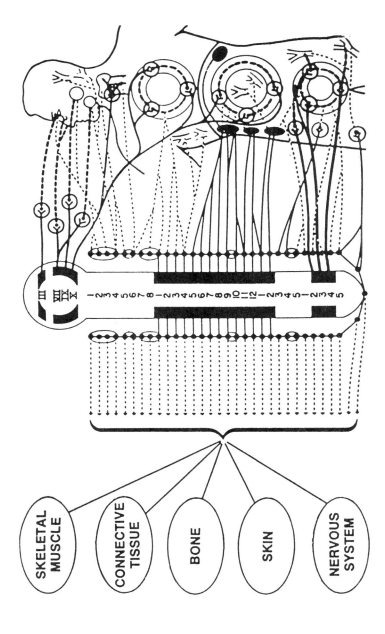

Figure 4 Schema of the peripheral autonomic nervous system, completed. (From Ref. 3.)

photostimulation (6, pp. 78–79). Furthermore, neurochemical and neurohormonal control is directly influenced by the superior cervical ganglion, which controls the pineal (6, p. 80). As Korr explains (6, p. 80): "The pineal controls the release of releasing factors for luteinizing hormone, follicle stimulating hormone, and prolactin inhibiting and releasing factors. This pineal control of releasing factors is mediated by the elaboration and secretion of melatonin and other polypeptide hormones which exert antigonadal action." Ultimately, all cerebral activity from blood flow to EEG and cognition is under sympathetic influence. Both spreading cortical depression and the "perturbation" of cells important in migraine and other types of headache are reflections of facilitated sympathetic neurons.

OSTEOPATHIC LESIONS

Many of the facilitated changes observed by Korr were initiated by "osteopathic lesions" of particular interest in headache patients, especially those who have suffered mechanical stress through whiplash injuries (7):

> The "osteopathic lesion," as identified by palpatory and other clinical criteria, is the local or regionally discrete somatic component of a reflexly organized and sustained response to stresses, irritations, and excessive demands placed upon specific tissues or organs by the environment and by the total activities, responses, and adaptations of the individual.

Shealy and colleagues (8) have emphasized that painful input from any limb elicits a generalized spinal state of hyperreactivity very similar to the state of spinal facilitation described by Korr. He has also noted that patients with cranial pain often present with nondermatomal "numbness" of a diffuse nature involving the entire arm. Furthermore, Shealy pointed out that painful stimulation of the trigeminal area elicits electrical hyperactivity at least as caudally as C5 (9):

1. Pain projections are diffuse throughout the spinal cord, except for dorsal columns, but particularly in the most primitive portion of the cord, the propriospinal tracts.
2. Once pain information enters the spinal cord, it projects caudally, ipsilaterally, contralaterally, and cephalad.
3. It appears that the entire propriospinal system is almost optimally activated by intense pain from one limb. Thus, when one limb evokes significant pain, relatively little additional stimulation from any other part of the body may maximally "fill" the pain pathways.

In addition, our clinical observations have included many patients with muscle trigger points at least as low as T10 eliciting headache. And patients with triggers at C2-3 commonly have referral to the ipsilateral eye.

The facilitated spinal segment reports of Korr are reinforced by clinical observations that pain tolerance is markedly lowered, often throughout the entire body, when there is a persistent pain syndrome. Thus, it is easy to propose that a cervical spinal cord, facilitated at least from C1 to C5 by a trigeminal stimulus, would be further facilitated or hyperresponsive if recruitment occurs from muscle tension anywhere in the cervical area.

Ultimately, even muscle tension from the sacrococcygeal area would facilitate the entire spinal cord and brain stem, including the trigeminal system. Thus, feedback, interrelating loops, and multiple subliminal stimuli may activate the entire primitive neural pathways subserving pain. Patients with whiplash injuries very commonly present with both headache and various degrees of generalized myofascial pain, as well as anxiety and depression.

MYOFASCIAL PAIN AND TRIGGER POINTS

Since voluntary or skeletal muscle represents 40% or more of body weight, it is not surprising that many pain syndromes involve either direct muscle pain or pain referred to muscles, fascia, tendons, or ligaments. The differential diagnosis of the remarkable variety of problems capable of causing soft-tissue pain is largely one of medical judgment. In general, the history and the physical exam will assist physicians in ruling out most of the wide variety of muscular and myofascial disorders. Ultimately, after one has ruled out all the other multiple factors that can cause pain, we are left with a group of patients who have what are variably called fibromyalgia, fibrositis, fibromyositis, or myofascial pain syndrome. In myofascial pain syndrome not only is there a myofascial trigger point with one or more specific trigger spots in a given muscle, but there is generally referred pain, numbness, or dysesthesia. Kellgren in 1938 (10) established the referral pain concept from tender points in muscle. Two German studies (11) reported on a total of 101 biopsies done on such trigger points, "characteristic nonspecific changes by light microscopy." Eventually, Awad from the United States and Fassbender and Wegner of Germany reported ultramicroscopic findings and biopsies of muscles having myofascial trigger points (12). These studies demonstrate that there are physical as well as symptomatic changes in myofascial pain syndrome.

The myofascial trigger point represents a specific, excessively irritable focus of pain within a given skeletal muscle that is identified by palpation.

There is always a general muscle spasm or contracture of that muscle with a focal, specifically triggered, more tender area. Pressure on such a trigger point evokes both referred pain and often autonomic dysfunction such as pilomotor contractures around hair follicles, making it look as if the individual has had a local chill. Trigger points are either active, which means they cause spontaneous pain, or latent, which means that they are tender and may have some restrictions of movement or weakness. Such latent trigger points often lead to recurrent acute episodes of pain after minor use, stretching, or chilling. It is important to emphasize that normal muscles are not tender, do not have spasm or contractures when the individual is in a position of rest, and have no tender or firm nodules within them, no local twitch response to minor pressure, and no referred pain or dysesthesias. On the other hand, a significant portion of individuals—54% of women and 45% of men—have latent trigger points, with about 25% of these individuals experiencing referred pain in response to pressure on their trigger points. Travell and Simons (13) believe that the likelihood of developing active trigger points increases with age from childhood into "the most active mental years." After age 60 or so, individuals are more likely to exhibit latent trigger points with stiffness and restrictive motion.

The spontaneous pain occurring in trigger points is not so much that of the trigger point itself, but a dull aching that is somewhat vague in distribution or referred to distant areas. Such pain may occur either at rest or with active contractions of the affected muscle. Incidentally, the finding of a specific trigger point that fulfills all the criteria for myofascial pain syndrome does not mean that it may not come from a referral origin from a more distant area. The subscapular pain of gallbladder disease is most typical of this particular problem.

The associated autonomic findings with trigger points include localized sweating, vasoconstriction, pilomotor activity, and at times tearing, nasal stuffiness, and stimulation. Trigger points and myofascial pain often lead to reflex changes, not only in the sympathetic nervous system but also in the sensory system with numbness that is generally of a nondermatomal nature, weakness such as "buckling knee syndrome," and problems with coordination such as difficulty with handwriting.

Certain symptoms are extremely characteristic of active trigger points, including those listed below:

1. Either passive or active stretching of the affected muscle increases pain.
2. The range of motion of such a muscle is restricted.
3. Significant pain occurs when the affected muscle is brought into active contracture.

4. The muscle is weakened even with maximal contraction.
5. Pressure on the myofascial trigger point not only induces deep tenderness but evokes dysesthesia to a specific referral area.
6. Autonomic dysfunctions occur in the area of referred pain or dysesthesia. These mostly include either increased sweating or pilomotor activation.
7. Small, firm, palpable nodules are felt in the vicinity of the trigger point.
8. Around the trigger point there is a palpable band that is sharply delineated and exquisitely tender.
9. Minor to moderate finger pressure over an active trigger point elicits an exaggerated response, with the patient moving or exclaiming loudly.
10. A rolling or snapping palpation of such a trigger point evokes a local twitch response.
11. Continuing even moderate pressure on a trigger point causes increasing pain, both locally and in the reference area.
12. There is often marked dermographia or panniculosis in the areas over active trigger points.

Laboratory diagnosis of myofascial pain is essentially negative, with one exception. A study (14) has shown normal serum enzyme concentrations but a shift in the distribution of LDH isoenzyme with the LD1 and LD2 fraction decreased and the LD3, LD4, and LD5 fractions increased. It is unfortunate that that particular work has apparently not been repeated by anyone else. Interestingly, it is also known that patients with myofascial pain tend to have decreases in serotonin, but such deficiencies are also present at times in patients with anxiety, insomnia, pseudodepression, hypothyroidism, etc. (I. J. Russell, unpublished observations). Further evaluation of neurochemicals remains to be done in patients with myofascial pain syndrome.

The major differential diagnosis of myofascial pain includes various myopathies, arthritides, and focal inflammation of musculoskeletal structures, such as tendonitis and bursitis. In the genetic myopathies there is very rarely any significant pain; if it is present, the pain is usually minor.

SLEEP DISTURBANCES

It would be inappropriate to conclude this discussion without mentioning the influence of interrupted stage IV—deep restorative—sleep in patients with myofascial pain syndrome. No one knows which comes first, the sleep disturbance or the myofascial pain, although it is known that individuals who have their sleep interrupted on a routine basis may develop myofascial pain. But many of the patients with myofascial pain have had it come on after surgery or after minor or moderate trauma that left them with acute pain, which might have interfered with sleep at the beginning of their disorder (15).

SEROTONIN

This loss of stage IV sleep, almost routine in patients with all types of chronic pain, opens the consideration of significant influences on the serotonin system, that neurochemical most often associated with headache. And, of course, depression is also often associated with serotonin dysfunction.

Sicuteri (16) has suggested that migraine represents a central, biochemical dysnociception. I suggest that the evidence in myofascial pain, so common in cervical/cranial pain states, both commonly associated with depression, suggests that all chronic pain may be associated with a generalized biochemical dysnociception (17), particularly involving catecholamines, serotonin, melatonin, and β-endorphin. In turn, these chemicals are intimately related to oxytocin, prolactin, testosterone, and estrogen.

Although serotonin receptors have been evaluated primarily in the central nervous system, the production of serotonin in the intestines and its widespread physiological effects on the vascular system suggest the possibility that serotonin receptors may be present throughout the body, most particularly in those muscles that become hypertonic in myofascial pain.

Jaeger (18) examined four myofascial trigger points and cervical spine dysfunction in 11 patients who had cervicogenic headaches. All patients had at least three myofascial trigger points on the symptomatic side, and in eight patients trigger-point palpation reproduced their headache. Overall, there were 70 myofascial trigger points in these individuals on the symptomatic side, and only 22 myofascial trigger points on the non-symptomatic side. Ten of the 11 patients had specific segmental dysfunction of the occiput or the atlas on the axis, and the other patient had some other form of cervical spinal dysfunction.

In a study of 27 patients with fibromyalgia and 29 healthy controls, Qiao and his coauthors (19) measured blood flow at the palmar skin during baseline, acoustic stimulation, and cold pressor tests. They also measured electrical conductance. They found increased cholinergic and decreased adrenergic activity in the hands of patients with fibromyalgia. Unfortunately, they did not measure sympathetic activity in the parascapular or cranial areas.

WHIPLASH/CERVICAL FLEXION–EXTENSION INJURY

Although many consider post-whiplash headache to be psychogenic, there are strong indications that psychogenic factors are much less important than direct physiological ones. Seventy-eight consecutive patients seen an average of 7.2 days after common whiplash accidents were evaluated for psychosocial stress, negative affectivity, personality traits, somatic complaints, and cognitive impairment. Six months later, 57 patients were fully recovered and 21 had persistent symptoms; the initial pain injury intensity, injury-related cognitive impairment, and age were significant factors predicting illness behavior. The authors conclude that psychosocial factors do not predict illness behavior in posttraumatic patients (20).

Although neurological examination, brain imaging, and clinical electrophysiological studies show no abnormality in individuals who have had minor whiplash injury, those patients who developed multiple somatic, affective, and cognitive dysfunction syndrome were found on neuropsychological evaluations to have impairment of cognitive flexibility, nonverbal reasoning, new learning/memory, psychomotor ability, and attention (21). And in 20 patients which chronic disabling symptoms after cervical spine injury, the velocity, accuracy, and pattern of eye movements were disturbed, whereas oculomotor function in 19 asymptomatic patients did not differ from that in members of a control group. This suggests a possible brain stem lesion in patients with chronic symptoms after a whiplash (22).

In addition to the less-defined headaches usually seen after whiplash injuries, Weiss and his coauthors (23) reported 35 adults with no prior history of headaches who developed recurrent common or classic migraine following minor head or neck injuries. None of these patients had significant injury to the head itself. Headaches began immediately or within a few days after the injury. In the long run, 78% of the patients did improve despite ongoing litigation. They were treated with propranolol or amitriptyline.

Of considerable interest in connecting cervicogenic headache to myofascial pain is the work of Oleson (24). He believes that in tension headache nociception is primarily myofascial, with vascular input being a secondary component, and that "supraspinal" facilitation may play a large and occasionally dominant role. He emphasizes that even between migraine attacks migraine patients have pericranial muscles that are much more tender than those in headache-free individuals. He feels that these myogenic nociceptive mechanisms are augmented by central sensitization or facilitation. He summarizes animal research data that certainly emphasize that supraspinal mechanisms have a net facilitating influence on nociceptive nucleus cordalis and other neurons. The entering extracranial blood vessels are surrounded by a dense network of nerve fibers that contain norepinephrine and neuropeptide Y, if they arose from the sympathetic nerves originating in the superior cervical ganglion. Nerve fibers containing acetylcholine, vasoactive intestinal polypeptide, and peptide histidine isoleucine were parasympathetic, originating from the sphenopalatine ganglion; those containing substance P, neurokinin A, and calcitonin gene–related peptide originated from the trigeminal ganglion. It is interesting that Oleson does not raise the possibility of facilitation of the peripheral sympathetic nervous system through direct traumatic stimulation of paravertebral muscles or of the tissue.

Postural Influences

As noted earlier, postural dynamics significantly influence the sympathetic hyperreactivity described by Korr. In this regard, I should like to report briefly our observations of postural abnormalities noted in 27 consecutive headache patients. There were 21 women aged 18 to 69 and six men aged 31 to 57. Eleven of the 27 patients had migraine. Sixteen had significant myofascial pain, often post-whiplash or post–cervical fusion. Twenty-six patients had various postural abnormalities, with only one migrainous patient exhibiting normal posture.

A wide variety of postural abnormalities were noted, a total of 131 postural deviations being found in 26 patients. The most common were:

Compressed or flattened thoracic spine	20
Head forward	17
Increased lordosis	11
Kyphosis	9
Scoliosis	9
Rotated pelvis	9

In addition, there were various and sundry rotations of head, shoulder, legs, and feet.

Thus, postural abnormalities undoubtedly contribute some degree of facilitation in almost all patients with headache.

Cervical Disarticulation Headache: Anatomical Changes After Whiplash

The initial response to a flexion–extension deceleration injury to the cervical spine virtually always includes muscle spasm and straightening of the cervical spine. Such changes are often maintained even many months later. Furthermore, more extensive ligamentous injury can often be demonstrated only with flexion and extension films or with cineradiography. Lastly, facet arthrosis may be rapidly accelerated after a whiplash injury.

Usually the extent of ligamentous pain is not extensive enough to require surgical fixation, and a ruptured disc is exceedingly rare after such injuries. The most commonly facilitated facets, C2-3, evoke referred pain into either the ipsilateral orbit and/or the occiput. On the other hand, a facilitated facet joint at least as low as C7-T1 may provide a major contribution to headache. The pain associated with facet arthrosis may be continuous or intermittent, steady or throbbing, and may mimic both vascular and tension headache. Headache may develop de novo after a cervical injury, or preexisting headaches may be exaggerated in frequency and/or intensity.

Indeed, even without a history of whiplash, careful consideration of cervical pathology should be part of the evaluation of every patient with headache, since at least some postural components are virtually universal.

HISTORY AND PHYSICAL EXAMINATION

In addition to the usual headache history, a number of questions specifically related to the spine should be asked, including:

1. Is your headache affected by positional changes or by bending, extending, or turning your neck?
2. Do you have any significant neck or shoulder-area pain:
   a. During headache?
   b. Even when you do not have headache?
3. Have you ever had a whiplash or motor vehicle accident? If so, did your headache change after that accident?
4. Do you recall a significant fall in which you injured your head or neck? (Remember that a head injury severe enough to require skull x-rays equally requires cervical spine x-rays.)
5. Have you or your family noted any changes in posture during headache or since the beginning of your headaches?
6. Do you have any pain, weakness, tingling, or numbness in arm(s) or hand(s) during a headache or otherwise?
7. Do you sleep soundly at least 6 or 7 hours, at least 6 nights a week?
8. Have you noticed any unusually tender spots in your neck or shoulder areas?

A nutritional history should also be done to check for adequacy of protein, vitamin, and mineral intake, as well as excessive caffeine consumption. Many chronic pain patients eat remarkably inadequate diets that deprive them of the essential amino acids for manufacture of neurotransmitters. Eighty-six percent of our depressed patients are deficient in taurine, with many of them having multiple essential amino acid deficiencies; at least 5% have six or more deficiencies. Well over 95% have at least one deficient essential amino acid.

Beyond a detailed neurological exam, headache patients should have an equally careful postural and musculoskeletal exam. Note posture both standing and sitting. Standing behind the patient, have the patient bend forward at the waist, without bending knees. Look for asymmetry of the lumbar or thoracic spine. While the patient is flexed at the waist, palpate by running two fingers along either side of the spine from sacrum to neck. Check extension, lateral bending, and rotation of the lumbar spine. Pay particular attention to muscle spasm.

Then have the patient lie flat, supine. Examine the length of the legs. If there is asymmetry, have the patient bend knees, lift buttocks, and then lie flat again while you recheck leg length. Flex each leg at the hip to 90 degrees and abduct the thigh; evaluate asymmetry of such hip motion, limitation of which may indicate either hip disease or sacral rotation. With the patient still supine, check for passive motion of the neck in all directions and palpate the neck from the occiput down to the scapulae, noting muscle spasm and/or tenderness and asymmetry of facets. Palpate especially the facets at C2-3 and check pressure there or over any tender area as a trigger of pain, tingling, or numbness into the head or arm. Palpate the sternocleidomastoids and pectoralis major for tender/trigger areas.

Check the temporomandibular joints (TMJs) in particular, as TMJ disorder is associated with neck pain and cervical muscle spasm as commonly as it is with headache or jaw pain.

One of the simplest tests for significant generalized hyperadrenergic activity is to check the pulse at rest and standing. If the pulse goes up 20 points or more, or above 100, or is consistently above 90, in the absence of thyroid or cardiac pathology, it may be worthwhile to check catecholamines after the patient has stood for 5 minutes. We have found a number of chronic pain patients to have remarkably excessive norepinephrine production (25).

Have the patient cup both hands and lie prone with the forehead resting in the palm of one hand. Observe for asymmetry of the spine at all levels. Palpate the inferior margins of the sacrum and the sacral base. Check for rotation, normal movement, and tenderness. Check the entire buttocks for trigger and/or tender areas or spasm. Palpate along the entire spine, one thumb on either side, checking at each spinal level for rotation, muscle spasm, asymmetry, pain, or trigger areas. Palpate the entire paraspinal musculature, especially the parascapular and suprascapular areas, up to the base of the skull.

Note any palpable temperature variations along the spine. The dorsum of the fingers can detect temperature changes of approximately 1°F and sympathetic changes associated with focal somatic dysfunction. Pain will usually produce sclerotomally associated skin coolness. I keep half a dozen small thermometers in my exam room to evaluate any suspicious areas. Thermometers taped to the skin with the outer side open to air should show normal skin temperature of 84 to 92°F. Differences of up to 10° can sometimes be noted in areas of sympathetic hyperactivity.

X-Ray and Laboratory Evaluations

If cervical pain or tenderness is found or if there are trigger areas in the neck, x-rays of the cervical spine should be obtained, including odontoid, PA, lat, obliques, and flexion and extension laterals. In patients who suffered an earlier whiplash or other neck injury, it is wise to repeat at least the three lateral films 12 to 18 months after the accident to look for subluxation that may have been missed earlier because of acute muscle spasm and to check for accelerated degenerative changes.

Unless there are neurological findings, cervical CT, MRI, and myelogram films are highly unlikely to add useful information. If there are subtle signs of atrophy or sensory change, an EMG and sensory nerve conduction tests may be indicated.

In patients with depression, a magnesium load test and amino acid profile are indicated (17). We have found that virtually all depressed patients are highly deficient in magnesium and in one or more essential amino acids, especially taurine. In chronic pain patients who are smokers, 80% will be deficient in vitamin B_6, which is essential for nerve function. Although there have been reports of CPK isoenzyme dysfunction in myofascial pain, we have not found it in a few patients tested.

Clinical judgment will determine whether it is wise to check for collagen disorders, muscle disease, or general inflammatory responses.

FORMULATING A DIAGNOSIS

Whatever the central or cranial findings, the contribution of postural and spinal pathology should be taken into account. Such abnormalities may be primary or aggravating features of the headache. Kyphosis and scoliosis or definitive facet tenderness/triggers are virtually always at least contributing factors, and treatment of these pathological conditions may lower the total mechanical stress enough to be therapeutic for the headache. Similarly, sleep disorders and nutritional deficiencies require attention and should be noted in one's overall diagnosis.

TREATMENT

Obviously nutritional deficiencies require specific treatment. When patients have magnesium and taurine deficiency, a series of 10 intravenous shots of magnesium chloride (2 g with 100 mg vitamin B_6 each), along with 3 g taurine orally at bedtime may provide highly therapeutic. For maintenance, magnesium taurate 250 mg plus taurine 1 to 2 g may be considered, if the initial 2 weeks of therapy is helpful.

When widespread essential amino acid deficiency is found, we recommend daily consumption of 1 quart of beef, chicken, or turkey broth, obtained by cooking 8 ounces of chopped meat in a slow-cooker, flavored with onion, soy sauce, carrot, and celery. This is very flavorful and can often be tolerable to patient who is otherwise quite negligent about diet.

When disturbed sleep is a problem, we prefer trazadone at bedtime, starting with 75–150 mg and building rapidly to 300 mg if needed. Although amitriptyline is widely used, we have found that many chronic pain patients become more agitated with tricyclics. If trazadone fails to induce sleep within 1 week, and magnesium and taurine replacement have not achieved this goal, amoxapine, up to 400 mg h.s., may be used temporarily.

Patients should generally not use extra-firm mattresses. For most patients with cervical contribution to their headache, a foam mattress or egg crate is best. They should not sleep prone, as this aggravates neck problems. Pillows should generally be very soft down. We have found that the special cervical pillows are rarely helpful.

Both manual and vibratory mechanical massage to neck and upper back may be most helpful for patients with neck and shoulder problems. Heating pads and hot tub soaks may also be useful at bedtime. Physical therapy is most helpful in passive and active soft-tissue work and in postural corrections.

Transcutaneous electrical nerve stimulation (TENS) should be tried with electrodes at the nape of the neck and at the C7-T1 area, with trials of vertical, horizontal, and crossed oblique current inputs and with both fast and 1 Hz frequencies, the latter at a borderline-painful intensity. Patients should be encouraged to use the stimulator for up to 16 hours per day and to try a variety of pulse variations before deciding that TENS is ineffective. And they should routinely receive relaxation/guided-imagery tapes to use at least twice a day while testing the effectiveness of TENS.

Cranial electrical stimulation (CES) using the Liss CES™ should be considered in all headache patients, including those with a spinal contribution. Current should be tried mid-forehead to inion, transtemporally, forehead to nape of neck bilaterally, forehead to nape of neck to the first dorsal interosseous area bilaterally. Application should be for 40 to 60 minutes in the morning, and then 10 to 20 minutes up to four times a day p.r.n. headache.

When TENS and CES fail, acupuncture should be tried. Needles at the occipital notch, the facets at C2-3 and at C7-T1, and the first dorsal interosseous, with electrical current 1 to 5 Hz for 20 to 30 minutes applied across the first interosseous needles, offer the best chance for successful acupuncture management of headache. Treatments may be done one to three times a week. If significant reduction in headache is not achieved within four treatments, acupuncture is unlikely to be helpful.

Trigger spots anywhere in the cervical or paraspinal areas should be anesthetized with local injections of 3–5 cm^3 0.25% bupivacaine. If headache relief is achieved, these may be repeated up to daily and up to 15 times, with expectation of progressively longer pain relief. Occasionally patients require intermittent trigger blocks for a prolonged period of time, but many find this approach quite therapeutic.

When any of the cervical facets is excessively tender or triggers appropriate headache pain, facet nerve blocks should be considered, under image-intensifier monitoring, by someone familiar with the anatomical concerns; this is especially important when injecting at C2, where it is possible to tap into the spinal canal. I have performed hundreds of cervical facet nerve blocks without a significant problem. The blocks should be done during a headache, as early as possible after its onset. If total headache relief is achieved on two occasions, then facet denervation has an 80% chance of long-term pain relief (26).

When the above approaches fail, or when patients are total invalids because of their spinally related headaches, they should enter an intensive, comprehensive pain-treatment program that offers all-day therapy including counseling, biofeedback training, intensive hands-on physical therapy, relaxation training, and therapeutic exercise, coupled with any or all of the other therapeutic modalities enumerated above.

In summary, spinal dysfunction is common in all headache patients, either as a primary cause or as one of the stressors contributing to the frequency and severity of various types of headache. Careful attention to comprehensive history and spinal mechanics, as well as to nutritional, sleep, and mood disturbances, will offer a variety of therapeutic options: nutritional, chemical, mechanical, and behavioral. Virtually all spinally mediated headache patients can be improved 50 to 100% using these approaches.

REFERENCES

1. Travell J, Rinzler SH. The myofascial genesis of pain. Postgrad Med 1952; 11:425–434.
2. Yamamoto M, Meyer JS. Hemicranial disorder of vasomotor adrenoceptors in migraine and cluster headache. Headache 1980; 20:321–335.
3. Nakashima K, Takahashi K. Exteroceptive suppression of the masseter, temporalis and trapezius muscles produced by mental nerve stimulation in patients with chronic headaches. Cephalalgia 1991; 11:23–28.
4. Cram JR. Clinical EMG: Muscle scanning and diagnostic manual for surface recordings. Seattle: Clinical Resources, 1986.
5. Korr IM. The neural basis of the osteopathic lesion. In: Peterson B, ed. The Collected Papers of Irvin M. Korr. Newark, Ohio: American Academy of Osteopathy, 1979.
6. Korr IM. Clinical significance of the facilitated state. In: Peterson B, ed. The Collected Papers of Irvin M. Korr. Newark, Ohio: American Academy of Osteopathy, 1979.
7. Shealy CN. A physiological basis for "hysterical" analgesia. Headache 1971; 11:102–106.
8. Kellgren J. A preliminary account of referred pains arising from muscle. Br Med J 1938; 1:325–327.
9. Glogowski G, Wallraff J. Ein beitrag zur klinik und histologie der muskelharten (myogelosen). Z Orthop 1951; 80:237–268.
10. Awad EA. Interstitial myofibrositis: Hypothesis of the mechanism. Arch Phys Med 1973; 54:440–453.
11. Travell J, Simons D. Myofascial pain and dysfunction: The trigger point manual. Baltimore: Williams and Wilkins, 1983.
12. Ibrahim GA, Awad EA, Kottke FJ. Interstitial myofibrositis: Serum and muscle enzymes and lactate dehydrogenase-isoenzymes. Arch Phys Med Rehabil 1974; 55:23–28.
13. Moldofsky J. Nonrestorative sleep and symptoms after a febrile illness in patients with fibrositis and chronic fatigue syndromes. J Rheum 1989; 16: 150–153.
14. Sicuteri F. Migraine, a central biochemical dysnociception. Headache 1976; 16:145–159.
15. Shealy CN, et al. The neurochemistry of depression. Amer J Pain Management 1992; 2:13–16.

16. Jaeger B. Are "cervicogenic" headaches due to myofascial pain in cervical spine dysfunction? Cephalalgia 1989; 9:157–164.
17. Qiao ZG, Vaeriy H, Markrid L. Electrodermal and microcirculatory activity in patients with fibromyalgia during baseline, acoustic stimulation and cold pressor tests. J Rheum 1991; 18:1383–1389.
18. Radanov BP, di Stefano G, Schnidrig A, Ballinari P. Role of psychosocial stress in recovery from common whiplash. Lancet 1991; 338:712–715.
19. Yarnell PR, Rossie GV. Minor whiplash head injury with major debilitation. Brain Injury 1988; 2:255–258.
20. Hildingsson C, Wenngren BI, Bring G, Toolanen G. Oculomotor problems after cervical spine injury. Acta Orthopaed Scand 1989; 60:513–516.
21. Weiss HD, Stern BJ, Goldberg J. Post-traumatic migraine: Chronic migraine precipitated by minor head or neck trauma. Headache 1991; 31:451–456.
22. Oleson J. Clinical and pathophysiological observations in migraine and tension-type headache explained by integration of vascular, supraspinal, and myo-fascial inputs. Pain 1991; 46:125–132.
23. Shealy CN. Neurochemical profiles in chronic pain and chronic stress. Complementary Medicine 1985; 1:22–23.
24. Cady RK, Cox R, Shealy CN, Wilkie RG. Facet rhizotomy/denervation: A fifteen year experience. J Neurolog Orthopaedic Med Surg 1988; 9(2):107–108.

15

Temporomandibular Disorders for the Primary-Care Physician

Michael L. Gelb

New York University College of Dentistry
New York, New York

INTRODUCTION

Temporomandibular disorder (TMD) is the current term used to describe a group of musculoskeletal disorders involving the masticatory musculature, the temporomandibular joints, and associated structures. Previously, used terms were temporomandibular joint pain dysfunction syndrome (TMJPDS), myofascial pain dysfunction syndrome (MPDS), craniomandibular disorders, and Costen's syndrome.

Costen (1), an otolaryngologist, first identified 11 posteriorly edentulous patients with headache and ear pain in 1934. He hypothesized that the pain was caused by mechanical impingement of the mandible against the auriculotemporal nerve due to the loss of posterior teeth. The condition, which he named Costen's syndrome, was later disproved anatomically and physiologically, yet restoration of the posterior edentulous space is still used by dentists to treat headache and facial pain. For the 50 years following Costen's hypothesis, dentists overtreated this condition by bite-raising and tooth-grinding.

In 1955, Lazlo Schwartz (2) replaced Costen's mechanical concept with a functional one. He coined the term temporomandibular joint pain dysfunction syndrome to explain how masticatory muscle pain accompanied by dysfunction could account for headache, facial pain, and limited opening of the mouth.

DIAGNOSIS

Laskin and Greene (3) identified the myofascial pain dysfunction syndrome in 1969 in a series of studies. They listed the four cardinal signs of MPDS as:

1. Masticatory muscle tenderness
2. Unilateral jaw pain
3. TM joint sounds with jaw movement
4. Limited opening with the following exclusion criteria:
   a. Absence of clinical or radiographic changes in the TMJs
   b. Lack of tenderness in the TMJ when this area is palpated through the external auditory meatus

Laskin and Greene found that myofascial pain dysfunction (MPD) was not a result of mouth and jaw misalignments. They advocated conservative treatment for MPD, which they believed has a psychophysiological etiology. This theory is still largely taught for acute myofascial pain problems; however, the relationship between MPDS and pathology of the temporomandibular joint remained unclear.

Farrar and McCarty (4), in 1978, defined internal derangement of the TMJ as an anterior displacement of the disc associated with a posterior superior displacement of the condyle in the closed-jaw position. They used arthrography and magnetic resonance imaging (MRI) to elucidate the anatomy and physiology of the disc in internal derangements of the TMJ. Dentists and oral surgeons focused largely on disc and condylar position throughout the 1980s.

Dworkin and leResche (5) recently advocated a biopsychosocial model for understanding the TMD patient. TMD as a chronic pain condition involves psychological, behavioral, and social factors in addition to physical pathology. Stress, depression, disability, and dysfunctional illness behaviors are seen in many patient profiles; many university TMD centers therefore have a psychologist as part of the management team.

In 1981 Reik and Hale (6), neurologists, reported that fourteen of 100 consecutive patients who presented to a headache clinic had TMD. None had previously been diagnosed. Four years later, Reik (7) published another study in which 20 of 100 headache patients had been referred or previously diagnosed with TMD; upon review, four of the 100 were determined to actually have the disorder. Many headache authorities now feel that TMD and related symptoms are "overstated and exaggerated as causes of pain and overtreated in general" (8).

Seventy-five percent of non-patient populations have at least one sign of TMJ dysfunction, such as limited movement, joint noise, and tenderness on palpation, according to cross-sectional epidemiological studies. About 33% have at least one symptom such as face pain or joint pain (9,10). Symptoms are most common in those between 15 and 45 years of age, and primarily in females, by a ratio of 5:1 (22).

Although a large percentage of the population has signs of TMD (50% have some form of joint noise), only 5–7% are estimated to be in need of treatment (11–15).

TMDs are commonly misdiagnosed and often improperly treated. Fricton (16) states:

> The variability of pain complaints in severity, location, description, and progression, coupled with frequent maladaptive behavioral and psychosocial sequelae, may lead a clinician to readily diagnose the problem as purely psychogenic. Occasional associated symptoms such as nausea, lacrimation, paresthesia, and sensitive teeth suggest such diverse diagnoses as cluster headache, migraine headaches, neuralgias, sinusitis, temporal arthritis, or hyperemic tooth pulps.

A diagnostic classification system for TMD must be clearly defined and simple to use, with inclusion and exclusion criteria to differentiate it from other diagnoses. Chief complaint and physical diagnosis should be differentiated from contributing factors, which can be predisposing, initiating, or perpetuating (Figure 1).

Numerous factors contribute to the functional equilibrium of the stomatognathic system. The masticatory system is very adaptable through physiological responses such as bony remodeling. However, after overt macrotrauma or more insidious microtrauma, pain or dysfunction may occur. Adverse loading of the masticatory system is usually a result of cofactors and may result in loss of structural integrity or altered function.

Maladaptive bite relationships, which may be genetic, developmental, or iatrogenic, have been downplayed as an etiological factor in recent

BEHAVIORAL Maladaptive behaviors	SOCIAL Adverse social situations	BIOLOGIC Biologic weakness
1. Diet 2. Sleep 3. Exercise level 4. Habits 5. Posture 6. Pacing problems 7. Bruxism and clenching 8. Smoking 9. Alcohol and drugs 10. Poor work habits 11. Poor hygiene 12. Lack of home activities 13. Medication use	1. Social support system 2. Work situation 3. Home situation 4. Social modeling 5. Avoidance of tasks 6. Operant learning 7. Cultural changes 8. Litigation 9. Disability compensation 10. Social dependencies 11. Secondary gain 12. Finances	1. Genetic predisposition 2. Developmental anomaly 3. Skeletal discrepancies 4. Hormonal changes 5. Past trauma 6. Other illnesses 7. Allergic hypersensitivity 8. Past surgery

ENVIRONMENTAL Imbalanced environmental stimuli	EMOTIONAL Prolonged negative emotions	COGNITIVE Counterproductive thought processes
1. Lighting 2. Air pollutants 3. Work chemicals 4. Weather 5. Water pollutants 6. Allergens 7. Food additives 8. Vibrations 9. Sound	1. Despair 2. Depression 3. Anxiety 4. Anger 5. Sadness 6. Guilt 7. Frustration 8. Nervousness 9. Worry 10. Irritability 11. Hatred 12. Apathy 13. Fear	1. Confusion 2. Negative self statements 3. Low intelligence 4. Low problem solving skills 5. Lack of proper understanding 6. Unrealistic expectations 7. Doubt about future 8. Negative body image 9. Low insight 10. Low motivation 11. Locus of control 12. Coping style

Figure 1 Diagnostic classification system for temporomandibular disorders. Contributing factors include all initiating, predisposing, or perpetuating factors for the development and maintenance of chronic illness. (From Ref. 10.)

years. The dental profession has historically viewed tooth-to-tooth discrepancies and malocclusion as a primary etiological factor for TMD, but these associations have not held up in the literature. Certain jaw displacements such as large midline discrepancies, severe overbite, skeletal open bite, slides greater than 2 millimeters, and lack of firm posterior support may be etiological cofactors.

Pathophysiological factors include degenerative, endocrine, infectious, metabolic, neoplastic, neurological, rheumatological, and vascular disorders. These factors can also predispose facial pain.

Chronic TMD patients have been found to have psychosocial characteristics similar to those of patients with headache and low back pain (16), although no "TMD personality" has been found.

The International Headache Society (IHS) has developed a classification for headache disorders, cranial neuralgias, and facial pain (Figure 2). The American Academy of Orofacial Pain has further subdivided the diagnostic categories for disorders of the TMJ and masticatory muscles (Figure 3).

Episodic and chronic tension-type headaches may be confused with myofascial pain of masticatory and cervical muscles. The IHS lists oromandibular dysfunction as a causative factor in tension-type headache. Oromandibular dysfunction is defined by the IHS as having three or more of the following diagnostic criteria:

1. TMJ noise on jaw movement
2. Limited or jerky jaw movements
3. Pain on jaw function
4. Locking of jaw on opening
5. Clenching of teeth
6. Gnashing of teeth (bruxism)
7. Other oral parafunction (biting or pressing of the tongue, lip, or cheek)

Oromandibular dysfunction can be a predisposing and perpetuating factor of tension-type headache. The trigeminal nerve innervates the TMJ as well as the muscles of mastication, teeth, and mandible, and may lead to headache.

The IHS narrowly defines TMJ disease with the following diagnostic criteria:

1. At least two of the following:
   a. Jaw pain precipitated by movement and/or clenching
   b. Decreased range of movement
   c. Noise during joint movement
   d. Tenderness of the joint capsule

Classification for Headache Disorders,
Cranial Neuralgias, and Facial Pain ᵗ

1. Migraine headache
2. Tension-type headache
3. Cluster headache and chronic
   paroxysmal hemicrania
4. Miscellaneous headaches, unassociated with structural lesion
5. Headache associated with head
   trauma
6. Headache associated with vascular
   disorders
7. Headache associated with non-
   vascular intracranial disorders
8. Headache associated with
   substances or their withdrawal
9. Headache associated with non-
   cephalic infection
10. Headache associated with
    metabolic disorder
11. Headache or facial pain associated
    with disorder of cranium, neck,
    eyes, ears, nose, sinuses, teeth,
    mouth, or other facial or cranial
    structures
12. Cranial neuralgias, nerve trunk
    pain, and deafferentation pain
13. Headache not classifiable

Recommended Diagnostic
Classification   for

11 Headache or facial pain associated
   with disorders of cranium, eyes,
   ears, nose, sinuses, teeth, mouth,
   or other facial or cranial structures

11.1   Cranial bones including
       mandible
11.2   Neck
11.3   Eyes
11.4   Ears
11.5   Nose and sinuses
11.6   Teeth and related oral
       structures
11.7   Temporomandibular joint
11.8   Masticatory muscles

Figure 2 International Headache Society classification. TMD is defined under item 11.7. (From Cephalalgia 1988; 8(suppl 7). Norwegian University Press, Publications Expediting Inc., P.O. Box 2459, Tolyen 0609, Oslo, Norway.)

   2. Positive x-ray (tomogram or MRI)
   3. Pain is mild to moderate and located to the TMJ and/or radiating
      from there

Most TMDs are not limited to the TMJ but involve the muscles of mastication, either primarily or secondarily.

Recommended Diagnostic Classification for

11.1 Cranial bones including the mandible
    11.1.1 Congenital and developmental disorders
        11.1.1.1 Aplasia
        11.1.1.2 Hypoplasia
        11.1.1.3 Hyperplasia
        11.1.1.4 Dysplasia
    11.1.2 Acquired disorders
        11.1.2.1 Neoplasia
        11.1.2.2 Fracture

Recommended Diagnostic Classification for

11.7 Temporomandibular joint disorders
    11.7.1 Deviation in form
    11.7.2 Disc displacement
        11.7.2.1 Disc displacement with reduction
        11.7.2.2 Disc displacement without reduction
    11.7.3 Dislocation
    11.7.4 Inflammatory conditions
        11.7.4.1 Synovitis
        11.7.4.2 Capsulitis
    11.7.5 Arthritides
        11.7.5.1 Osteoarthrosis
        11.7.5.2 Osteoarthritis
        11.7.5.3 Polyarthritides
    11.7.6 Ankylosis
        11.7.6.1 Fibrous
        11.7.6.2 Bony

Recommended Diagnostic Classification for

11.8 Masticatory muscle disorders
    11.8.1 Myofascial pain
    11.8.2 Myositis
    11.8.3 Spasm
    11.8.4 Protective splinting
    11.8.5 Contracture
    11.8.6 Neoplasia

Figure 3 IHS classification for disorders involving cranial bones, the TMJ, and masticatory muscles. (From Ref. 15.)

The primary-care physician should add the recommended screening questionnaire (Figure 4) to his or her intake form. Six simple screening-examination procedures for TMD can also be used for those who present with positive responses to the screening questionnaire (Figure 5). The comprehensive history format for TMD patients is shown in Figure 6. This is similar to a headache and chronic pain history.

TREATMENT

Treatment for TMD has changed significantly in the last 10 years, from a heavy occlusal-structural emphasis to a more conservative, chronic pain management approach. Of the myriad approaches to treatment, only five therapies have been scientifically validated (17–19):

1. Behavioral therapy
2. Pharmacological therapy
3. Interocclusal appliances
4. Physical therapy (physical medicine)
5. TMJ surgery

Recommended Screening Questionnaire for TMD

1. Do you have difficulty, pain, or both when opening your mouth, for instance, when yawning?
2. Does your jaw get "stuck," "locked," or "go out"?
3. Do you have difficulty, pain, or both when chewing, talking, or using your jaws?
4. Are you aware of noises in the jaw joints?
5. Do your jaws regularly feel stiff, tight, or tired?
6. Do you have pain in or about the ears, temples, or cheeks?
7. Do you have frequent headaches and/or neckaches?
8. Have you had a recent injury to your head, neck, or jaw?
9. Have you been aware of any recent changes in your bite?
10. Have you previously been treated for a jaw-joint problem? If so, when?

Figure 4 All patients should be screened for TMD through a questionnaire such as this. The decision to refer to a trained clinician for a comprehensive history and clinical examination will depend on the number of positive responses and the severity of the chief complaint. (From Ref. 15.)

Recommended Screening Examination Procedures for TMD

1. Measure range of motion of the mandible on opening and right and left laterotrusion. (Note any incoordination in the movements.)
2. Palpate for preauricular or intrameatal TMJ tenderness.
3. Auscultate and/or palpate for TMJ sounds (ie, clicking or crepitus).
4. Palpate for tenderness in the masseter and temporalis muscles.
5. Note excessive occlusal wear, excessive tooth mobility, buccal mucosal ridging, or lateral tongue scalloping.
6. Inspect symmetry and alignment of the face, jaws, and dental arches.

Figure 5 Tension-type headache patients should be screened for TMD during the clinical exam along with the cranial nerve exam. (From Ref. 15.)

Behavioral Therapy

Cognitive and behavioral therapy involves biofeedback, relaxation therapy, and stress management to decrease tension in the masticatory muscles and decrease the adverse load on the masticatory system.

Pharmacological Therapy

NSAIDs are the first line of treatment to decrease the pain and inflammation of myositis and capsulitis.

Short-term benzodiazepines such as diazepam or alprazolam may be helpful for tension-related acute pain episodes. Muscle relaxants such as cyclobenzaprine and metaxalone are useful following motor vehicle accidents and similar events to promote sleep and reduce muscle tension.

Tricyclic antidepressants are excellent for patients with nonrestorative sleep and generalized muscle pain as in fibromyalgia. "In dosages of 10mg through 75mg, the tricyclics are beneficial in the treatment of chronic or facial pain, various oral dysesthesisas, which include glossodynia and idiopathic intraoral burning" (15, p. 87). Cyclobenzaprine shares some properties, especially antimuscarinic effects, with the tricyclic agents.

Interocclusal Appliances

Acrylic biteplates are used for the reduction of parafunctional activity, pain, and muscle tension. Both stabilization and repositioning appliances can decrease the adverse loading on the TMJs. After 6 weeks to 3 months of appliance use, when symptoms have subsided, the prescription is

---

Comprehensive History Format for TMD Patients

Chief complaint

History of present illness

    Date and event of onset
    Location of signs and symptoms
    Character, intensity, duration, frequency of signs and symptoms
    Remissions or change over time
    Modifying factors (alleviate, precipitate, or aggravate)
    Previous treatment results

Medical history

    Current or pre-existing relevant physical disorders or disease (specifically systemic
        arthritides or other musculoskeletal/rheumatologic conditions)
    Previous treatments, surgeries, and/or hospitalizations
    Trauma (specifically to head, face, or neck)
    Medications (prescription, nonprescription)
    Allergies
    Alcohol and other substances of abuse

Dental history

    Current or pre-existing relevant physical disorders or disease
    Previous treatments including patient's attitude toward treatment
    History of trauma to the jaw, teeth, or supporting tissues (including iatrogenic trauma)
    Parafunctional history, both diurnal and nocturnal

Personal history

    Social, behavioral, and psychologic
    Occupational, recreational, and family
    Litigation, disability, or other secondary gain issues

Figure 6 Comprehensive history for TMD patients is similar to that for headache patients. Attention should be focused on trauma to the teeth and jaws, recent dental work or orthodontics, and evidence of diurnal or nocturnal parafunction. (From Ref. 15.)

changed to nighttime use only. Many patients with nocturnal parafunction use upper stabilization appliances on an as-needed basis.

Physical Therapy (Physical Medicine)

Physical therapy is useful for relieving musculoskeletal pain and restoring function. It is most often an adjunct to other therapy. Posture training, exercise, mobilization, and physical modalities are an integral part of treatment.

TMJ Surgery

The American Association of Oral and Maxillofacial Surgeons (20) has developed criteria that should be satisfied before considering TMJ surgery:

1. Documented TMJ internal derangement or other structural joint disorder with appropriate imaging
2. Positive evidence suggesting that the symptoms and objective findings are a result of a structural disorder
3. Pain and/or dysfunction of such magnitude as to constitute a disability to the patient
4. Prior unsuccessful nonsurgical treatment
5. Prior management, to the extent possible, of bruxism, oral parafunctional habits, other medical or dental conditions, and other contributing factors that may affect the outcome of surgery
6. Patient's consent after a discussion of potential complications, goals, success rate, timing, postoperative management, and alternative approaches including no treatment

TMDs and orofacial pain conditions constitute a significant health problem, with a prevalence comparable to that of other headache disorders. Serious disability can result from acute and chronic pain and dysfunction of the orofacial region. There is debate over whether TMD is underdiagnosed by the primary-care physician, but most agree that there has been misdiagnosis and overtreatment from the dental community. A scientifically supported data base will help improve understanding of the pathophysiology, epidemiology, etiology, diagnosis, and management of these disorders.

REFERENCES

1. Costen JB. Syndrome of ear and sinus symptoms dependent upon disturbed function of the temporomandibular joint. Ann Otol Rhin Laryngol 1934; 43.
2. Schwartz LL. Disorders of the Temporomandibular Joint. Philadelphia: WB Saunders, 1959.
3. Laskin DM, Greene CS. Etiology of the pain–dysfunction Syndrome. J Am Dent Assoc 1969; 79:147–153.
4. Farrar WB, McCarty WL. A Clinical Outline of Temporomandibular Joint Diagnosis and Treatment. 7th ed. Montgomery, AL: Normandie Publications, 1983.
5. Dworkin S, leResche L. Research diagnostic criteria for temporomandibulars disorders: review, criteria, examinations and specifications, critique. J Orofac Pain 1992; 6:301–355.

6. Reik L, Hale M. The temporomandibular joint pain-dysfunction syndrome: A frequent cause of headache. Headache 1981; 21:151–156.
7. Reik L. Unnecessary dental treatment of headache patients for temporomandibular joint disorders. Headache 1985.
8. Saper J. Handbook of Headache Management. Baltimore: Williams and Wilkins, 1993.
9. Rugh JD, Solberg WK. Oral health status in the United States: Temporomandibular disorders. J Dent Educ 1985; 49:398–404.
10. Schiffman E, Fricton JR. Epidemiology of TMJ and craniofacial pain. In: Fricton JR, Kroening RJ, Hathaway KM, eds. TMJ and Craniofacial Pain: Diagnosis and Management. St. Louis: IEA Publishing, 1988:1–10.
11. Solberg WK. Epidemiology, incidence and prevalence of temporomandibular disorders: A review. In: The President's Conference on the Examination, Diagnosis, and Management of Temporomandibular Disorders. Chicago: American Dental Association, 1983:30–39.
12. Schiffman E, Fricton JR, Haley D, Shapiro BL. The prevalence and treatment needs of subjects with temporomandibular disorders. J Am Dent Assoc 1989; 120:295–304.
13. Dworkin SF, et al. Epidemiology of signs and symptoms in temporomandibular disorders: 1. Clinical signs in cases and controls. J Am Dent Assoc 1990; 120:273–281.
14. Greene CS, Marbach JJ. Epidemiologic studies of mandibular dysfunction: A critical review. J Prost Dent 1982; 48:184–190.
15. American Academy of Orofacial Pain. McNeil C, ed. Temporomandibular Disorders: Guidelines for Classification, Assessment and Management. Chicago: Quintessence, 1993.
16. Fricton JR. TMJ and craniofacial pain: Diagnosis and management. St. Louis: IEA Publishing, 1988.
17. Laskin DM, Greene CS. Technological methods in the diagnosis and treatment of temporomandibular disorders. Quintess Intl 1992; 23:95–102.
18. Mohl N, Ohrbach R. Clinical decision making for temporomandibular disorders. J Dent Educ 1992; 56:12.
19. Travell J, Symons D. The Trigger Point Manual. Baltimore: Williams and Wilkins, 1983.
20. American Association of Oral and Maxillofacial Surgeons. Position paper on TMJ Surgery, 1984.
21. Howard JA. Temporomandibular joint disorders, facial pain and dental problems of performing artists. In: Sataloff R, et al., eds. Textbook of Performing Arts Medicine. 1990:111–169.

16

Psychological Aspects of Headache

Randall E. Weeks and Steven Baskin

New England Institute for Behavioral Medicine
Stamford, Connecticut

INTRODUCTION

The recorded history of head pain dates back thousands of years, evidenced by written annals from the Sumerian era (circa 4000 B.C.) (1). Presently, over 50 million Americans suffer head pain. They spend more than $4 billion on over-the-counter analgesics each year (2), with an annual cost to business estimated at $57 billion (3). Despite its long history and significant impact, there is no clear consensus as to the underlying pathophysiology of headaches. Similarly, there is no consensus as to the role psychological factors play in the etiology and maintenance of head pain.

Headache is a disorder surrounded by myths and misconceptions from both a cultural and a medical perspective. Our culture uses *headache* to refer not only to head pain but also to an unpleasant task or individual (4); it is also an often cited reason for not having sex. Medically, although it is the most common pain complaint, physician training in this area is limited (5), and psychological explanations are often assumed when traditional treatments fail. Such attributions are deeply rooted in history; for example, trepanation, the first known headache remedy, was done to relieve headache pain by supposedly releasing demons and evil spirits. Present-day clinicians struggle to identify to what extent psychological "demons" play a role in the onset and maintenance of head pain.

Subtle cultural and psychological factors also deter headache sufferers from seeking treatment because, "after all, it's only a headache." It has been estimated that at least 50% of headache sufferers do not bother to seek medical care (3) due to misperceptions and cultural and medical attitudes.

This chapter reviews the role psychological factors may play in the headache process. It assumes that primary headache disorders involve complex central and peripheral mechanisms that can be influenced by a number of factors, not limited to but including psychological factors (6). The contribution of psychological factors occurs on a continuum. A rare minority of patients manifest purely psychological etiology for their headache syndrome, but the vast majority of patients may have psychological symptoms that coexist or are a result of the headache process itself.

The chapter first reviews studies that have examined psychological factors in headache patients. Next, the rare occurrence of primary psychiatric diagnoses in which headache can be a part of the psychiatric symptom complex are examined. Finally, the psychobiological factors involved in headache treatment are reviewed.

PSYCHOLOGICAL FACTORS AFFECTING HEADACHE

Most headache specialists agree that there is an underlying biological/ biochemical abnormality that serves as a triggering mechanism for the onset and maintenance of head pain. Areas of current research include 5-hydroxytryptamine receptors (7), central neuronal hyperexcitability (8), and the trigeminovascular system (9). Despite the proliferation of studies, there is still no universal agreement as to the specific underlying biological mechanism for head pain.

Few would disagree that psychological factors are important treatment considerations for headache patients. What is unclear, however, is exactly how these psychological variables interact with biological/physiological factors in the headache process. While psychiatric and psychological factors are the primary "causes" in only a small number of headache patients, it is widely accepted that they interact with biological factors to help precipitate, exacerbate, and maintain headache (10).

Depression

Headache is the most common somatic symptoms of patients presenting for the treatment of depression (10). In a study of 160 depressed patients, headache was present in 51.9%, but the data argued against a specific association between type of headache and depressive disorder (11). This is consistent with other recent research that has noted an independence between headache diagnosis and psychological variables (12) and suggests that the frequency of headache may be a confounding factor in such research (13). One study, however, reports to have found a significant relationship between personality characteristics and headache diagnosis—but only for women (14). Hence, there does not seem to be a predictable association between specific headache subtype and psychological variables such as depression.

A primary role of depression has been suggested for headache patients (15–19). Weekend headache sufferers were found to have greater dysphoric mood and psychological distress than non-weekend headache sufferers (20). Other studies have failed to confirm the existence of depression as a primary variable or even as a covariate in such individuals (21–24).

Research has examined the role of chronic pain and how it might impact on individual personality changes. One study examined duration of illness, personality traits, and diagnostic category of headache and failed to find any correlation between personality variables, duration of illness, and headache diagnosis (25). In fact, chronic headache patients have been found to have personality alterations, but within the range of normalcy and with no specific, predictable change in psychological status (26). This suggests the importance of individual differences across headache subtypes. Some patients may feel more helpless than others early in the pain process (27). For such patients, helplessness and depression improved following nondrug treatment and was independent of degree of headache relief (28).

In summary, although emotional state contributes to the development of headache in some patients, there are others in whom comparable headaches are unlikely to be due to emotional factors. When head pain is persistent, some patients will be increasingly concerned or depressed while others will develop tolerance and seek active coping mechanisms (29).

Anxiety

Various studies have found headache patients to manifest higher levels of anxiety (16,18,30) as well as to be more anxiety-prone (31) than non-headache controls. A psychological distress hypothesis has been offered for chronic headache sufferers (32), and a proposed association between psychic tension and vascular headache for the weekend headache sufferer (33). Headache patients have been found to be more sensitive and shy (34) as well as have a heightened sensitivity to pain (35).

Other studies, however, failed to find an association between anxiety and headache, either from self-report measures (21) or from psychometric data (36). Studies have failed to support the hypothesis of an intense, perfectionist migraine personality (37). Further, children with migraine are not more anxious than their non-headache friends (38). In such patients, normal amounts of stress and anxiety appeared to lead to the expression of migraine, with anxious children suffering more frequent and severe attacks (38).

In summary, as with the studies on depression, there is no consistent trend in the literature that headache patients manifest higher levels of anxiety than controls. It appears that these patients also have a great variety of mechanisms to cope with pain. Certainly, it is likely that anxious individuals may be more susceptible to difficulties in coping with head pain and therefore manifest psychological changes that may serve to help maintain the pain syndrome.

Stress

Andrasik (10) has found that stress can trigger headaches in three ways: 1) by initiating the headache in a biologically prone individual, 2) by indirectly potentiating or intensifying an ongoing headache, or 3) by prolonging headache, which in turn can exert a psychological toll on the patient. The role of stress in headache may be one of the most confusing issues for headache patients and physicians.

Typically, headache sufferers fall in one of two groups with respect to the association of stress and head pain. The first group consists of patients who readily identify stressors as related to their headaches (with a clear understanding that pain itself may be a stressor). The other group contains patients who are extremely defensive about the contribution of stress. They are constantly bombarded with the charge that "if you weren't so 'stressed out,' your headaches would disappear."

In a 6-month longitudinal study examining migraine and stress, increased stress was generally not found for days 2 and 3 before an attack, but often for day 1, and on the migraine day itself (39). Other authors note that in various types of headache, especially migraine, the effect of a low degree of daily annoying stress may be associated much more with headache than the occurrence of a major stress event (major stress, in fact, may prevent a headache in some patients) (40).

Lifestyle factors and coping abilities may differ in individuals with different headache types (41). One study found that 53% of migraine patients were classified as "type-A personalities" compared to only 23% of tension-type headache subjects (42). There also seemed to be a difference in reactivity patterns between the two groups. Those with tension-type headache reacted more selectively to negative emotional arousal (anger or anxiety) and reported more frequent attacks precipitated by emotional states. Migraine sufferers reported a more uniform distribution of attacks among different emotional precipitants (43). This highlights the role that cognitive mediation plays with respect to appraisal and coping with stress and its impact on head pain. Other authors, however, propose a dysregulation model of headache across headache subtypes (44) in which sudden increases in the frequency and magnitude of stressful life events (in association with an emotional appraisal of their negative impact on life patterns) contribute to the onset and maintenance of headache (45).

Anger

Headache patients, in general, have been shown to differ relative to control patients with respect to degree of anger and anger expression (16,18). Migraine patients have demonstrated a trend toward more repression of their emotions and more self-aggression (46), with less reactivity to negative emotional arousal (anger/anxiety), when compared to tension-type headache patients (43). Repression of feelings and inhibition of aggressiveness may develop early in life, as children with migraine seem to demonstrate similar responses (47).

The data need to be viewed cautiously because other studies have failed to support a consistent "migraine personality" that includes perfectionism and anxiety, as well as repressed feelings (36,37). Future research needs to operationalize a precise definition of anger and assess whether such anger may be a precipitant or a result of having to live with frequent and unpredictable attacks of intense pain (48).

Family Issues

Recent epidemiological data indicate that as many as 78% of individuals with chronic pain come from families in which at least one other family member has chronic pain (49). This suggests that children of individuals with chronic pain may be especially at risk for developing chronic pain conditions. Other studies examined interaction patterns in headache patients versus controls and found that headache couples reported greater differences in consensus, cohesion, affection, and sexual relationships than did non-headache control couples (50). Other data, however, failed to find a strong link between family factors and recurrent headache (51).

Coping Skills and Reaction to Pain

Headache sufferers have been found to be more sensitive to pain than headache-free persons, but the heightened sensitivity is not specific to the head (35). Tension-type headache sufferers felt themselves to be more anxious, depressed, and angry than they were during non-headache states and felt themselves to be more hassled by external stressors (52). Avoidance behavior has been noted in patients with migraine with aura (53). There is evidence that avoidance behavior becomes persistent even during pain-free states (54).

Occasionally, when a patient has described a headache as being a "really good one," it is found that it somehow helped the patient to avoid a more unpleasant emotional situation (55). When headaches are described as "good," there may well be something in the person's life that could be worse. Similarly, coping strategies that overpredict future pain by remembering a previous episode as having been more painful than it was may serve a protective function (56).

Active rather than passive coping strategies have been suggested (57), including an understanding that a patient's distress is likely to be a consequence of having to live with frequent and unpredictable episodes of intense pain (48). Head pain of increased severity seems to be associated with a cognitive shift whereby the patient's primary concern moves from situational and interpersonal distress to distress associated with the disorder itself (58,59). Cognitive treatment should target pain management to achieve a greater degree of internal locus of control as well as less helplessness.

Summary

From the above review, it is obvious that much of the data are contradictory with respect to psychological factors as they relate to headache patients. One of the issues that may confound research results has been the lack of consistent classification criteria with respect to group membership across studies. In addition, factors such as analgesic overuse, use of anxiolytics and beta-blockers, and reaction to pain medications can affect psychological states of headache patients. Finally, few studies have examined patients longitudinally to more clearly ascertain whether psychological factors exist as a cause of the pain, a result of the pain, or a coexisting symptom due to apparent underlying biochemical mechanisms.

The Minnesota Multiphasic Personality Inventory (MMPI) appears to be the most often used personality measure in such studies. Although its utility has been noted recently (60), results from MMPI test data purporting to measure similar patient groups are quite contradictory. One needs to be reminded of issues that our group raised several years ago with respect to interpreting MMPI data cautiously, as the differences in profile configuration may be more reflective of frequency of head pain rather than any type of underlying psychopathology (61). Proper use of the MMPI would include reporting the percentage of patients that have meaningful psychological profiles (a configured analysis) versus merely reporting group means of selected scale scores (an average analysis). Unfortunately, most research simply averages scale scores, which limits the interpretation of data. MMPI data should also be corroborated by self-report data as well as behavioral assessment so a more meaningful, multimodal clinical picture may emerge.

PSYCHIATRIC FACTORS INVOLVED IN HEADACHE

The *Diagnostic and Statistical Manual of Mental Disorders* (Third Edition, Revised) (62) offers a listing of primary psychiatric disorders that may include headache as part of the symptom complex. The most common psychiatric diagnoses that may account for or elicit head pain are described below. It should be noted that psychiatric "causes" of headache are rare and probably too often cited when patients fail with therapy. The criteria for psychiatric diagnosis are included to assist practitioners in assessing patients' psychiatric status and, when significant psychiatric disease is present, to direct treatment appropriately.

Factitious disorders with physical symptoms involve the intentional production or feigning of physical symptoms or the exacerbation/exaggeration of preexisting physical conditions. In such individuals, there is a psychological need to assume a sick role with no apparent secondary gain. Such patients often present their medical history with a great dramatic flair but are vague or inconsistent when questioned in more detail.

Malingering is the intentional production of false or grossly exaggerated physical or psychological symptoms with evidence of external incentives. Such patients rarely present symptoms in the context of emotional conflict, and the symptoms are not likely to be symbolically related to an underlying emotional need. Secondary gain issues are apparent if pain symptoms persist.

A *somatomform disorder* is defined by an individual's preoccupation with pain in the absence of adequate physical findings to account for the pain or its intensity. The description of the pain symptom is inconsistent with the anatomical distribution of the nervous system or cannot adequately be accounted for by organic pathology. Other characteristics include frequent physician visits to obtain medical reassurance, excessive use of analgesics without relief of the pain, requests for surgery, and the development of "sick role behavior" to the point of potentially becoming an invalid.

Head pain may also serve as part of the symptom constellation of other psychiatric diagnoses. In a *conversion disorder*, pain may occur in addition to other purely psychological symptoms such as paralysis and coordination disturbances. These are produced unconsciously and may be temporally related to psychosocial stressors that represent a psychological conflict or need. Symptoms presenting in conversion disorders often have symbolic meaning. *Hypochondriasis* exists when there is a preoccupation with a determinate belief that headache is part of a serious disease process based on the patient's interpretation of the physical signs and in spite of complete medical workup results and reassurance to the contrary. *Delusional (paranoid) disorder* occurs when a predominant theme emerges that the person has some physical defect, disorder, or disease, and often occurs as part of a psychotic process.

Headache may exist as part of *major depression*, in which the affective state may serve as a trigger for the underlying headache mechanism. Differential diagnosis is difficult because, for example, the concept of transformational migraine (63) and drug-induced headache (64) have clinical correlates and behavioral markers that are consistent with depression.

Reaction to head trauma may also involve a primary psychiatric diagnosis. In a recent study (65), 19 of 20 patients referred for posttraumatic headache were found to fit the criteria for a specific psychiatric diagnosis, including 15 who were diagnosed as having *posttraumatic stress disorder*. This involves the development of characteristic symptoms following a psychologically distressing event that has been experienced with intense fear, terror, and helplessness. Such symptoms involve reexperiencing the traumatic event, avoidance of stimuli associated with the event, and apparent increased arousal.

Adjustment disorders with differing affective states (depression, anxiety, mixed) may result from major life stressors that tax coping skills. These may be common situations such as major life changes, but can also include difficulties in the adjustment to the experience of pain itself.

Diagnoses of dependency and withdrawal are relevant because chronic headache patients may become dependent on pain medication, anxiolytics, or other agents, eventually requiring detoxification. It is important that substances not be used in the absence of pain; most patients do not resist withdrawal from pain medications when the concept of analgesic rebound and analgesic habituation is explained to them. Substance abuse patients (or patients with a primary addiction disorder) typically present with a great deal of drug-seeking behavior regarding pain medication. They have a tendency to "lose" prescriptions for pain medications, have difficulty sticking to detoxification limits, and are often receiving pain medications from numerous physicians. Obviously, such individuals require a more psychiatric rehabilitation program, unlike the vast majority of headache patients who merely need to be detoxified from an overuse of abortive headache medications.

These are the primary psychiatric disorders in which headache may manifest itself as part of the symptom complex. Shulman (66) suggests that the practitioner ask himself the following questions should he suspect that psychodynamic factors play a primary role in the headache pattern:

What role does the headache play in the patient's life?
Is the invalid role useful to the patient?
What other person is most affected by the headaches?
Is the pain used to influence someone else's behavior?
What does the pain allow the patient to avoid?
What does the pain permit the patient to do (e.g., make demands on others)?
Is the patient angry, and at whom?
Is the patient playing a martyr role? (p. 712)

In summary, we view headache as a biological/physiological disorder in which psychological factors may contribute to the initiation of exacerbation of head pain. Practitioners often use the code "Psychological Factors Affecting Physical Condition" to highlight the interaction of psychological factors with the headache process itself.

PSYCHOBIOLOGICAL TREATMENT OF HEADACHE

Assessment

Headache is believed to be a biochemical manifestation that may be triggered by psychological variables as well as any type of chronobiological dyssynchrony (63). Only after a thorough history is obtained that considers the diverse factors that can precipitate and maintain headache can a proper treatment program be implemented. Due to the complexity of the disorder as well as the need to treat headache from an interdisciplinary approach, specialty clinics have been established to better serve headache patients.

An initial evaluation should include, minimally, a complete headache and medical history, complete neurological exam, investigational testing when appropriate (e.g., EEG, evoked potentials, or MRI scan of the brain), and a psychophysiological evaluation. As the first three components are somewhat commonplace (and described elsewhere in this text), they will not be reviewed here. A description follows of the psychophysiological evaluation that we have used over the past 15 years in treating headache patients as part of our treatment program.

This consultation is typically performed by a behavioral specialist, usually a psychologist or psychiatrist, who has an in-depth knowledge of headache pathogenesis and treatment. The evaluation usually lasts 60 to 90 minutes, and occurs after an initial medical and headache history is taken by one of our staff nurses. The initial part of the session is devoted to reviewing the headache history that has been taken previously. A significant number of patients will modify information that was obtained in the initial nurse interview (apparently independent of the previous interviewer's skills). By performing such a review, the history can be clarified and made more valid.

Other medical history is reviewed with special attention to present and past medication usage, dosage levels, side effects, and degree of headache relief. A great deal of time is taken to assess whether the patient may have habituated to or be rebounding from overuse of analgesic or ergotamine compounds. This is a critical part of the assessment, as traditional pharmacological and nonpharmacological treatments have been shown to be compromised by the overuse of such agents. Therefore, it is important to assess not only whether medications and nonpharmacological strategies have been ineffective, but also whether the patient may have been rebounding during such treatment.

Lifestyle issues such as cigarette and caffeine consumption and intake of alcohol (as well as other recreational drugs) are also an important part of this assessment. Factors such as sleep-pattern changes and insomnia (initial, middle, or terminal) are examined. Patients are asked whether they miss meals and have appetite changes (either weight gain or loss), constipation difficulties, decreased libido, decreased concentration or memory, tearfulness, decreased energy, recurring nightmares, rapid heart rate, panic attacks, bruxism, cervical tightness, or cold extremities. Such symptoms are behavioral correlates of underlying affective disorders but can also be side effects of medication (e.g., beta-blockers or pain medication) or the result of pain itself.

A family history is taken with respect to interpersonal dynamics. It is important to try to establish the impact of the patient's pain experiences on the family unit. Similarly, it is useful to note the reaction of significant others to the patient's pain experience (e.g., are they supportive/empathic or critical/punitive). One must also assess the degree of "guilt" that a patient may feel should they become compromised with respect to the family responsibilities and involvement. Finally, family history with respect to headache, affective, and psychological issues, as well as substance abuse issues is taken.

Psychological factors are evaluated through the above behavioral assessment, which indicates affective issues such as anxiety or depression. It is important to elicit self-report data with respect to the patient's view about his or her mood state. Similarly, one tries to assess whether any acknowledged affective problem may be primary or secondary to the pain experience and, if appropriate, whether it could relate to medication.

Finally, patients' perceptions about their headache problems are important to ascertain. Important questions include: Do you believe your headaches are related to stress? How do other people react to your headaches? Do you think your headaches are all psychologically based? What works best for you to reduce head pain? When appropriate, interviews with significant others may also take place.

Patients are required to complete a battery of self-administered psychological tests prior to this interview. These typically include the MMPI, a depression inventory (Beck, Zung, or Lubin), an anxiety questionnaire, and the Holmes Life Change Index (67). These offer a rather efficient assessment of overall possibility status as well as an index of stress and adjustment. Once again, interpretation of test results must take into account that chronic pain can affect performance on such measures and that symptoms of depression and/or anxiety must be viewed within this context. Results are reviewed with the patient during this session.

Physiological data are gathered as the final part of the evaluation. Such an assessment may be structured in a variety of formats (68,69). A physiological profile is obtained in a structured assessment utilizing muscle scanning (70) and photoplethysmographic measures of vascular lability. Data are gathered both statically and dynamically across conditions of baseline, relaxation, mental stressors, and recovery. Results are presented to the patient with respect to the absolute magnitude of the responses as well as relative changes across conditions.

In summary, such a comprehensive assessment provides a complete analysis of the headache pattern as well as an introduction to the biofeedback instrumentation (for those who are candidates for such treatment). A discussion takes place regarding behavioral management of headache and the patient's responsibilities in treatment. Time is allotted for questions posed by the patient and/or significant others.

Treatment

The purpose of the program is to combine behavioral and medical treatments to provide a comprehensive, multifaceted treatment for headaches. The program's goals are:

Education—teaching the patient current concepts regarding the causes and treatment of headaches

Dietary and behavioral restriction—altering certain lifestyle patterns that could cause headache

Self-Regulation—teaching the patient to control various physiological responses to abort and prevent headaches

Cognitive behavior modification—examining and changing certain actions, thoughts, attitudes, and expectations that could cause heightened levels of physiological arousal that might lead to headaches

Participation—involving the patient as an active participant in the treatment program through education and acquisition of the skills mentioned previously

The program is built on the premise that it is important for the patient to take some responsibility for headache improvement rather than professionals having total control and responsibility.

Education

This portion of the program includes a complete examination of the pathophysiology of the different types of headache. Genetic predispositions for headache, the physiology of stress, and the relationship between stress and headaches are other topics.

Information regarding different classes of headache medications, their therapeutic mechanisms of action, and potential side effects is presented. The rationale for the selection of abortive or prophylactic medications is explained.

Traditionally accepted myths regarding personality factors and headache are examined and exposed as unfounded. Questions about biofeedback are answered. The anticipated course of treatment is explained regarding detoxification from medications and "time lags" before therapeutic levels of daily medication are reached.

Finally, patients are taught how to keep a headache calendar, which is brought to each treatment appointment. Such a calendar should include the intensity of the pain, the time of day the headache begins, the duration of the headache, types and amounts of medication taken, degree or relief from the medication, and any other particular dietary or emotional factors that may have triggered the headache. If applicable, women should note their menstrual days. Although the calendar may sound complicated, formats have been established to record these data efficiently and easily (71).

Dietary and Behavioral Restrictions

When appropriate, patients are put on an elimination diet to limit foods that have been shown to trigger headaches. The diet is reviewed and questions are answered. Patients are advised that if they slip and eat one of the restricted foods, they should note this on this headache calendar. They are also requested to decrease their caffeine consumption, and are given an explanation as to why this is necessary.

Some medications need to be discontinued, and patients are given structure and/or support with regard to reduction schedules and discontinuation. The rational for the elimination of frequent ergotamine and analgesic usage as it relates to rebound headaches is presented, with a description of the time period before the "washout effect" is complete. Patients need a great deal of support and education regarding these factors.

Sleep is also an important consideration in headache treatment. Patients are advised to get enough sleep but to avoid oversleeping. Changes in sleep patterns may precipitate headaches, so patients are advised to keep to their usual sleep patterns, even on weekends and vacations. Sleep problems (initial, middle, and/or terminal insomnia) are noted and treated pharmacologically and/or behaviorally.

Self-Regulation

Biofeedback facilitates the self-regulation process as patients learn what must be done to achieve the desired responses and become aware of internal feelings that accurately reflect a relaxed system. As biofeedback is discussed in Chapter 17, our program will not be presented here.

Generalization strategies are discussed to encourage the patient to use the self-regulation strategies on an ongoing basis. Patients learn mini-exercises that are to be utilized throughout the day to heighten body awareness and reduce physiological arousal. Booster biofeedback sessions are held on an infrequent basis to ensure continued maintenance of acquired responses.

Cognitive Behavior Modification

This portion of the program is often referred to as the "stress management" aspect of treatment. Behavioral issues such as time management, overscheduling, and the need to increase pleasurable activity are discussed. Indices of type A behavior are reviewed with attempts at modification (72).

A variety of cognitive styles have been shown to affect levels of stress. Maladaptive styles of thinking and irrational beliefs are believed to enhance and sustain high levels of arousal, anxiety, or depression (73,74). Coping strategies are discussed to help eliminate traditional styles of thinking that perpetuate stress (75).

An analysis of the patient's life is made to determine the degree of these maladaptive behavioral patterns and thoughts as well as to discover particular areas of stress in the patient's life. Significant others may be interviewed at this point to provide additional input regarding the patient's status. Often, they present with misunderstandings of the patient's level of stress. All stress-management strategies are designed to promote more effective coping skills and facilitate acquisition of a more adaptive, pain-free lifestyle.

This stress-management course serves as a forum in which to begin to explore the role of underlying psychological factors in patients for whom there is a need to do so. A more formal type of psychotherapy (individual, couples, or family therapy) can be initiated at that point.

SUMMARY

Headache is a complex, biological, biochemical disorder that can be further complicated by psychological and lifestyle habits. Effective treatment incorporates these factors into the treatment process. As can be seen from the above review, there is no simple relationship between psychological variables and head pain, but the skilled clinician needs to be aware of the importance of such factors as well as individual differences between patients.

REFERENCES

1. Ziegler DK. Headache: Public health problem. In: Matthew NT, ed. Neurologic Clinics—Headache 1990; 8:781–792.
2. National Headache Foundation statistics, 1992.
3. Siegelman S. Headache hurts millions. Buss Health 1992; 8–12.
4. American Heritage Dictionary. New York: Houghton Mifflin, 1969.
5. Anderson B. Clinical perspectives on patient needs. In: Proceedings: Headache in the Canadian Clinical Setting: An Inclusive Look at Epidemiology, Diagnosis and Treatment. Canadian Headache Society, 1990:76–91.
6. Sheftell FD. Psychological considerations in evaluation and treatment of headache disorders. In: Rapoport A, Sheftell FD, eds. Headache. New York: PMA Publishing. In press.
7. Peroutka SJ. Developments in 5-hydroxytryptamine receptor pharmacology in migraine. In: Mathew NT, ed. Neurologic Clinics—Headache 1990; 8:829–839.
8. Welch KMA, D'Andrea G, Tepley N, et al. The concept of migraine as a state of central neuronal hyperexcitability. In: Mathew NT, ed. Neurologic Clinics—Headache 1990; 8:817–828.
9. Moskowitz MA. Basic mechanisms in vascular headache. In: Mathew NT, ed. Neurologic Clinics—Headache 1990; 8:801–816.
10. Andrasik F. Psychologic and behavioral aspects of chronic headache. In: Mathew NT, ed. Neurologic Clinics—Headache 1990; 8:961–976.
11. Marchesi C, DeFerri A, Petrolmi N, et al. Prevalence of migraine and muscle tension headache in depressive disorders. J Affect Disorder 1989; 16:33–36.
12. Pfaffenrath V, Hummelsberger J, Pollmann W, et al. MMPI personality profiles in patients with primary headache syndromes. Cephalalgia 1991; 11:263–268.
13. Rappaport NB, McAnulty DP, Waggoner CD, et al. Cluster analysis of Minnesota Multiphasic Personality Inventory (MMPI) profiles in a chronic headache population. J Behav Med 1987; 10:49–60.
14. Shulman BH. Psychological factors affecting migraine. Clin J Pain 1989; 5:23–28.
15. Formisano R, Carletto F, Assenza S, et al. Tension-type headache: A neuropsychological and neurophysiological study. Ital J Neurolog Sci 1992; 13: 331–336.
16. Kinder BN, Curtis G, Kalichman S. Affective differences among empirically derived subgroups of headache patients. J Pers Dis 1992; 58:516–524.
17. Ellersten B, Klove H. MMPI patterns in chronic muscle pain, tension-type headache, and migraine. Cephalalgia 1987; 7:65–71.
18. Hatch JP, Schoenfeld LS, Boutros NN, et al. Anger and hostility in tension-type headache. Headache 1991; 31:302–304.
19. Brandt J, Celentano D, Stewart W, et al. Personality and emotional disorder in a community sample of migraine headache sufferers. Am J Psychiatry 1990; 147:303–308.
20. Nattero G, DeLorenzo C, Biale L, et al. Psychological aspects of weekend headache sufferers in comparison with migraine patients. Headache 1989; 29:93–99.

21. Morrison DP, Peck DF. Do self-report measurers of affect agree? A longitudinal study. Br J Clin Psychol 1990; 29:395–400.
22. Guidetti V, Fornara R, Ottaviano S, et al. Personality inventory for children and childhood migraine: A case-controlled study. Cephalalgia 1987; 7:225–230.
23. Hundleby JD, Loucks AD. Personality characteristics of young adult migraneurs. J Pers Assess 1985; 49:497–500.
24. Mathew NT. Cluster headache. Neurology 1992, 42:22–31.
25. Invernizzi G, Gala C, Buono M, et al. Neurotic traits and disease duration in headache patients. Cephalalgia 1989; 9:173–178.
26. Mongini F, Ferla E, Maccagnani C. MMPI profiles in patients with headache or craniofacial pain: A comparative study. Cephalalgia 1992; 12:91–98.
27. Spinhoven P, Jochems PA, Linssen AC, et al. The relationship of personality variables and patient recruitment to pain coping strategies and psychological distress in tension headache patients. Clin J Pain 1991; 7:12–20.
28. Blanchard EB, Steffek BD, Jaccard J, et al. Psychological changes accompanying non-pharmacological treatment of chronic headache: The effects of outcome. Headache 1991; 31:249–253.
29. Mersky H, Brown J, Brown A, et al. Psychological normality and abnormality in persistent headache patients. Pain 1985; 23:35–47.
30. Blanchard EB, Appelbaum KA, Radnitz CL, et al. The refractory headache patient. I. Chronic, daily, high intensity headache. Behav Ther 1989; 27:403–410.
31. Levi R, Edman GV, Ekbom K, et al. Episodic cluster headache—personality and some neuropsychological characteristics in male patients. Headache 1992; 32:119–125.
32. Ahles TA, Martin JB. The relationship of electromyographic and vasomotor activity to MMPI subgroups in chronic headache patients: The use of the original and contemporary MMPI norms. Headache 1989; 29:584–587.
33. Nattero G, DeLorenzo C, Biale L, et al. Psychological aspects of weekend headache sufferers in comparison with migraine patients. Headache 1989; 29:93–99.
34. Kowal A, Pritchard DW. Psychological characteristics of children who suffer from headache: A research note. J Child Psychol Psychiatry Allied Disc 1990; 31:637–649.
35. Marlowe NI. Pain sensitivity and headache: An examination of the central theory. J Psychosom Res 1992; 36:17–24.
36. Schmidt FN, Carney P, Fitzsimmons G. An empirical assessment of the migraine personality type. J Psychosom Res 1986; 30:189–197.
37. Kohler T, Kosanic S. Are persons with migraine characterized by a high degree of ambition, orderliness, and rigidity? Pain 1992; 48:321–323.
38. Cooper PJ, Bawden HN, Camfield PR, et al. Anxiety and life events in childhood migraine. Pediatrics 1987; 79:999–1004.
39. Kohler T, Haimerl C. Daily stresses as a trigger of migraine attacks: Results of thirteen single-subject studies. J Consult Clin Psychol 1990; 58:870–872.
40. Sjaastad O. Headache and the influence of stress. A personal view. Am Clin Res 1987; 19:122–128.

41. Jensen J. Life events in neurological patients with headache and low back pain (in relation to diagnosis and persistence of pain). Pain 1988; 32:47–53.

42. Kowal A, Pritchard D. Psychological characteristics of children who suffer from headache: A research note. J Child Psychol Psychiatry 1990; 31:637–649.

43. Donias SH, Peioglou-Harmoussi S, Georgiadis G, et al. Differential emotional precipitation of migraine and tension-type headache attacks. Cephalalgia 1991; 11:47–52.

44. Hovanitz CA, Chin K, Warm JS. Complexities in life stress–dysfunction relationships: A case in point—tension headache. J Behav Med 1989; 12:55–75.

45. DeBenedittis G, Lorenzetti A, Pieri A. The role of stressful life events in the onset of chronic primary headache. Pain 1990; 40:65–75.

46. Passachier J, Goudswaard P, Orlebake JF, et al. Migraine and defense mechanisms: Psychophysiological relationships in young females. Soc Sci Med 1988; 26:343–350.

47. Guidetti V, Mazzei G, Ottaviano S, et al. The utilization of the Rorschach test in a case—controlled study. Cephalalgia 1986; 6:87–93.

48. Andrasik F, Kabela E, Quinn S, et al. Psychological functioning of children who have recurrent migraine. Pain 1988; 34:43–52.

49. Mikail SF, von Baeyer CL. Pain, somatic focus, and emotional adjustment in children of chronic headache sufferers and controls. Soc Sci Med 1990; 31:51–59.

50. Basolo-Kunzer M, Diamond S, Maliszewski M, et al. Chronic headache patients' marital and family adjustment. Iss Ment Health Nurs 1991; 12:133–148.

51. Stevenson J, Simpson J, Bailey V. Recurrent headaches and stomachs in preschool children. J Child Psychol Psychiatry Allied Disc 1988; 29:897–900.

52. Murphy AI, Lehrer PM. Headache versus nonheadache state: A study of electrophysiological and affective changes during muscle contraction headaches. Behav Med 1990; 16:23–30.

53. Spierings EL, Reinders MJ, Hoogdvin CA. The migraine aura as a cause of avoidance behavior. Headache 1989; 29:255–256.

54. Lacroix R, Barbaree HE. The impact of recurrent headaches on behavior lifestyle and health. Behav Res Ther 1990; 28:235–242.

55. Packard RC, Andrasik F, Weaver R. When headaches are good! Headache 1989; 29:100–102.

56. Rachman S, Eyrl K. Predicting and remembering recurrent pain. Behav Res Ther 1989; 27:621–635.

57. van den Bree MB, Passchier J, Emmon HH. Influence of quality of life and stress coping behavior on headaches in adolescent male students: An explorative study. Headache 1990; 30:165–168.

58. Demjen S, Bakal DA, Dunn BE. Cognitive correlates of headache intensity and duration. Headache 1990; 30:423–427.

59. Demjen S, Bakal D. Subjective distress accompanying headache attacks: Evidence for a cognitive shift. Pain 1986; 25:187–194.

60. Ellertsen B. MMPI profiles (editorial). Cephalalgia 1992; 12:68.

61. Weeks R, Baskin S, Rapoport A, et al. A comparison of MMPI personality data and frontalis electromyographic readings in migraine and combination headache patients. Headache 1983; 23:75–82.
62. American Psychiatric Association. Diagnostic and Statistical Manual of Mental Disorders. 3rd ed., revised. Washington D.C., 1987.
63. Saper JR. Help for Headaches. New York: Warner Books, 1987.
64. Mathew NT. Drug-induced headaches. In: Mathew NT, ed. Neurologic Clinics—Headache. 1990, 8:903–912.
65. Hickling EJ, Blanchard EB, Silverman DJ, et al. Motor vehicle accident, headache, and post-traumatic stress disorder: assessment findings in a consecutive series. Headache 1992; 32:147–151.
66. Shulman BH. Psychiatric aspects of headache. Med Clin North Am 1991; 75:707–715.
67. Aero R, Weiner E. The Mind Test. New York: William Morrow, 1981.
68. Weeks RE. Behavioral medicine approach to headache. In: Rapoport A, Sheftell FD, eds. Headache. New York: PMA Publishing. In press.
69. Boudewyns PA. Assessment of headache. In: Keefe FJ, Blumenthal JA, eds. Assessment Strategies in Behavioral Medicine. New York: Grune & Stratton, 1982:67–180.
70. Cram JR. Clinical EMG: Muscle Scanning and Diagnostic Manual for Surface Recordings. Seattle: Clinical Resources, 1986.
71. Rapoport AM, Sheftell FD. Headache Relief. New York: Simon & Schuster, 1990.
72. Friedman M, Ulmer D. Treating Type A Behavior and Your Heart. New York: Knopf, 1984.
73. Beck AT. Cognitive Therapy and the Emotional Disorders. New York: International Universities Press, 1976.
74. Ellis A, Grieger R. RET: Handbook of Rational-Emotive Therapy. New York: Springer Publishing, 1977.
75. Meichenbaum D. Cognitive Behavior Modification. Morristown, N.J.: General Learning Press, 1974.

17

Biofeedback and the Treatment of Headache

Kathleen Farmer

*Shealy Institute for Comprehensive Health Care
Springfield, Missouri*

INTRODUCTION

Biofeedback is a process that refines a living organism's physiological responses to change or stress. Sweating, shivering, satiation, thirst, hunger, pressured, strained, at ease, tight, and restless are messages that speak to mechanisms regulating physiological equilibrium or homeostasis. The body's response occurs more or less automatically unless specific change is redirected toward a new physiological response. As a therapeutic modality, biofeedback utilizes technology to "feed back" at a cognitive level specific information that enhances a desired physiological response.

Pain is a message that something is wrong and that immediate corrective action is necessary. When the cause of pain can be identified, the individual learns to avoid future painful experiences. But with recurrent or persistent pain that does not reenforce an appropriate reaction, desperation sets in. The longer the discomfort lasts, the greater the fear until the environment itself becomes a source of fear and uncertainty (1).

Biofeedback can help an individual reinterpret this physiological confusion by translating the body's messages into understandable terms. Specifically, the response of fear and desperation is redirected into a new response that can be understood as "taking better care of myself."

REVIEW OF BIOFEEDBACK RESEARCH

More than 20 years ago, Green et al. (2) made the seminal observation that headache sufferers tended to have finger temperatures around 70°F. By contrast, individuals without severe headaches recorded finger temperatures of about 85°F. The investigators designed a biofeedback treatment for migraine by combining finger-warming with autogenic training (repeating phrases such as "My hands are warm and heavy"). They reported that 74% of the 75 patients had fewer and less severe migraine attacks after biofeedback training.

Since then, researchers have attempted to uncover mechanisms underlying temperature biofeedback that account for this observation. Many researchers have experimentally demonstrated the functional similarity of pain and anxiety (3), which may in part account for the success of temperature biofeedback. However, treatment of anxiety alone does not account entirely for this observation. Other types of biofeedback techniques (EMG and EEG) have been studied and found to be useful as therapeutic modalities for headache sufferers.

Since 1972, over 500 published studies have assessed biofeedback and other behavioral treatment for headache (4). Even though several have questioned the usefulness of nonpharmacological treatment of headache (5), the vast majority have reported successful trials. Typically, more than 50% of headache sufferers enrolled in behavioral treatment experience at least a 50% decrease of headache frequency, intensity, duration, and medication needs (6–12).

In one typical study, Blanchard et al. (13) reported that the behavioral treatment of 116 patients with vascular headache (migraine or migraine and tension) reduced frequency, intensity, and duration of attacks by 51%, compared to those who merely monitored their headaches; of those in the active treatment group, thermal biofeedback produced higher improvement rates (51%) than a meditation technique (37.5%). There were no significant differences between a group that practiced thermal biofeedback with adjunctive relaxation training compared to thermal biofeedback with cognitive therapy. Blanchard et al. (14) commented:

Table 1 Indicators for Success with Biofeedback

1. The migraineur is female (55,56).
2. Migraine has existed less than 2 years (20).
3. The migraineur is less than 60 years of age (14); the younger, the more responsive to biofeedback (57).
4. The headache sufferer is motivated to practice finger warming at home (48).
5. The individual is not unusually anxious (14,58)—although biofeedback is a highly effective treatment for anxiety and panic.
6. The individual can warm the finger during the first thermal biofeedback session.
7. The migraineur has received 7 to 15 thermal biofeedback sessions (19,20,23,59).
8. Headaches are preceded by a physiological cue or a warning (60).
9. The individual achieves a finger temperature of 96°F sometime during the training.
10. The Minnesota Multiphasic Personality Inventory (MMPI) falls within normal limits (14,61).

It should be remembered that all of these patients were treated according to a specified protocol which allowed only minimal attention in treatment to other issues in the patient's life, such as marital problems, depression, etc. We would expect the practicing clinician to attend to the "whole patient," that is, to treat not only the presenting headache problem but also the other psychological problems of the patient which might be contributing to the headache problem. Thus, in our opinion, the practicing clinician's patients should be able to do as well as our results, and probably better.

Blanchard's specific focus was to measure the efficacy of biofeedback and/or relaxation training for the treatment of headache. To ensure objectivity, there was minimal contact from a psychotherapist and a reliance primarily on audio and visual feedback. Blanchard et al. added (14):

Our previous research has shown the percent improvement score to be a very conservative measure in comparison to the patient's global estimate of degree of improvement at the end of treatment. For example, the regression analysis showed that a patient who had a 50% improvement based on the Headache Diary would, on average, rate her improvement as 85%.

Other research confirms that biofeedback therapy is highly effective (15–18). Olson (19) found that 75% of 524 patients improved as a result of biofeedback therapy. Symptom frequency decreased by 54%, severity by 30%, and 54% reported a decreased need for medication. No therapist-dependent effects were noted, which, as in the study by Blanchard and colleagues (14), controlled for procedural variables and measured the results of biofeedback treatment as directly as possible.

Reich (20) treated 703 adults who suffered from vascular/migraine headaches or muscle contraction headaches with four methods: relaxation training, biofeedback, microelectrical therapy, or multimodal treatment. All treatments significantly reduced the frequency and intensity of head pain over a period of 3 years. However, of the four techniques, biofeedback was the most successful.

Long-term studies indicate that the benefits of biofeedback for the treatment of headache extend over a period of 5 or 6 years (21,22). Smith (23) found that 86% of 318 patients diagnosed with muscle contraction, migraine, or mixed headache who attended seven or more biofeedback training sessions maintained a 75–100% reduction in headache frequency over 25 or more months. Of these subjects, 65.5% reported a reduction in associated symptoms such as neck pain, back pain, shoulder pain, dizziness, and fatigue. Of patients who never attended a biofeedback session, 31% reported a reduction in headache frequency and 16.3% reported a reduction in associated symptoms. Lastly, 11% of those in the no-biofeedback group reported an increase in associated symptoms over time.

Blanchard et al. (24) followed 21 chronic headache patients (nine tension and 12 vascular) over a period of 5 years after the successful completion of biofeedback and/or relaxation training, documenting that 78% of tension and 91% of vascular headache subjects reported continued improvement of headache frequency. There can be no doubt that patients who respond to biofeedback maintain their response for prolonged periods of time.

TYPES OF BIOFEEDBACK

Thermal Biofeedback

By learning to increase finger temperature, patients gain voluntary control of sympathetically mediated vascular tone. This effect appears to impart voluntary control of the sympathetic nervous system—broadly, not simply restricted to the upper limb. Finger temperature can be viewed as

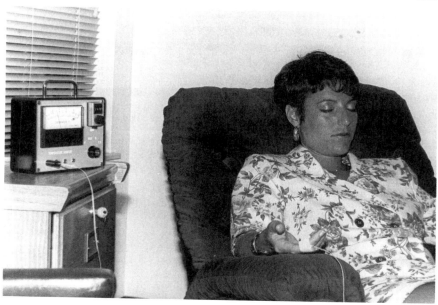

Figure 1 During thermal biofeedback, the patient is instructed to warm the finger temperature to 96°F.

an index of sympathetic arousal and correlates with the level of stress experienced by the subject: a lower finger temperature is associated with sympathetic arousal and peripheral vasoconstriction while higher finger temperature is due to vasodilation and is associated with decreased sympathetic arousal (25).

Several studies validate the observation that migraineurs have finger temperatures of approximately 70°F (26–28). Few subjects have baseline finger temperatures above 90°F. The therapeutic end point of thermal biofeedback training is considered to be 96°F. A simple thermometer or temperature probe can provide the necessary feedback to monitor circulatory response. Voluntary attainment of finger temperature elevation to 96° implies control of sympathetically mediated vascular response. The technique has also been shown to be of value in Raynaud's syndrome.

A comparison of thermal biofeedback, frontalis EMG biofeedback, and relaxation training has been carried out in a group of 27 migraine patients. Improvement (reduction) of migraine frequency in all three treatment groups was observed. However, thermal biofeedback was superior, nearly eliminating migraine attacks by the end of training (28).

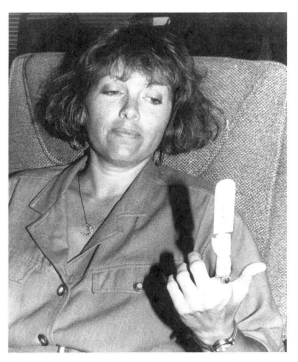

Figure 2 By raising the finger temperature, the individual gains control over the physiological response to stress.

Cephalic Vasomotor Response (CVMR) Feedback

Building on the findings with finger-warming, biofeedback researchers were encouraged to focus volitional control of the vasculature more directly on the putative cerebral vascular mechanism of headache. Subjects were trained to self-regulate vasomotion in the superficial temporal artery. Once again, focusing on the superficial temporal artery instead of the finger had a beneficial effect on headache frequency (29).

The next step was to compare finger-temperature feedback and temporal artery vasomotion feedback. The two techniques were equally effective in controlling headaches and produced more benefits than experienced by a control group who received no biofeedback training (30). These findings have been confirmed, and the improvement has been documented to be as high as a 70% reduction in daily headache frequency and a 45% decrease in headache severity which lasted through the 21 months of the study (31).

One complexity is that subjects trained to constrict the temporal artery appear to do just as well as those trained to dilate the temporal artery. In addition, while changes in headache activity and medication were associated with changes in vasomotor variability (32), they were not controlled by CVMR feedback. As Litt (15) pointed out, temporal artery constriction as trained in CVMR feedback requires increased sympathetic activity, whereas hand-warming calls for decreased sympathetic activity. Yet both produce beneficial results. It would appear that migraine headache is more complex than advocates of CVMR feedback would imply. Over the past five years, CVMR feedback research has dwindled in popularity, probably because thermal biofeedback produces similar results and is simpler to teach and more practical to incorporate in daily life.

Electromyographic (EMG) Biofeedback

Electrical output from specific muscle(s), such as the frontalis muscle of the forehead, can be used as an afferent for a feedback loop that teaches patients how to reduce muscle tension. The feedback may be visual (converting the microvolt current to a digital or analog readout) or auditory (amplifying the current and its frequency and passing to a speaker). The individual is instructed to reduce the afferent signal.

Typically, three electrodes (one being a ground) are placed over the muscle group targeted for relaxation. The frontalis muscle is usually the first muscle chosen because of its easily observed tightening in response to stress and its accessibility for electrode placement. Reduction of the afferent to 1 μV or less is a measure of successful control. Other muscle groups can then be trained if sore or tense. A common application is for tension headache sufferers, who can benefit from relaxation of the upper girdle (33).

EMG is probably the most effective treatment in reducing muscle tension in headache suffers (34–36), and has been shown to be effective for the treatment of tension headaches. Sargent (37) compared nondrug treatments, specifically autogenic phrases, EMG, and thermal biofeedback, in 136 migraineurs. A substantial reduction in headache frequency occurred in all but the no-treatment group.

The effectiveness of EMG biofeedback extends to tension headaches. Billings (38) compared 42 migraine subjects with 42 tension headache individuals; all were treated with frontal EMG feedback and thermal biofeedback. On study entry, the migraineurs had longer headache

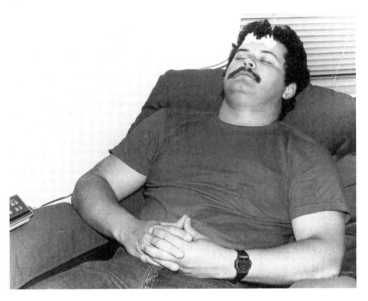

Figure 3 EMG biofeedback involves applying three electrodes to a muscle group (the frontalis in this photograph) to measure the microvoltage. By decreasing the microvolt reading, the person learns to relax the muscles.

histories than the tension headache group. Yet the tension headache group recorded higher frontal muscle tension while the migraine group had significantly lower peripheral hand temperature. EMG feedback showed significant decreases in frontal muscle tension for both groups. However, thermal biofeedback resulted in a more significant reduction in migraine frequency than did EMG feedback.

Electroencephalographic Biofeedback or Brain Wave Training

An electroencephalogram (EEG) records the aggregate electrical activity of huge numbers of neurons. Software is available that analyzes traces for patterns in wave frequency or amplitude and changes thereof, in real time, for immediate feedback. Unlike EEG interpretation oriented to pathological electrical activity, EEG biofeedback interpretation is oriented toward identifying and then amplifying brain wave activity associated with relaxation.

A brain map is a computerized, 19-electrode lead EEG that displays types of brain wave activity in the five major areas of the brain (frontal,

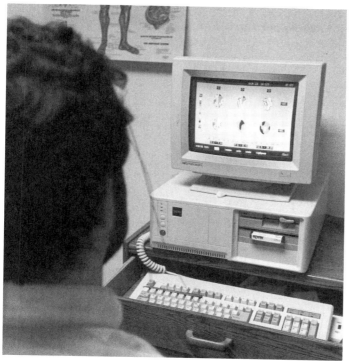

Figure 4 EEG biofeedback trains the brain to produce alpha, which produces relaxation and a sense of well-being.

temporal, parietal, central, and occipital). Brain waves are divided into four ranges, according to frequency (cycles per second—Hz). These ranges are beta, alpha, theta, and delta.

Beta rhythm appears on an EEG record as fast waves, of 13 Hz or higher, with small amplitude. These are indicative of arousal. Beta brain waves are associated with problem-solving, concept formation, new learning, being attentive, alert, and concentrating. Chronic headache patients typically display a predominance of beta activity, especially in the temporal area.

Alpha activity is slower than beta (8–13 Hz). These traces are often symmetrical, with larger amplitude than beta. Simply closing the eyes produces an increase of alpha activity in the occipital area of the brain in about 90% of individuals. Alpha activity is associated with reduction of arousal and relaxation.

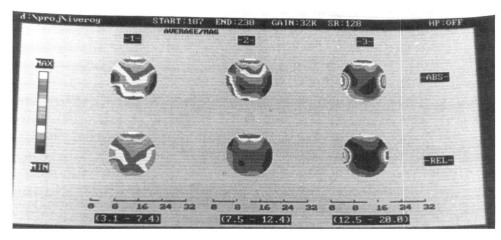

Figure 5 These topographs are analyses of the relative concentrations of brain waves produced during a specific task or condition. (Left, theta; center, alpha; right, beta.) In this case, the migraineur is solving block design problems. Our studies demonstrate that those suffering from migraine have a high level of beta activity in the temporal areas, as shown in the lower right circle.

Theta rhythm (4–8 Hz) commonly occurs spontaneously just before sleep or immediately upon awakening. These traces are irregular and with lower amplitude than alpha. Theta activity is said to be associated with creativity, as in composing a story, painting a portrait, or solving a complicated problem.

Delta rhythm is seen in sleep. The traces have slow frequency (0.5–4 Hz), and are irregular and asymmetrical. The delta rhythm is associated with the periods of sleep in between REM periods: a more beta-type rhythm is associated with dreaming.

The seminal demonstration of volitional alterations of the EEG was made in 1958 by Kamiya. This paved the way for the use of the EEG as an afferent for biofeedback. Initially, the inconvenience of attaching electrodes to the scalp reduced clinical utility. However, with the invention of the electrocap—a cap into which the electrodes are sewn—the entire procedure for recording a valid and reliable EEG was greatly simplified.

Recently, computerized interpretations and real-time feedback has reduced the computational expenses of the large amounts of data that these recordings can generate. A brain map can be constructed to depict the proportions of each trace that falls within the four frequency ranges at each electrode site. The computer's algorithm also has to edit out potentials from overlying muscle, as well as more gross, extraneous skeletal muscle movement. The rhythm proportions are then displayed as a topograph. The record is analyzed for symmetry and characterization of each rhythm in each area of the brain. For example, a predominance of beta activity in the temporal area, which is common in headache patients, can be used as the target for EEG biofeedback, and the goal would be for the individual to produce alpha rhythm frontally. An increase in alpha would produce greater relaxation and shift the focus away from pain.

The process of EEG biofeedback for headaches, specifically alpha training, may require only two or three electrodes to a site shown on topographic analysis to lack alpha rhythm. Auditory feedback tells the individual whether the alpha state is being attained. However, with highly cognitive or controlled people, visual feedback—that is, the actual topographs that the brain is producing—can also be a very effective feedback signal.

EFFICACY OF BIOFEEDBACK

Thermal biofeedback is therapeutic for 70% of headache patients, EMG biofeedback for 20%, and EEG biofeedback (alpha training) for 10%. EMG biofeedback (39) is effective for patients with a strong muscular or myofascial component to headache. EEG biofeedback is suited to individuals who have extreme difficulty with relaxation and who are highly cognitive, controlling, and relatively suspicious of treatment measures that fail to address the complexity of the problem.

Despite the multiple, well-controlled studies demonstrating efficacy (40,41), a survey of 465 physicians indicated that over 62% admitted to knowing little about biofeedback in headache. Only 22% had referred patients for biofeedback, and 47% were undecided about whether insurance coverage should be provided for biofeedback treatment (42). Many complications noted with management styles relying primarily on pharmacological interventions can be avoided by proper early psychological interventions. Biofeedback and relaxation therapy are effective, have no side effects, and produce significant positive cognitive changes.

Mizener et al. (43) found that migraineurs who received biofeedback training realized the control they had achieved over their own health and refocused away from pain, toward more positive activities. The tendency to catastrophize ("Things can't get worse than this") was replaced by self-talk that encouraged coping ("I can handle this"). These significant changes occurred during the first half of treatment (between pre- and

Table 2 The Role of Psychological Treatment of Headaches

1. Educating the headache sufferer about:
   a. The stress reaction that occurs as part of the pain/headache cycle
   b. How to transform the stress reaction into the relaxation response
   c. Changing anticipatory behaviors and medication misuse patterns
   d. The headache-prone environment, which is identified through 4 weeks of recording life events with a headache diary
   e. The headache-protective environment, which is created by eliminating stressors and precipitating factors and learning self-care
2. Cognitive restructuring of negative self-talk
3. Through biofeedback, beginning the process of retraining the person's physiology to relax
4. Teaching behavior management that identifies alternative responses to present and future problems
5. Through psychotherapy, helping the person reconcile emotional responses arising from past hurts, faults, mistakes, disappointments, and failures

mid-measures), which deemed the last half of treatment as a testing ground of what was learned.

Prophylactically, both propranolol and relaxation-biofeedback training yielded a 43–63% reduction in migraine frequency in 2445 migraine subjects studied (44). There were no differences between the treatment groups.

In a 3-year study that compared the effectiveness of ergotamine tartrate and relaxation-biofeedback training, both methods reduced headache activity by 50% or more (45). However, over time, the subjects treated with ergotamine were more likely to a) have obtained additional medical treatment for headaches and b) use either prophylactic or narcotic medications. Both groups reported that daily headaches occurred less frequently at the 3-year follow-up than prior to treatment.

Another study (46) found similar improvement in headache frequency among 37 subjects, half treated with ergotamine tartrate (41% lessening of headache frequency) and half with relaxation-biofeedback training (52% reduction in headache activity). The study encouraged home-based behavioral treatment.

Typically, home practice of finger-warming is needed at least twice a day for the technique to become reliable. Weekly sessions with a psychologist are not frequent enough to reinforce the internal physiology; finger-warming needs to become a habit that the individual learns to use, instantly, at the first signs of tension (47). The technique probably also reinforces the notion that the responsibility for the headache sufferer's health ultimately rests on himself, and not on the medical system. Success with the finger-warming regimen, with active and regular participation, may also indicate a motivated patient (48). If a person raises the temperature of the fingers through home practice, the probability of controlling headaches likewise increases.

Some authors (49,50) have suggested that relaxation-biofeedback training by a psychologist is expensive. However, a 1985 study (51) demonstrated that headache sufferers who underwent relaxation-biofeedback training experienced a drop in medical expenses from $955 prior to treatment to $52 after completion of the self-regulation process. The cost of treatment is an investment in the person's future medically, socially, and financially.

During the physiological relaxation that necessarily accompanies finger-warming (52), issues, especially unresolved emotional conflict, may surface (21,53). For this reason, psychological support needs to be available on a regular basis, for at least 6 weeks. Many times, unresolved issues perpetuate an internal environment conducive to migraine activity. Ongoing support helps the person identify, explore, and bring resolution to these unexpressed emotions and fears. This is particularly true for anticipatory behaviors influencing medication use and coexisting psychological disturbance such as anxiety and depression.

The acknowledgment of headache disorders as chronic conditions justifies a treatment plan that combines pharmacological and nonpharmacological modalities. Educating patients to participate in the management of headache and utilize effective, internal-based therapies reduces the disability of headache for many sufferers. Promises of "cures" implied when only pharmacological therapies are given to patients have limitations, including reliance on polypharmacy to treat behavior problems. By incorporating biofeedback and appropriate psychological intervention, the physician facilitates the process of treating the multifaceted dilemma of headache (54).

REFERENCES

1. Isler H, Solomon S, Spielman AJ, Wittlieb-Verpoort E. Impaired time perception in patients with chronic headaches. Headache 1987; 27:261–265.
2. Sargent JD, Green EE, Walters ED. The use of autogenic feedback training in a pilot study of migraine and tension headaches. Headache 1972; 12:120–125.
3. Philips HC, Jahanshahi M. Chronic pain: An experimental analysis of the effects of exposure. Behav Res Ther 1985; 23:281–290.

4. Martin PR, Marie GV, Nathan PR. Behavioral research on headaches: A coded bibliography. Headache 1987; 27:555–570.
5. Holmes DS, Burish TG. Effectiveness of biofeedback for treating migraine and tension headaches: A review of the evidence. J Psychosom Res 1983; 27:515–532.
6. Andrasik F, Pallmeyer TP, Blanchard EB, Attanasio V. Continuous vs interrupted schedules of thermal biofeedback: An exploratory analysis with clinical subjects. Biofeedback Self-Reg 1984; 9:291–298.
7. Blanchard EB. Three studies of the psychologic changes in chronic headache patients associated with biofeedback and relaxation therapies. Psychosom Med 1986; 48:73–83.
8. Blanchard EB, Hillhouse J, Appelbaum KA, Jaccard J. What is an adequate length of baseline in research and clinical practice with chronic headaches? Biofeedback Self-Reg 1987; 12:323–329.
9. Cheren S, ed. Psychosomatic Medicine: Theory, Physiology, and Practice. Vols. 1 and 2. Madison, Conn.: International Universities Press, 1989.
10. Diamond S, Dalessio DJ. The Practicing Physician's Approach to Headache. 3rd ed. Washington, D.C.: Williams and Wilkins, 1982:180–191.
11. Engel JM, Rapoff MA, Pressman AR. Long-term follow-up of relaxation training for pediatric headache disorders. Headache 1992; 32:152–156.
12. Daly EJ, Zimmerman JS, Donn PA, Galliher MJ. Psychophysiological treatment of migraine and tension headaches: A 12-month follow-up. Rehab Psych 1985; 30:3–10.
13. Blanchard EB, Appelbaum KA, Radnitz CL. A controlled evaluation of thermal biofeedback and thermal biofeedback combined with cognitive therapy in the treatment of vascular headache. J Consult Clin Psych 1990; 58:216–224.
14. Blanchard EB, Andrasik F, Evans DD, Neff DF, Appelbaum KA, Rodichok LD. Behavioral treatment of 250 chronic headache patients: A clinical replication series. Behav Ther 1985; 16:308–327.
15. Litt MD. Mediating factors in non-medical treatment for migraine headache: Toward an interactional model. J Psychosom Res 1986; 30:505–519.
16. Chapman SL. A review and clinical perspective on the use of EMG and thermal biofeedback for chronic headaches. Pain 1986; 27:1–43.
17. Blumenthal JA. Relaxation therapy, biofeedback, and behavioral medicine. Psychotherapy 1985; 22:516–530.
18. Sternbach RA. Psychological management of the headache patient. In: Diamond S, Dalessio DJ, eds. The Practicing Physician's Approach to Headache. 3rd ed. Washington, D.C.: Williams and Wilkins, 1982:159–165.
19. Olson RP. A long-term single-group follow-up study of biofeedback therapy with chronic medical and psychiatric patients. Biofeedback Self-Reg 1988; 13:331–346.
20. Reich BA. Non-invasive treatment of vascular and muscle contraction headache: A comparative longitudinal clinical study. Headache 1989; 29:34–41.
21. Libo LM, Arnold GE. Relaxation practice after biofeedback therapy: A long-term follow-up study of utilization and effectiveness. Biofeedback Self-Reg 1983; 8:217–227.

22. Lisspers J, Ost LG. Long-term follow-up of migraine treatment: Do the effects remain up to six years? Behav Res Ther 1990; 28:313–322.
23. Smith WB. Biofeedback and relaxation training: The effect on headache and associated symptoms. Headache 1987; 27:511–514.
24. Blanchard EB, Appelbaum KA, Guarnieri P, Morrill B. Five-year prospective follow-up on the treatment of chronic headache with biofeedback and/or relaxation. Headache 1987; 27:580–583.
25. Danskin DG, Crow MA. Biofeedback, an Introduction and Guide. Palo Alto, Calif.: Mayfield Publishing, 1981.
26. Green E, Green A. Beyond Biofeedback. Fort Wayne, Ind.: Knoll Publishing, 1977.
27. Blanchard EB, Morrill B, Wittrock DA, Scharff L. Hand temperature norms for headache, hypertension, and irritable bowel syndrome. Biofeedback Self-Reg 1989; 14:319–331.
28. Lacroix JM. Biofeedback and relaxation in the treatment of migraine headaches: Comparative effectiveness and physiological correlates. J Neurol Neurosurg Psych 1983; 46:525–532.
29. Falkenstein M, Hoormann J. Psychophysiological correlates of vasomotor self control mediated by biofeedback. J Psychophysiol 1987; 4:383–392.
30. Gauthier J, Lacroix R, Cote A, Doyon J. Biofeedback control of migraine headaches: A comparison of two approaches. Biofeedback Self-Reg 1985; 10:139–159.
31. Hoelscher TJ, Lichstein KL. Blood volume pulse biofeedback treatment of chronic cluster headache. Biofeedback Self-Reg 1983; 8:533–541.
32. Gauthier J, Doyon J, Lacroix R, Drolet M. Blood volume pulse biofeedback in the treatment of migraine headache: A controlled evaluation. Biofeedback Self-Reg 1983; 8:427–442.
33. Cram JR, Steger JC. EMG scanning in the diagnosis of chronic pain. Biofeedback Self-Reg 1983; 8:229–241.
34. Reading C. Psychophysiological reactivity in migraine following biofeedback. Headache 1984; 24:70–74.
35. Daly EJ, Donn PA, Galliher MJ, Zimmerman JS. Biofeedback applications of migraine and tension headaches: A double-blinded outcome study. Biofeedback Self-Reg 1983; 8:135–152.
36. Arena JG, Blanchard EB, Andrasik F, Appelbaum K, Myers PE. Psychophysiological comparisons of three kinds of headache subjects during and between headache states: Analysis of post-stress adaptation periods. J Psychosom Res 1985; 29:427–441.
37. Sargent J. Results of a controlled, experimental, outcome study of nondrug treatments for the control of migraine headaches. J Behav Med 1986; 9:291–323.
38. Billings RF. Differential efficacy of biofeedback in headache. Headache 1984; 24:211–215.
39. Weinman ML, Semchuck KM, Gaebe G. The effect of stressful life events on EMG biofeedback and relaxation in the treatment of anxiety. Biofeedback Self-Reg 1983; 8:191–205.

40. Middaugh SJ. On clinical efficacy: Why biofeedback does and does not work. Biofeedback Self-Reg 1990; 15:191–208.
41. Gamble EH, Elder ST. Multimodal biofeedback in the treatment of migraine. Biofeedback Self-Reg 1983; 8:383–392.
42. Weinman ML, Mathew RJ, Claghorn JL. A study of physician attitude on biofeedback. Biofeedback Self-Reg 1982; 7:89–98.
43. Mizener D, Thomas M, Billings RF. Cognitive changes of migraineurs receiving biofeedback training. Headache 1988; 28:339–343.
44. Holroyd KA, Penzien DB. Pharmacological versus non-pharmacological prophylaxis of recurrent migraine headache: A meta-analytic review of clinical trials. Pain 1990; 42:1–13.
45. Holroyd KA, Holm J, Penzien DB, Cordingley GE. Long-term maintenance of improvements achieved with (abortive) pharmacological and nonpharmacological treatments for migraine: Preliminary findings. Biofeedback Self-Reg 1989; 14:301–308.
46. Holroyd KA, Holm J, Hursey KG, Penzien DB. Recurrent vascular headache: Home-based behavioral treatment versus abortive pharmacological treatment. J Consult Clin Psych 1988; 56:218–223.
47. Stout MA. Homeostatic reconditioning in stress-related disorders: A preliminary study of migraine headaches. Psychotherapy 1985; 22:531–541.
48. Gallagher RM, Warner JB. Patient motivation in the treatment of migraine: A non-medicinal study. Headache 1984; 24:269–271.
49. Attanasio V, Andrasik F, Blanchard EB. Cognitive therapy and relaxation training in muscle contraction headache: Efficacy and cost-effectiveness. Headache 1987; 27:254–260.
50. Primavera JP, Kaiser RS. Non-pharmacological treatment of headache: Is less more? Headache 1992; 32:393–395.
51. Blanchard EB. Reduction in headache patients' medical expenses associated with biofeedback and relaxation treatments. Biofeedback Self-Reg 1985; 10:63–68.
52. Goldstein DS. Neurotransmitters and stress. Biofeedback Self-Reg 1990; 15:243–271.
53. Wolff HG. Headache. New York: Oxford University Press, 1963:399–431.
54. Lake AE. Behavioral treatment of headache: Practical applications. Update on Headache: American Association for Study of Headache, Scottsdale, Ariz., Jan 24–26, 1992.
55. Stewart WF, Lipton RB, Celentano DD, Reed ML. Prevalence of migraine headache in the United States: Relation to age, income, race, and other sociodemographic factors. JAMA 1992; 267:64–69.
56. Morrill B, Blanchard EB. Two studies on the potential mechanisms of action in thermal biofeedback treatment of vascular headache. Headache 1989; 29:169–176.
57. Diamond S, Montrose D. The value of biofeedback in the treatment of chronic headache: A four-year retrospective study. Headache 1984; 24:5–18.
58. Blanchard EB, Taylor AE, Dentinger MP. Preliminary results from the self-regulatory treatment of high-medication-consumption headache. Biofeedback Self-Reg 1992; 17:179–202.

59. Lake AE, Pingel JD. Brief versus extended relaxation: Relationship to improvement at follow-up in mixed headache patients. Med Psychother 1988; 1:119–129.
60. Gauthier J, Fradet C, Roberge C. The differential effects of biofeedback in the treatment of classical and common migraine. Headache 1988; 28:39–46.
61. Ellerton B, Klve H. MMPI patterns in chronic muscle pain, tension headache, and migraine. Cephalalgia 1987; 7:65–71.

18

Headache Specialists and Headache Clinics

Robert Smith

University of Cincinnati College of Medicine
Cincinnati, Ohio

It is now possible for primary care physicians to provide more effective care for headache patients than at any time in the past (1). It is essential to good primary care to know when to consult or refer a headache specialist.

HEADACHE SPECIALIZATION

Headache specialization is a relatively new field. There are increasing numbers of headache clinics and centers throughout the country. National and international headaches societies are actively stimulating interest in this field through journals and regular scientific meetings. A recent review (2) shows that growth in the headache field represents one of the fastest-growing areas in the neurosciences.

TREATMENT OR REFERRAL

Many factors influence whether the practitioner treats or refers a headache patient. These factors include the practitioner's level of comfort in dealing with headache patients and the ease with which patients can be referred locally. In more isolated communities, practitioners assume more responsibility for the care of their patients and refer less. Financial considerations—for example, lack of insurance coverage for specialty treatment—can also be a barrier.

Reasons for referring cases of headache include:

1. Inadequate physician comfort level in treating headache and/or patient request for referral
2. Uncertainty in diagnosis—fear of underlying pathology
3. Failure to respond to treatment
4. Chronic daily headache

Inadequate Physician Comfort Level in Treating Headache and/or Patient Request for Referral

Headaches are considered a trivial matter because so many headaches are mild or respond well to simple analgesics. This attitude toward headache is shared by some doctors. Studies show that many headache patients are unhappy because of this (3). Many cases of disabling headache are missed or misdiagnosed in practice (4), and the problem is aggravated by the increasing prevalence of migraine, which, according to the Centers for Disease Control and Prevention, has risen during the period 1980–1989 from 25.8 per thousand to 41 per thousand, an increase of nearly 60%. Inadequate care—real or perceived—results in many patient requests for referral.

Characteristic of many patients with chronic headache is the continuous changing from one physician to another, forever seeking a cure. Repeated treatment failure generates frustration and a request for treatment at the specialist level. Some practitioners provide the referral with relief, hoping that the specialist will not only provide treatment but also assume the ongoing care. This may not always be practical because of distance or the cost involved. The optimal arrangement is for the physician to refer for the purpose of guidance yet be willing to continue the needed long-term care. Here the primary care physician and the specialist play complementary roles.

There is no official register of headache specialists or headache clinics or centers. As the field develops, it should eventually mature into a recognized specialty with accredited training programs and treatment centers.

In the meantime, referrals will be made to those who by reputation have gained the confidence of their colleagues as experts in the field.

Uncertainty of Diagnosis

Most patients who seek medical help for headache consult a primary care physician (5). They do so either during an acute attack or between attacks when they need a prescription. In either circumstance, making an accurate headache diagnosis may not be easy. Ambiguities in headache classification add to the practitioner's problems.

The first attempt to clarify headache diagnosis was made by a National Institutes of Health ad hoc committee in 1966 (6), and their definitions became the standard for many years. Recently this classification has been criticized as being too imprecise and unclear, and leaving too much discretion to the physician making the diagnosis. In 1988 the International Headache Society (IHS) published a more detailed and explicit classification (7) listing over 125 different types of headache, face, and neck pains. Many of the conditions listed are very rare; primary care physicians are unlikely to see them. A recent primary care headache study involving many practices in the United States and Canada (8) reported that the IHS classification was too cumbersome for use in office practice. A more practical classification is necessary for daily use by busy practitioners.

Headaches represent about 2% of all primary care problems, amounting to over 10 million cases annually (9). Although the great bulk of these problems fall into a small group of frequently occurring headaches, within the scope of the primary care practitioner there is the ever-present threat of a hidden serious headache problem.

A Practical Headache Classification

A practical headache classification for primary care is to divide all headaches into primary or secondary types. This difference is important not only diagnostically but for patient management in general practice.

Primary headaches are benign recurring headaches that have no underlying pathology. These include migraine, tension-type headache, cluster headache, and rarer forms such as benign cough headache, ice-cream headache, and coital headache. These are fully described in other chapters and will not be dealt with here.

Secondary headaches are caused by underlying disease and may be a signal of dangerous pathology requiring immediate action by the primary care physician. Patients seen in primary care with headache should always be approached with secondary headache in mind. Further investigation or referral is clearly indicated if secondary headache cannot be firmly excluded. It is noteworthy that a patient with a correctly diagnosed primary headache may present with a superimposed secondary headache on a subsequent visit. Edmeads (10) has developed a helpful checklist for primary care physicians to exclude the likelihood of secondary headache:

1. All first headaches in patients over 50 years old. Primary headaches typically begin in younger patients and continue through middle age. A first headache in a patient over 50 may herald an intracranial lesion that requires investigation or referral.
2. Headache of extraordinary severity. The patient reporting "my worst headache ever" may be experiencing the severe pain of meningeal irritation due to a subarachnoid hemorrhage needing immediate investigation. Headache sufferers are quick to recognize change in their headache and report it as "not my usual headache."
3. Nuchal rigidity. A patient with severe migraine typically lies on the headache side curled in a fetal position. The patient who lies on the back and has a stiff neck may have meningitis or cerebral hemorrhage.
4. Onset of headache with exertion. This may occur due to increased intracranial pressure or cerebral hemorrhage.
5. Headache worsening under observation. When acute headache due to migraine is seen in the office or emergency room, the attack will usually have been under way for several hours and has probably reached a plateau. Headaches worsening under observation are probably caused by some progressive pathological process.
6. Decreased alertness or cognition. Headaches associated with these symptoms may be caused by abnormal processes interfering with cerebral function and require investigation or referral.
7. Abnormality in vital signs, including fever. Changes in blood pressure, temperature, and respiration associated with headache require investigation. Systemic illnesses such as colds or influenza frequently precipitate migraine in migraineurs.

Physical Examination to Exclude Secondary Headache

Although the history is most important in making a headache diagnosis, all headache patients should be physically examined. The following examination falls within the scope of primary care practice and can be carried out within the time usually allotted to a routine visit.

Cognitive State The patient who is alert, coherent, and behaving reasonably does not have impairment of cognition. This can be judged easily at the onset of the examination.

Vital Signs Temperature, blood pressure, pulse, and respiration are taken routinely. Abnormalities in these require further evaluation, and the relationship to the headache needs consideration.

Neck Nuchal rigidity, a cardinal sign for meningism, must always be looked for. Positive Kernig and Brudzinki signs will help to confirm the likelihood of underlying neurological pathology.

Cranial Nerves Examination of pupil size, light and accommodation reflexes, fundi and facial symmetry (for presence of nystagmus), and of the other cranial nerves will help screen for possible headache-related intracranial lesions.

Power Deltoids, handgrip, hip movements, and flexor and ankle dorsiflexion should be tested for motor power. Biceps tendon reflexes, knee jerks, and flexor responses should be tested, and the finger–nose test should be performed. The patient should be watched walking to test for gait abnormality. Abnormality in any of the above requires further investigation and calls for considering referral or consultation.

Radiodiagnosis in Primary Care

With the increased availability to primary care physicians of computed tomography (CT) scanning and magnetic resonance imaging (MRI), these diagnostic procedures are increasingly being used to investigate headaches. They are often performed as an alternative to referral. The yield of useful data from these procedures is very low. Because of the ever-present threat of serious disease, pressure from patients requesting these diagnostic procedures, and physicians' malpractice anxiety over the disastrous effect of missing a serious lesion, CT scans and MRI of the head will continue to be performed too frequently in the evaluation of headache.

A study involving 58 primary care practices in the United States and Canada on the use of CT scan for headache diagnosis showed that the investigation was carried out in 3% of all headache patients (8). The clinicians made careful selective use of the scans. Most were ordered because the clinician felt that a tumor (48.8%) or a subarachnoid hemorrhage (8.8%) might be present. Of the 293 reports reviewed, 14 (4.8%) indicated a significant lesion, two of which were false-positive. Forty-four (15%) noted incidental findings of no significance. Many of these were accompanied by hedging statements by the radiologist suggesting repeat testing, angiography, or MRI scans if "clinical findings indicated" such tests. The authors reported that these recommendations tended to delay treatment, increase the anxiety of patients, and raise the cost of treatment.

In a separate study of 624 headache patients seen in two emergency departments over a 13-month period, a CT scan was done in 145 (23.2%) of patients (11). In nine cases (6.2%) a relevant lesion was diagnosed. Although there was a sevenfold increase in CT scanning compared with the previous study, the diagnostic yield remained very low, increasing only from 4.8% to 6.2%. In the primary care study, one-half of patients with intracerebral lesions had no neurological abnormalities or headache. Guidelines for the use of imaging studies are presented in Table 1.

CT Scan in Primary Care

Should an acute subarachnoid hemorrhage be suspected, a CT scan without contrast is the preferred investigation and is able to identify

Table 1 Guidelines for the Use of Imaging Studies for Acute Headache in Primary Care Practice

---

CT or MRI indicated

When *any* of the following is present:
1. Unaccountable abnormality in vital signs
2. Decreased alertness or cognition
3. Onset with exertion
4. Worsening under observation
5. Nuchal rigidity
6. Focal neurological signs
7. First headache in patient over 50 years
8. "My worst headache ever."

CT or MRI not indicated

When *all* of the following are present:
1. Previous identical headaches
2. Normal vital signs
3. Alertness and cognition intact
4. Supple neck
5. No neurological signs
6. Improvement in headache without analgesics or abortive medications

---

Source: Based on Ref. 10.

85–90% of cases (12). It is speedier to perform than an MRI, which may be important if the patient is unstable. A CT scan is more sensitive in detecting blood in the first several hours of subarachnoid hemorrhage and is less costly (13). Both CT scan and MRI can reveal hydrocephalus and most lesions large enough to produce headache as a result of increased intracranial pressure (14). Lumbar puncture will detect meningitis as well as the 10–15% of subarachnoid hemorrhages missed in imaging. It is indicated only if there are no focal neurological signs or papilledema suggesting a mass lesion. A sedimentation rate should be determined to exclude giant-cell arteritis in the older patient with headaches and tenderness over the temporal artery.

Magnetic Resonance Imaging

MRI is used increasingly in diagnosing central nervous system disorders (15). Its high cost requires very careful selection for its appropriate use. MRI provides better soft-tissue contrast than plain radiography or CT. CT scans use iodine contrast material whereas MRI contrast media contain magnetically active substance such as gadolinium, a rare-earth metal with excellent biodistribution in the tissues and a better margin of safety than iodine contrast.

The MRI is superior to the CT scan in detecting smaller lesions, especially those in the brain stem and cerebellum. If vascular lesions such as aneurysms are suspected, an MRI can be performed in conjunction with an MR angiogram for vascular visualization, avoiding the need for vascular catheterization.

Because of the magnetic basis of the method, it should not be used in patients with cardiac pacemakers, implanted neurotransmitters, cochlear implants, metal in the eye, and ferromagnetic intracranial aneurysm clips, which might be displaced by the magnetic field.

Failure to Respond to Treatment

It is not uncommon for patients with primary headache to experience recurrent periods of increased frequency of headaches although still maintaining previously effective treatment regimens. The reason for this is unclear; it may be due to the nature of the headache condition itself or to environmental or psychophysiological changes. An increase in the intensity and frequency of headaches, developing into chronic daily headaches, is a major reason for headache referral.

Chronic Daily Headache

The IHS classifies chronic daily headache as chronic tension-type headache present for at least 15 days a month for at least 6 months. The headache is usually pressing/tightening in quality, mild or moderate in severity, and bilateral, and does not worsen with routine physical activity. Nausea, photophobia, and phonophobia may occur.

A more severe chronic daily headache with many of the features of chronic tension headache may develop in patients who have migraine. The daily headache periodically becomes severe and indistinguishable from an acute migraine with nausea. Mathew et al. (15) call this condition "transformed" or "evolutive" migraine caused by headache rebound associated with analgesic abuse.

The condition should be suspected when there is overuse of headache medications for long periods of time. Use of 100 or more analgesics a month signals overuse, but any quantity of daily analgesic accompanying the complaint of chronic daily headache requires careful review by the physician. Use of combination analgesics containing barbiturate sedatives or ergotamine preparations more often than three times a week for long periods is an indication of drug overuse. Effectiveness of preventive medication is nullified and, when attempts are made to stop the medication, withdrawal symptoms (nausea, vomiting, and headache closely mimicking migraine) prompt the patient to restart the medication. It has been shown that nonnarcotic over-the-counter analgesics, if overused, can also produce this condition (16). These patients complain "I've tried everything and nothing works." This not unfamiliar statement in primary care practice frequently results in referral.

To prevent chronic daily headache, all medications should be carefully prescribed and monitored. Prescribing records should be strictly maintained, and telephone requests for medication should be discouraged and approved only after a check has been made to ensure that the request falls within the agreed-upon prescribing limits.

In treating chronic daily headache on an outpatient basis, Mathew recommends cessation of all offending analgesic/sedative drugs and replacing them with valproic acid (Depakote 1000 mg daily) and nonsteroidal analgesics.

Controlling analgesic use in primary care is not always an easy matter. If control cannot be achieved on an outpatient basis, it may be necessary to admit these patients to hospital for treatment, as advocated by Raskin (17). He has shown that intravenous dihydroergotamine (DHE-45 0.5–1.0 mg, with intravenous metoclopramide given beforehand to reduce nausea) at

8-hour intervals for 4–7 days is effective. Before admission, patients are pretreated for 2 weeks with valproic acid to counteract withdrawal effects of the analgesics. During hospitalization, patients require counseling regarding drug overuse. Silberstein et al. (18) have reported favorably on this method in a study involving 300 patients with refractory headache. Not all patients respond favorably, and some patients revert to analgesics overuse. In such cases, Saper (19) advocates referral for more prolonged treatment in specialized behavior-modification inpatient units.

THE MULTIDISCIPLINARY APPROACH TO REFRACTORY HEADACHE

Multidisciplinary programs for the treatment of refractory headache are highly structured and require a 2–3 week hospitalization or intense out-patient program. Many programs include patients suffering from chronic pain due to causes other than headache.

Admission to such a program requires an initial evaluation by a multi-disciplinary team so that the potential for progress can be determined beforehand. It is wise to ensure beforehand that insurance carriers, worker's compensation, and/or employers will support the approach being taken. At the initial evaluation, the program is fully explained to the patient, who is usually required to sign a consent form so that there is no misunderstanding regarding the nature of the program and the roles to be played by the patient and the treatment team. Family members are involved in this initial preparation and are encouraged to be supportive.

Although no promises are made to rid the patient entirely of the headache, important gains can be made that will make the pain and discomfort more tolerable. With education and guidance by the team of specialists, a sense of real hope and direction is generated, and dependence on narcotic or other medication is eliminated. As a result of such programs, many individuals whose lives were changed by the headache learn to return to a socially and economically effective level of functioning.

Patients are admitted in small treatment groups. The program is continuous on a daily basis, throughout the day 5 days a week and for several hours on weekends. Patients are responsible for their individual schedules, which are charted daily. Working individually and in small groups, they participate in relaxation techniques, including biofeedback, deep-breathing exercises, hypnosis, stress management, assertiveness-training, and personal goal management. Special attention is paid to relapse prevention with follow-up visits.

Occasionally a patient resists this intensive program and is asked to leave. In general, though, the success rate is high, and even patients with intractable long-standing headaches report improvements in their lives and in coping with the pain.

The bonding within the group, through the sharing of pain and their gradual improvement as they progress through the program, creates a form of therapeutic networking, which has a positive effect on the individual members of the group.

Ideally, the primary care physician remains a key player in such programs. Patients should not feel isolated from their long-term source of care. Contact between the therapeutic team and the primary care physician should be maintained to generate the necessary mutual respect and understanding of each other's role necessary in complex treatments. This is particularly important in relation to future prescribing of medication. Much useful work can be undone if patients are allowed to resume their previous drug-taking habits after completing the programs.

The number of controlled studies demonstrating the value of the behavioral approach to controlling intractable headache is increasing (20). The combined medical and behavioral approach offers new hope for these patients.

Diagnostic skill, knowledge of treatment options, and sound judgment in making referrals are the hallmarks of good primary care practice. Appreciation of the role played by the primary care physician and sensitivity to the problems of a busy practice are the signs of a good specialist. Referral is a two-way process, and when it works well the patient is the greatest beneficiary.

SUMMARY

The primary care physician's first duties are to take a history, examine the patient thoroughly, and decide whether there is a possibility of a significant secondary headache disorder. If secondary headache is suspected, then radiologic and/or specialist consultation may be indicated. Chronic daily headaches are often maintained by pharmacological measures initiated to treat headache and the condition may go unrecognized if the diagnosis is not kept in mind. Intensive multidisciplinary treatment programs may be necessary to adequately manage the needs of such patients.

REFERENCES

1. Smith R. Headaches: An area of special responsibility for family practice. J Fam Pract 1993; 37(2):126–127.

2. Smith R. The Migraine Trust: headache research 1965-1990. In: Rose FC, ed. New Advances in Headache Research. London: Smith-Gordon, 1989; 1:1–10.
3. Klassen AC, Berman M. Medical care for headache: a consumer survey. Cephalalgia 1991; 11(suppl):85–86.
4. Lipton RB, Stewart WF, Celentano DC, Reed ML. Undiagnosed migraine headaches: a comparison of symptom-based and reported physician diagnosis. Cephalalgia 1991; 11(suppl):89–90.
5. Linet MS, Stewart WF, Celentano DD, Ziegler D, Sprecher M. An epidemiologic study of headache among adolescents and young adults. JAMA 1989; 261:2211–2216.
6. Ad Hoc Committee on Classification of Headache. Classification of headache. JAMA 1962; 179:717–718.
7. Headache Classification Committee of the International Headache Society. Classification and diagnostic criteria for all headache disorders, cranial neuralgias and facial pain. Cephalalgia 1988; 8(suppl 7):1–96.
8. Becker LA, Green LA, Beaufait D, Kirk J, Froom J. Use of CT scans for the investigation of headache: a report from ASPN. Part 1. J Fam Pract 1993; 37:129–134.
9. Stewart WF, Lipton RB, Celentano DD, Reed ML. Prevalence of migraine headache in the United States. JAMA 1992; 267:64–69.
10. Edmeads J. Challenges in the diagnosis of acute headache. Headache 1990; 30(suppl):537–540.
11. Singal BM, Succop PA, Huber D. The outcome of patients treated for headache in the Emergency Department. In press.
12. Prager M, Mikulis DJ. The radiology of headache. Med Clin North Am 1991; 75(3):525–544.
13. Mitchell CS, Osborn RE, Gross Kreutz SR. Computed tomography in the headache patient. Headache 1993; 33:82–86.
14. Weingarten S, Kleinman M, Elperin EB. The effectiveness of cerebral imaging in the diagnosis of chronic headache. Arch Intern Med 1992; 152:2457–2462.
15. Matthew NT, Reuveni U, Perez F. Transformed or evolutive migraine. Headache 1987; 27:102–106.
16. Kudrow L. Paradoxical effects of frequent analgesic use. Adv Neurol 1982; 33:335–341.
17. Raskin NH. Repetitive intravenous dihydroergotamine as therapy for intractable migraine. Neurology 1986; 36:995–997.
18. Silberstein SD, Schulman EA, Hopkins MM. Repetitive intravenous DHE in the treatment of refractory headache. Headache 1990; 30:334–339.
19. Saper JR. Drug treatment of headache: changing concepts and treatment strategies. Sem Neurol 1981; 7:178–191.
20. Psychological aspects. 5th International Headache Congress. Cephalalgia 1991; 11(suppl):296–312.

19

Future Developments in Headache Therapy

Roger K. Cady

Shealy Institute for Comprehensive Health Care
Springfield, Missouri

Donna L. Gutterman

Glaxo Inc. Research Institute
Research Triangle Park, North Carolina

INTRODUCTION

From evil spirits and trepanation to intricate biochemical models and dreams of the perfect drug, headache has offered much to the study of medicine! Many great minds have offered insights and observations in hopes of freeing mankind from this disease.

Over a century ago, Thomas Willis opened the door to rational therapy when he offered his brilliant clinical insights and proposed the vascular theory of migraine. This theory, elaborated by Wolfe and Graham through scientific methodology, became the standard by which headache was measured for the next 50 years. In 1908 Paul Ehrlich, corecipient of the

Nobel Prize for medicine in physiology, postulated the existence of cell receptors, and that their interaction with specific agents was a mechanism for disease. Ehrlich's work laid the foundation for receptor biochemistry, launching the odyssey of pharmacological treatment of disease—his concept of "magic bullets" regulating cellular function remains central to medicine today.

Technological advancements now allow scientists to study the very molecular underpinnings of human disease. Refinements of pathophysiological mechanisms involved in headache are occurring at an extraordinarily rapid pace. One can only stand in awe of the technological wizardry that elaborates the intricate receptor mechanisms being offered as explanations of headache. Receptor biochemists now define human receptors by their amino acid sequence and function, and genetically clone specific receptors for study. Specific therapeutic intervention from these endeavors is already available to patients. Despite these marvelous advancements, the quest to understand headache is far from complete. With each answer, more questions emerge. The possibilities for future research appear endless.

DIAGNOSIS

Headache remains one of the few disorders that has no confirmatory diagnostic test and relies for diagnosis on a good history and examination. The International Headache Society (IHS) has been instrumental in defining migraine and other headache disorders, but the need for a confirmatory laboratory test remains paramount. Researchers have explored the multiple biochemical pathways searching for such a marker but, to date no defined, clinically useful test exists.

Secondary headaches are rare but may be catastrophic, and they require rapid differentiation from benign headache disorders. This continues to be a source of concern to the clinician. A simple, cost-effective, diagnostic test to differentiate primary and secondary headache disorders is clearly needed.

Further, with respect to the benign headache disorders, the tightly defined clinical criteria of IHS do not adequately differentiate the subtle boundaries of headache diagnoses. Diagnostic tests to distinguish relevant primary headache disorders would allow clinicians to more effectively target therapy and ease the diagnostic burden of the practicing physician.

Finally, there is the ever-present concern of the drug-seeking patient. How can one ever be sure that someone is suffering a migraine? The drug-seeking patient is a common problem in emergency medicine, when the clinician may not be familiar with the patient, and reliable diagnostic tests are needed to differentiate this disease from headache.

TREATMENT

Acute

The development of sumatriptan has been heralded by many as a major breakthrough for the acute treatment of migraine. It is efficacious and offers relief from disabling migraine to millions of sufferers. The advent of sumatriptan has shifted the therapeutics of acute management to the patient.

However, 20–30% of migraineurs do not experience adequate response to sumatriptan. Nor do all headaches, even in the responsive patient, respond completely to this drug. Extracranial vessels appear devoid of $5\text{-}HT_1$-like receptors, suggesting that a therapeutic differentiation between extracranial and intracranial migraine is responsible for variations in response. Further, only a minority of patients experience an abortive response to a single injection of sumatriptan. Perhaps future drugs with more specific receptor specificity or longer duration of action at the $5\text{-}HT_1$ receptor will be more efficacious.

Specific therapeutic interventions at other receptor sites have yet to be explored. The presence of other 5-HT receptors, α-2 receptors, μ-opioid receptors, and somatostatin receptors, which are also found in the trigeminal vascular system, offer possibilities for future therapy. Inflammatory peptides such as substance P, neurokinin A, and calcitonin gene–related peptide are thought to be integral aspects in the genesis of migraine pain. The possibility of specific inhibitors of these peptides offers potential avenues of therapy. Although there are undoubtedly many receptor mechanisms yet to be discovered, the perfect "magic bullet" that can relieve migraine in all patients without producing adverse effects remains to be found.

Prophylaxis

Many medications are available for the prophylactic treatment of migraine. Most of these, discovered fortuitously on clinical grounds, are poorly understood. The mechanism by which prophylactic agents protect migraineurs requires further elaboration. The only drug specifically for migraine prophylaxis is methysergide, and, while often effective, it has been used cautiously by physicians because of its rare but significant potential side effects. Researchers have proposed that many prophylactic drugs act by antagonizing the 5-HT$_2$ receptor system. To date, no new specific antagonists for this site have been developed for clinical use. Almost all the prophylactic medications in current use frequently cause significant side effects with long-term use. Problems such as weight gain, lethargy, impotence, sedation, and subtle disturbances in the central nervous system are often ignored by physicians but are of concern to patients. Often, patients require several different prophylactic drugs, which compounds potential side effects. Clearly, there is a need to develop specific efficacious prophylactic therapies for migraine that have none of these adverse outcomes.

With the development of better acute therapies, the current indications for using prophylactic medications may change. When acute therapy is successful, the fear and anxiety of future migraine attacks diminish, and the frequency of migraine may decrease as well. Indications for prophylactic therapy will need to be reassessed in light of these advances.

Pharmacologically Maintained Headaches

Perhaps one of the most important advances in migraine has been the recognition that daily use of many symptomatic medications can transform episodic migraine into daily headache. The mechanism(s) by which this occurs, and the reason migraineurs are susceptible, are still subjects of scientific scrutiny. Educating patients and physicians about treatment strategies that minimize this possibility will decrease morbidity of this iatrogenic disease. Treatment medications with low risk of migraine transformation have yet to be completely defined.

Behavioral Therapy

Nowhere is the relationship to pathophysiology of headache as misunderstood as in behavioral therapies, and nowhere is there greater potential to safely advance migraine therapy. How do clinicians provide appropriate education and ensure compliance with therapy? Behavioral therapy has demonstrated therapeutic value in many other chronic conditions. However, in the limited time for which physicians encounter patients in the primary-care setting, how can behavioral dynamics be initiated, and which patients are likely to benefit from them? Models of health-care delivery that include behavioral therapy need to be defined and expanded.

Outcome-based research with biofeedback has demonstrated its efficacy; nonetheless it is underutilized by primary-care physicians. Even though the mechanisms of biofeedback are still unclear, future partnerships between physician and psychologist can approach headache patients more holistically and address not only headache but the patier.t's response to secondary complications. Psychology should be integrated into medical care early in the headache disease process rather than as a last resort. Behavioral intervention offered in this manner may reduce migraine morbidity and lessen the risk of developing migraine-associated disorders such as depression.

Considerable research into physiological mechanisms explaining behavioral therapy remains to be done. If pain is memory, then chronic headache should be viewed as a centrally maintained pain disease. How is it that perception of pain exists beyond stimulation of nociceptive pathways? Why, in our most difficult chronic headache patients, does minor perturbation of pain pathways lead to devastating migraine? Mechanisms involving c-phos, NMDA receptors, and the endogenous opioid system may provide answers in the future. Researchers will likely develop drugs to interact with these systems, and explore the role of therapies such as biofeedback on these pain-memory systems. It is observed clinically, as well as in the laboratory, that as headaches become more chronic, the degree of stimulation required to disrupt the protective threshold mechanisms diminishes. Biofeedback and cognitive therapies have been shown to decrease the frequency of headaches, but the mechanism by which they protect the headache threshold is poorly understood.

Serotonin

Serotonin is involved in many physiological responses. Many subclasses of serotonin receptor have now been described, but their role in disease is only beginning to be hypothesized. The potential to understand the interrelationship of these diseases and find specific treatment for them is enormous. Are disorders such as migraine early clinical markers for a larger spectrum of serotonergic dysfunction? Epidemiological studies suggest that, over time, migraine becomes associated with many other medical conditions. Would early interventions and rational therapies that manipulate serotonin metabolism protect patients from future disease? If serotonin, CGRP, and other neurotransmitters are shown to be involved in fibromyalgia, etc., then headache may be reframed into one of a constellation of problems rather than a discrete entity. Future pharmacological advancement and lifestyle adjustment may ultimately help patients to maintain health rather than disrupt disease.

MEDICAL MANAGEMENT MODELS

Perhaps one of the most important fundamental changes in headache therapy comes with the recognition that headache is a chronic disorder. Recent epidemiological data suggest that there is a natural history to headache and that physicians must change the emphasis from managing recurrent acute attacks to managing a chronic disease state. Obvious steps in this management would include early screening; quality patient education; the development of concise, understandable, rational treatment plans; and long-term management. While relief of acute migraine is available for most patients, it is not likely to be cured; its impact does not end with the resolution of the acute attack. Patients need to be educated in this regard and encouraged to participate with their physician and/or other health-care professionals in managing the multiple dynamics of this disease.

MEDICAL–SOCIAL CONCERNS

One of the most important developments in clinical research today is the concept of quality of life as an endpoint. The endpoint for successful therapy of migraine is ambiguous. Traditionally, it has been defined as the resolution of headache pain, but clearly the consequences of migraine extend beyond the disability of an acute attack. It is essential to design therapeutic interventions that affect the patient's overall lifestyle, day in and day out. Does adequate management of acute attacks allow people to live more productive lives? If so, how do we measure the effectiveness of this adequate management? In many diseases, the endpoint for adequate management is clearly defined catastrophic pathology. This is not the case in headache, necessitating this shift in emphasis of medical outcome management. Much of the epidemiological data already gathered have focused on economic concerns, direct and indirect costs, and other parameters generated by migraine, but little emphasis has been given to whether therapies and treatments actually change these outcomes. Quality-of-life issues will be increasingly important in the future as justification for specific therapeutic interventions. Exactly what defines quality of life and how to study the impact of therapies on quality of life remain to be defined.

POLITICAL–SOCIAL CONCERNS

Unquestionably the practice of medicine is changing. The concept of medical care centering on the physician–patient relationship is affected by many external forces. Directing this changing relationship are third-party payers, hospital administrators, and the government. Often their focus of concern is quite different from that of the physician or the patient. One likely change is that many approaches will be far more generic to a general population, which could negatively affect care for headache patients. Social myths and biases about headache and its sufferers abound in our culture, and so it is often not deemed worthy of aggressive treatment and management. These feelings are shared by many third-party payers. Those removed from the plight of the suffering patient may support financial constraints as a means of managing an "annoyance" such as headache. It will be up to physicians—in particular, primary-care physicians, who will be the "gatekeepers" in the new hierarchy—to justify adequate treatment and humanly address the suffering of the headache patient.

FUTURE CLINICAL RESEARCH

Much of the research done in the United States, both clinically and scientifically, is ultimately funded by the pharmaceutical industry with the hope of developing therapies that will be profitable. It is, in fact, those profits that are largely responsible for many of the scientific, clinical, and educational advances going on in medicine today. Clearly there needs to be a responsible partnership among the medical, pharmaceutical, and third-party industries. The threat of overregulation leading to declining research funding and medical education is significant. If cost becomes the driving concern of medical care, medical advancement as we know it may be irrevocably changed. It will be crucial that both physicians and representatives of the pharmaceutical industry behave responsibly in the changing social structure facing medicine today. It is equally essential that we be advocates of quality in patient care and maintain the needs of the patient at the center of health reform.

Currently the cost of developing a new drug can exceed $300 million, and the cost continues to escalate. The pharmaceutical industry is under increasing regulation, and their role in funding research may change. Future funding may need to come from the profits of the insurance industry or other profitable third-party systems. It is essential that all concerned in medicine today strive to be advocates for responsible progress in medicine.

Appendix

International Headache Society Classification Criteria

1. MIGRAINE

Comment: If a patient fulfils criteria for more than one type of migraine all types should receive a diagnosis. This is in contrast to tension-type headache and cluster headache where the different types at any given time are mutually exclusive. If migraine occurs for the first time in close temporal relation to one of the disorders listed in groups 5–11 code to that group. If migraine is aggravated by 100 per cent or more (headache days) in close temporal relation to one of the disorders listed in groups 5–11, this may be mentioned in parentheses, but the patient is still coded to group 1.

The terms common migraine and classic or classical migraine have been widely confused and convey no information. Therefore, they have been replaced by "migraine without aura" and "migraine with aura." The aura is the complex of focal neurological symptoms which initiates or accompanies an attack. Most patients will exclusively have attacks without aura. It seems that patients who have frequent attacks with aura

Reprinted from Headache Classification Committee, International Headache Society, Classification and diagnostic criteria for headache disorders, cranial neuralgias, and facial pain, Cephalalgia 1988; 8(suppl 7):19–42.

would usually also have attacks without aura (classify 1.2 and 1.1). Premonitory symptoms occur hours to a day or two before a migraine attack (with aura or without aura). They usually consist of hyperactivity, hypoactivity, depression, craving for special foods, repetitive yawning and similar atypical symptoms. The term prodromes has been used with different meanings, most often synonymous with aura. It should therefore not be used and the same is true of the ambiguous term "warning symptoms."

1.1 Migraine Without Aura

Previously used terms: Common migraine, hemicrania simplex.
Description: Idiopathic, recurring headache disorder manifesting in attacks lasting 4–72 hours. Typical characteristics of headache are unilateral location, pulsating quality, moderate or severe intensity, aggravation by routine physical activity, and association with nausea, photo- and phonophobia.
Diagnostic criteria:

A. At least 5 attacks fulfilling B–D.
B. Headache attacks lasting 4–72 hours* (untreated or unsuccessfully treated).
C. Headache has at least two of the following characteristics:
   1. Unilateral location
   2. Pulsating quality
   3. Moderate or severe intensity (inhibits or prohibits daily activities)
   4. Aggravation by walking stairs or similar routine physical activity
D. During headache at least one of the following:
   1. Nausea and/or vomiting
   2. Photophobia and phonophobia
E. At least one of the following:
   1. History and physical and neurological examinations do not suggest one of the disorders listed in groups 5–11
   2. History and/or physical and/or neurological examinations do suggest such disorder, but it is ruled out by appropriate investigations
   3. Such disorder is present, but migraine attacks do not occur for the first time in close temporal relation to the disorder

---

* In children below age 15, attacks may last 2–48 hours. If the patient falls asleep and wakes up without migraine, duration of attack is until time of awakening.

Comment: The separation of migraine without aura from episodic tension-type headache may be difficult. Therefore at least 5 attacks are required. Patients rarely seek a doctor before they have had many attacks, and this requirement therefore probably excludes very few who should be coded 1.7. The mechanisms of the attack are as yet poorly understood. Regional cerebral blood flow remains normal or is perhaps slightly increased during an attack. Changes in blood composition and platelet function initiated endogenously or by environmental influences may play a triggering role. The pathophysiological process of the attack is presumed to occur in the brain, which via the trigemino-vascular and other systems interacts with intra- and extracranial vasculature and perivascular spaces. This form of migraine accounts for most cases debilitated by migraine.

Migraine without aura may occur almost exclusively at a particular time of the menstrual cycle—so-called menstrual migraine. Generally accepted criteria for this entity are not available. It seems reasonable to demand that 90 per cent of attacks should occur between two days before menses and the last day of menses, but further epidemiological knowledge is needed.

1.2 Migraine with Aura*

Previously used terms: Classic migraine, classical migraine; ophthalmic, hemiparesthetic, hemiplegic or aphasic migraine; migraine accompagnée; complicated migraine.

Description: Idiopathic, recurring disorder manifesting with attacks of neurological symptoms unequivocally localizable to cerebral cortex or brain stem, usually gradually developed over 5–20 minutes and usually lasting less than 60 minutes. Headache, nausea and/or photophobia usually follow neurological aura symptoms directly or after a free interval of less than an hour. The headache usually lasts 4–72 hours, but may be completely absent (1.2.5).

Diagnostic criteria:

A. At least 2 attacks fulfilling B.
B. At least 3 of the following 4 characteristics:
   1. One or more fully reversible aura symptoms indicating focal cerebral cortical and/or brain stem dysfunction.
   2. At least one aura symptom develops gradually over more than 4 minutes or 2 or more symptoms occur in succession.

---

*
Aura as herein used does not necessarily imply that it precedes the headache, nor does it imply any relationship with epilepsy.

3. No aura symptom lasts more than 60 minutes. If more than one aura symptom is present, accepted duration is proportionally increased.

4. Headache follows aura with a free interval of less than 60 minutes. (It may also begin before or simultaneously with the aura.)

C. At least one of the following:
   1. History and physical and neurological examinations do not suggest one of the disorders listed in groups 5–11
   2. History and/or physical and/or neurological examinations do suggest such disorder, but it is ruled out by appropriate investigations
   3. Such disorder is present, but migraine attacks do not occur for the first time in close temporal relation to the disorder

Comment: Before or simultaneously with onset of aura symptoms, regional cerebral blood flow is decreased corresponding to the clinically affected area and often including an even wider area. Blood flow reduction usually starts posteriorly and spreads anteriorly. It is above or at the ischemic threshold, but not infrequently below it. After one to several hours, gradual transition into hyperemia occurs in the same region. It has been reported that hyperemia is not related to headache, which usually begins during ischemia, and may disappear during hyperemia. Cortical arteriolar vasospasm and/or spreading depression of Leao have been implied. Relationship to the headache phase and mechanisms of the headache phase are uncertain (see comment to 1.1). The cerebral blood flow changes are not fully studied in all the subforms, but for several (1.2.1, 1.2.2, 1.2.3 and 1.2.5) there seems to be only quantitative differences. Systematic studies have demonstrated that most patients with visual auras occasionally have symptoms in the extremities. Conversely, patients with symptoms in the extremities virtually always also suffer visual aura symptoms. A distinction between ophthalmic migraine and hemiparesthetic/hemiparetic migraine is therefore probably artificial and is not recognized in this classification.

1.2.1 Migraine with Typical Aura

Previously used terms: Ophthalmic, hemiparesthetic, hemiparetic, hemiplegic, or aphasic migraine; migraine accompagnée.
Description: Migraine with an aura consisting of homonymous visual disturbances, hemisensory symptoms, hemiparesis or dysphasia or combinations thereof. Gradual development, duration under 1 hour and complete reversibility characterize the aura which is associated with headache.
Diagnostic criteria:

A. Fulfils criteria for 1.2 including all four criteria under B.

B. One or more aura symptoms of the following types:
 1. Homonymous visual disturbance
 2. Unilateral paresthesias and/or numbness
 3. Unilateral weakness
 4. Aphasia or unclassifiable speech difficulty

Comment: This is the commonest form of migraine with aura, and the diagnosis is evident after a careful history alone. Visual aura is most common, usually as a fortification spectrum i.e. a star shaped figure near the point of fixation gradually spreading right or left and assuming a laterally convex shape with angulated scintillating edge, leaving a variable degree of absolute or relative scotoma in its wake. In other cases it is a scotoma without positive phenomena which often is perceived as being of acute onset, but on scrutiny enlarges gradually. Next in frequency are sensory disturbances in the form of pins and needles moving slowly from the point of origin and affecting a greater or smaller part of the one side of the body and face. Numbness occurs in its wake, but numbness may also be the only symptom. Less frequent are speech disturbances, usually dysphasia but often hard to categorize, and unilateral weakness. Symptoms usually follow one another in succession beginning with visual, followed by sensory symptoms, dysphasia and weakness, but the reverse and other orders have been noted. Patients often find it hard to describe their symptoms in which case they should be instructed how to time and record their symptoms. After such prospective observation the clinical picture often becomes more clear. Common mistakes are incorrectly reported lateralization of headache, report of sudden onset when it is gradual, of monocular visual disturbances which are homonymous, as well as incorrect duration of aura.

1.2.2 Migraine with Prolonged Aura

Previously used terms: Complicated migraine, hemiplegic migraine.
Description: Migraine with one or more aura symptoms lasting more than 60 minutes and less than a week. Neuroimaging is normal.
Diagnostic criteria:

A. Fulfils criteria for 1.2, but at least one symptom lasts more than 60 minutes and ≤ 7 days. If neuroimaging reveals relevant ischemic lesion, code 1.6.2 migrainous infarction regardless of symptom duration.

Comment: Rare patients have only this form. The majority who experience prolonged aura have it rarely and intermingled with much more frequent attacks of typical aura. Prolonged acute onset aura is difficult to separate from TIA or small strokes and not sufficiently validated.

1.2.3   Familial Hemiplegic Migraine

Description: Migraine with aura including hemiparesis and where at least one first-degree relative has identical attacks.
Diagnostic criteria:

A.   Fulfils criteria for 1.2.
B.   The aura includes some degree of hemiparesis and may be prolonged.
C.   At least one first-degree relative has identical attacks.

Comment: This disorder probably has the same pathophysiology as migraine with typical aura. The reason for still keeping it separate is that families have been described where attacks are strikingly identical and sometimes long lasting. The term familial hemiplegic migraine has been abused since in most families different forms of migraine occur, and most patients with hemiplegic attacks have these intermingled with more frequent attacks of migraine without hemiparesis.

1.2.4   Basilar Migraine

Previously used terms: Basilar artery migraine, Bickerstaff's migraine, syncopal migraine.
Description: Migraine with aura symptoms clearly originating from the brain stem or from both occipital lobes.
Diagnostic criteria:

A.   Fulfils criteria for 1.2.
B.   Two or more aura symptoms of the following types:
Visual symptoms in both the temporal and nasal fields of both eyes
Dysarthria
Vertigo
Tinnitus
Decreased hearing
Double vision
Ataxia
Bilateral paresthesias
Bilateral pareses
Decreased level of consciousness

Comment: Many of the symptoms listed under diagnostic criteria are subject to misinterpretation as they may occur with anxiety and hyperventilation.

Originally the term basilar artery migraine was used, but since spasm of the basilar artery may not be the mechanism of the attacks, the term basilar migraine should be preferred. Many cases have basilar attacks intermingled with attacks with typical aura. Basilar attacks are mostly seen in young adults.

1.2.5 Migraine Aura Without Headache

Previously used terms: Migraine equivalents, acephalgic migraine.
Description: Migrainous aura unaccompanied by headache.
Diagnostic criteria:

A. Fulfils criteria for 1.2.
B. No headache.

Comment: It is common for migraine with aura that headache occasionally is absent. As patients get older, headache may disappear completely even if auras continue. It is less common to have always suffered exclusively from migraine aura without headache. When the onset occurs after the age of forty and for other reasons the distinction between this entity and thromboembolic transient ischemic attacks may be difficult and require extensive investigation. Acute onset aura without headache is not sufficiently validated.

1.2.6 Migraine with Acute Onset Aura

Description: Migraine with aura developing fully in less than 5 minutes.
Diagnostic criteria:

A. Fulfils criteria for 1.2.
B. Neurological symptoms develop within 4 minutes.
C. Headache lasts 4–72 hours (untreated or unsuccessfully treated).
D. Headache has at least two of the following characteristics:
   1. Unilateral location
   2. Pulsating quality
   3. Moderate or severe intensity (inhibits or prohibits daily activities)
   4. Aggravation by walking stairs or similar routine physical activity
E. During headache at least one of the following:
   1. Nausea and/or vomiting
   2. Photophobia and phonophobia
F. Thromboembolic TIA and other intracranial lesion ruled out by appropriate investigations.

Comment: Inaccurate history is the most common explanation of acute onset aura. Acute onset should be confirmed by repeated close questioning and preferably by prospective observation. Presence of a typical headache phase is required and the diagnosis is supported by previous migraine attacks of other type or a strong family history. Extensive investigations are usually necessary to rule out thromboembolic TIA.

1.3 Ophthalmoplegic Migraine

Description: Repeated attacks of headache associated with paresis of one or more ocular cranial nerves in the absence of demonstrable intracranial lesion.
Diagnostic criteria:

A. At least 2 attacks fulfilling B.
B. Headache overlapping with paresis of one or more of cranial nerves III, IV, and VI.
C. Parasellar lesion ruled out by appropriate investigations.

Comment: Whether ophthalmoplegic migraine in fact has anything to do with migraine is uncertain since the headache often lasts for a week or more. Association with other forms of migraine has often been noted, but a relationship to the Tolosa-Hunt syndrome has also been suggested. The condition is extremely rare.

1.4 Retinal Migraine

Description: Repeated attacks of monocular scotoma or blindness lasting less than an hour and associated with headache. Ocular or structural vascular disorder must be ruled out.
Diagnostic criteria:

A. At least 2 attacks fulfilling B–C.
B. Fully reversible monocular scotoma or blindness lasting less than 60 minutes and confirmed by examination during attack or (after proper instruction) by patient's drawing of monocular field defect during an attack.
C. Headache follows visual symptoms with a free interval of less than 60 minutes, but may precede them.
D. Normal ophthalmological examination outside of attack. Embolism ruled out by appropriate investigations.

Comment: The monocular nature of the visual disturbances has been documented in only a few cases. Some cases without headache have been reported, but their migrainous nature cannot be ascertained.

1.5 Childhood Periodic Syndromes That May Be Precursors to or Associated with Migraine

Previously used terms: Migraine equivalents.
Comment: It is not possible to propose criteria for delineation of the multiple heterogeneous and undefined disorders comprised under the terms

periodic syndromes, abdominal migraine and cyclical vomiting, and it is unlikely that any progress will be made in this uncertain area until markers are found. At the present time, therefore, these syndromes of childhood cannot be included in the classification despite the generally accepted view that some presentations are indeed headache free "equivalents" of migraine.

1.5.1 Benign Paroxysmal Vertigo of Childhood

Description: This probably heterogeneous disorder is characterized by brief attacks of vertigo in otherwise healthy children.
Diagnostic criteria:

A. Multiple, brief, sporadic episodes of disequilibrium, anxiety, and often nystagmus or vomiting.
B. Normal neurological examination.
C. Normal electroencephalogram.

1.5.2 Alternating Hemiplegia of Childhood

Description: Infantile attacks of hemiplegia involving each side alternately. Is associated with other paroxysmal phenomena and mental impairment.
Diagnostic criteria:

A. Onset before 18 months of age.
B. Repeated attacks of hemiplegia involving both sides of the body.
C. Other paroxysmal phenomena, such as tonic spells, dystonic posturing, choreoathetoid movements, nystagmus or other ocular motor abnormalities, autonomic disturbances associated with the bouts of hemiplegia or occurring independently.
D. Evidence of mental or neurological deficits.

Comment: The nature of the disorder is not clear. A relationship with migraine is suggested on clinical grounds. The possibility that the disorder is an unusual form of epilepsy cannot be ruled out.

Benign recurrent vertigo in adults has been regarded as a migraine equivalent, but is not sufficiently validated.

1.6 Complications of Migraine (code for previous migraine type plus the complication)

1.6.1 Status Migrainosus

Description: Attack of migraine with headache phase lasting more than 72 hours despite treatment. Headache-free intervals of less than 4 hours (sleep not included) may occur.

Diagnostic criteria:

A. The patient fulfils criteria for 1.1 or 1.2.
B. The present attack fulfils criteria for one form of migraine except that headache lasts more than 72 hours whether treated or not.
C. Headache is continuous throughout the attack or interrupted by headache-free intervals lasting less than 4 hours. Interruption during sleep is disregarded.

Comment: Migraine with prolonged aura and headache lasting > 72 hours is coded 1.2.2, ophthalmoplegic migraine is coded 1.3. Status migrainosus is usually associated with prolonged drug use. See also group 8.

1.6.2 Migrainous Infarction

Previously used terms: Complicated migraine
Description: One or more migrainous aura symptoms not fully reversible within 7 days and/or associated with neuroimaging confirmation of ischemic infarction.
Diagnostic criteria:

A. Patient has previously fulfilled criteria for 1.2.
B. The present attack is typical of previous attacks, but neurological deficits are not completely reversible within 7 days and/or neuro-imaging demonstrates ischemic infarction in relevant area.
C. Other causes of infarction ruled out by appropriate investigations.

Comment: No causal relationship has been established between migraine without aura and cerebral infarction. Ischemic stroke in a migraine sufferer may be categorized as a) cerebral infarction of other cause coexisting with migraine, b) cerebral infarction of other cause presenting with symptoms resembling migraine or c) cerebral infarction occurring during the course of a typical migraine attack. Applying strict criteria, only category (c) should be coded as migrainous infarction. In so doing, it is recognized that patients with stereotyped migrainous aura may suffer, although rarely, cerebral infarction possibly due to migraine mechanisms during the course of migraine-like symptoms that are not typical for that patient. Nevertheless, because of uncertainty as to mechanism, cerebral infarction under those circumstances should be designated under category b. Increased risk for stroke in migraine patients has not been found in population-based studies, indicating that stroke is a rare complication of migraine.

1.7 Migrainous Disorder not Fulfilling Above Criteria

Description: Headache attacks which are believed to be a form of migraine, but which do not quite meet the operational diagnostic criteria for any of the forms of migraine.
Diagnostic criteria:

A. Fulfils all criteria but one for one or more forms of migraine (specify type(s)).
B. Does not fulfil criteria for tension-type headache.

Comment: Patients who do not have sufficient numbers of otherwise typical attacks to fulfil criteria should be coded here, as should patients with sufficient numbers of attacks which fulfil all criteria but one.

Cyclic migraine, lower-half headache, facial migraine, hemicrania continuat and cervical migraine are not sufficiently validated.

Coexisting Migraine and Tension-Type Headache—A Comment

Previously used terms: Mixed headache, tension-vascular headache, combination headache.

Migraine and tension-type headache often coexist in the same patient. Previously the diagnosis "combination headache" has been used, but it has never been defined. Patients represent a continuum varying from those having pure migraine over those with migraine and moderate amounts of tension-type headache, those with half of each, those with preponderance of tension-type headache to those with pure tension-type headache. The concept of combination headache is therefore arbitrary, and it has been judged impossible to single out a suitable group of patients who should receive this diagnosis. Patients should instead be coded for migraine and for tension-type headache if they have both forms. Since it is a general rule that number of headache days per year should be given in brackets after each diagnosis, the evaluation of the relative importance of the two conditions is easy.

If a patient has attacks/episodes each of which fulfil criteria for migraine without aura and for episodic tension-type headache, the general rule applies according to which the attacks should be coded as the type listed first in this classification, i.e. migraine without aura.

2. TENSION-TYPE HEADACHE

Previously used terms: Tension headache, muscle contraction headache, psychomyogenic headache, stress headache, ordinary headache, essential headache, idiopathic headache and psychogenic headache.

Comment: If tension-type headache occurs for the first time in close temporal relation to one of the disorders listed in groups 5–11 code to that group. If tension-type headache is aggravated by 100 per cent or more (headache days) in close temporal relation to one of the disorders listed in groups 5–11, it is still coded to group 2. The aggravating factor may be coded for using the fourth digit 9. At a given time a patient can only have one form of tension-type headache. Another type may have been present before. The subgrouping of tension-type headache into an episodic and a chronic form is introduced because patients with daily or almost daily headache constitute a large group in specialized practices and hospital clinics. Their treatment and perhaps also their pathogenic mechanisms vary to a considerable extent from the episodic form.

The subgrouping in forms with and without a muscular factor is a novel creation. For decades dispute has prevailed concerning the importance of muscle contraction mechanisms, but conclusive studies are still lacking. The classification committee believes that the diagnostic subdivision according to presence or absence of a muscular factor will stimulate research in this field. In view of the poor scientific basis for the subdivision, it should, however, be regarded as optional.

2.1 Episodic Tension-Type Headache

Previously used terms: See above.
Description: Recurrent episodes of headache lasting minutes to days. The pain is typically pressing/tightening in quality, of mild or moderate intensity, bilateral in location and does not worsen with routine physical activity. Nausea is absent, but photophobia or phonophobia may be present.
Diagnostic criteria:

A. At least 10 previous headache episodes fulfilling criteria B–D listed below. Number of days with such headaches < 180/year (< 15/month).
B. Headache lasting from 30 minutes to 7 days
C. At least 2 of the following pain characteristics:
    1. Pressing/tightening (non-pulsating) quality

2. Mild or moderate intensity (may inhibit, but does not prohibit activities)
3. Bilateral location
4. No aggravation by walking stairs or similar routine physical activity

D. Both of the following:
   1. No nausea or vomiting (anorexia may occur)
   2. Photophobia and phonophobia are absent, or one but not the other is present

E. At least one of the following:
   1. History and physical and neurological examinations do not suggest one of the disorders listed in groups 5–11
   2. History and/or physical and/or neurological examinations do suggest such disorder, but it is ruled out by appropriate investigations
   3. Such disorder is present, but tension-type headache does not occur for the first time in close temporal relation to the disorder

Comment: The exact mechanisms of tension-type headache are not known. Involuntary tightening in muscles induced mentally or physically is important as are purely psychogenic mechanisms.

2.1.1 Episodic Tension-Type Headache Associated with Disorder of Pericranial Muscles

Previously used terms: Muscle contraction headache.
Description: Episodic tension-type headache with increased levels of tenderness and/or EMG of pericranial muscles.
Diagnostic criteria:

A. Fulfils criteria for 2.1.
B. At least one of the following:
   1. Increased tenderness of pericranial muscles demonstrated by manual palpation or pressure algometer
   2. Increased EMG level of pericranial muscles at rest or during physiological tests

Comment: There is not yet sufficient evidence available regarding the limits of normality of pericranial muscle tenderness. Neither has sufficient attention been given to the methodology of pericranial palpation. Evidence concerning normal EMG levels of pericranial muscles is similarly deficient. Until evidence accumulates concerning tenderness on palpation and pericranial EMG, each investigator must judge as best he can on the basis of experience with non-headache sufferers and by comparing symmetrical sites. Estimation of tenderness by palpation is evidently subject to large bias. Reliable quantitation requires experience and systematic approach. Then, judgement of tenderness is no more subjective than other elements of the sensory neurological examination. For research purposes, blinding of the observer remains mandatory.

2.1.2 Episodic Tension-Type Headache Unassociated with Disorder of Pericranial Muscles

Previously used terms: Idiopathic headache, essential headache, psychogenic headache.
Description: Episodic tension-type headache with normal levels of tenderness and/or EMG of pericranial muscles.
Diagnostic criteria:

A. Fulfilling criteria for 2.1.
B. No increased tenderness of pericranial muscles. If studied, EMG of pericranial muscles shows normal levels of activity.

Comment: It is not known how often episodic tension-type headache is unassociated with pericranial muscle tenderness. That such cases exist is, on the other hand, well known. Mechanisms of headache are unknown in such cases, but psychogenic etiologies are suspected.

2.2 Chronic Tension-Type Headache

Previously used terms: Chronic daily headache. See also [beginning of Section 2].
Description: Headache present for at least 15 days a month during at least 6 months. The headache is usually pressing/tightening in quality, mild or moderate in severity, bilateral and does not worsen with routine physical activity. Nausea, photophobia or phonophobia may occur.
Diagnostic criteria:

A. Average headache frequency $\geq$ 15 days/month (180 days/year) for $\geq$ 6 months fulfilling criteria B–D listed below.
B. At least 2 of the following pain characteristics:
    1. Pressing/tightening quality
    2. Mild or moderate severity (may inhibit, but does not prohibit activities)
    3. Bilateral location
    4. No aggravation by walking stairs or similar routine physical activity
C. Both of the following:
    1. No vomiting

2. No more than one of the following:
   Nausea, photophobia or phonophobia
D. At least one of the following:
   1. History and physical and neurological examinations do not suggest one of the disorders listed in groups 5–11
   2. History and/or physical and/or neurological examinations do suggest such disorder, but it is ruled out by appropriate investigations
   3. Such disorder is present, but tension-type headache does not occur for the first time in close temporal relation to the disorder

Comment: Sometimes migraine is gradually transformed into chronic tension-type headache, but more frequently it is the episodic tension-type headache which becomes chronic. In both instances, overuse of drugs frequently plays a role in aggravating the disorder. Discontinuation of daily drug intake often results in improvement.

2.2.1 Chronic Tension-Type Headache Associated with Disorder of Pericranial Muscles

Previously used terms: Chronic muscle contraction headache.
Description: Chronic tension-type headache associated with increased levels of tenderness and/or EMG of pericranial muscles.
Diagnostic criteria:

A. Fulfils criteria for 2.2.
B. At least one of the following:
   1. Increased tenderness of pericranial muscles demonstrated by manual palpation or using pressure algometer
   2. Increased EMG level of pericranial muscles at rest or during physiological tests

2.2.2 Chronic Tension-Type Headache Unassociated with Disorder of Pericranial Muscles

Previously used terms: Chronic idiopathic headache, chronic psychogenic headache.
Description: Chronic tension-type headache with normal levels of tenderness and/or EMG of pericranial muscles.
Diagnostic criteria:

A. Fulfils criteria for 2.2.
B. No increased tenderness of pericranial muscles. If studied, EMG of pericranial muscles shows normal levels of activity.

2.3 Headache of the Tension-Type Not Fulfilling Above Criteria

Description: Headache which is believed to be a form of tension-type headache, but which does not quite meet the operational diagnostic criteria for any of the forms of tension-type headache.
Diagnostic criteria:

A. Fulfils all but one criterion for one or more forms of tension-type headache (specify type(s)).
B. Does not fulfil criteria for migraine without aura.

Comment: Coded to this number are cases who have had < 10 typical episodes of tension-type headache or with many episodes which fail one of the criteria. Also patients who are not chronic, but who have episodes lasting longer than 7 days or with headache for more than 15 days a month which has not yet lasted for 6 months.

Fourth digit code number for group 2 indicates most likely causative factor(s). If third digit has not been coded, a zero should be inserted prior to the fourth digit.

0. No identifiable causative factor
1. More than one of the factors 2–9 (list in order of importance)
2. Oromandibular dysfunction

Previously used terms: Myofacial pain-dysfunction syndrome, temporo-mandibular-joint pain dysfunction syndrome, Costen's syndrome, cranio-mandibular dysfunction.
Diagnostic criteria: Three or more of the following: temporo-mandibular-joint noise on jaw movements, limited or jerky jaw movements, pain on jaw function, locking of jaw on opening, clenching of teeth, gnashing of teeth (bruxism), other oral parafunction (tongue, lips or cheek biting or pressing).
Comment: Tenderness of pericranial muscles was part of the previously used syndromes. This is not logical and has not been used in this classification, since tenderness may be part of a generalized muscle hyperactivity or caused by other factors not related to the function of the mandible or the temporo-mandibular joint. It was therefore necessary to create the new term "oromandibular dysfunction."

3. Psychosocial stress (DSM-III-R criteria)

Diagnostic criteria: Associated with psychosocial stressors rated 4–6 on a 1–6 scale (1 no stress, 2 mild, 3 moderate, 4 severe, 5 extreme, 6 catastrophic).

Comment: In rating, pay attention to the amount of change in the individual's life caused by the stressor, the degree to which the change is desired and under the individual's control, and to the number of stressors. Stressors may be grouped as follows: conjugal (marital and non-marital), parenting, other interpersonal, occupational, living circumstances, financial, legal, developmental (for children), physical disorder or injury, other.

4. Anxiety—fulfilling DSM-III-R criteria for one of the anxiety disorders
5. Depression—fulfilling DSM-III-R criteria for one of the depressive disorders
6. Headache as a delusion or an idea

Previously used terms: Psychogenic headache, conversion cephalalgia.
Diagnostic criteria: Fulfilling DSM-III-R criteria for somatic delusion or somatoform disorder.
Comment: The previously used term psychogenic headache is now coded as 2.1.2.6 or 2.2.2.6 i.e. episodic- or chronic tension-type headache unassociated with a muscular factor but associated with somatic delusion or somatoform disorder.

7. Muscular stress—associated with at least one of the following types of muscular stress: Unphysiological working position, long-lasting tonic muscular contraction for other reasons, lack of rest and/or sleep
8. Drug overuse for tension-type headaches—associated with one or more of the following:
   Monthly weak analgesics exceeding 45 g of aspirin or equivalent
   Morphinomimetic drugs more than twice a month
   Monthly diazepam exceeding 300 mg or equivalent of other benzo-diazepines
9. One of the disorders listed in groups 5–11 of this classification (specify). Use the fourth digit code only when preexisting tension-type headache is aggravated by 100 per cent or more (headache days) in close temporal relation to the organic disorder. If headache occurs for the first time in close temporal relation to the organic disorder, code to group 5–11

3. CLUSTER HEADACHE AND CHRONIC PAROXYSMAL HEMICRANIA

Comment: If cluster headache or chronic paroxysmal hemicrania occur for the first time in close temporal relation to one of the disorders listed in groups 5–11, code to that group. If cluster headache or chronic paroxysmal hemicrania are aggravated by 100 per cent or more (headache days) in close temporal relation to one of the disorders listed in groups 5–11, this may be mentioned in parentheses, but the patient is still coded to group 3. At a given time a patient can only have one type of cluster headache. Another type may have been present before.

Cluster headache and chronic paroxysmal hemicrania share the following characteristics: 1) the unilaterality of the pain, 2) the severe intensity of the pain, 3) the location of the pain, 4) the accompanying autonomic phenomena, 5) the temporal pattern of the attacks. Similarities also exist with regard to the course of the diseases (episodic or chronic pattern/stage) and other changes indicating autonomic involvement. A number of features, however, distinguish between the two: sex preponderance, frequency and duration of attacks, night preponderance, drug effects (both symptomatic and prophylactic).

So-called cluster variants and combined forms are not included in the present classification as they are considered not to be sufficiently validated.

Cluster-like headaches have occasionally been reported in patients presenting with evidence of cephalic (intra or extracranial) lesions of vascular or neoplastic type. The relationship of these lesions to the pathogenesis of cluster headache is at present not clear.

3.1 Cluster Headache

Previously used terms: Erythroprosopalgia of Bing, ciliary or migrainous neuralgia (Harris), erythromelalgia of the head, Horton's headache, histaminic cephalalgia, petrosal neuralgia (Gardner), sphenopalatine, Vidian and Sluder's neuralgia, hemicrania periodica neuralgiformis.

Description: Attacks of severe strictly unilateral pain orbitally, supraorbitally and/or temporally, lasting 15–180 minutes and occurring from once every other day to 8 times a day. Are associated with one or more of the following: conjunctival injection, lacrimation, nasal congestion, rhinorrhea, forehead and facial sweating, miosis, ptosis, eyelid edema. Attacks occur in series lasting for weeks or months (so-called cluster periods) separated by remission periods usually lasting months or years. About 10 per cent of the patients have chronic symptoms.

Diagnostic criteria:

A. At least 5 attacks fulfilling B–D.

B. Severe unilateral orbital, supraorbital and/or temporal pain lasting 15 to 180 minutes untreated.

C. Headache is associated with at least one of the following signs which have to be present on the pain side:
   1. Conjunctival injection

2. Lacrimation
3. Nasal congestion
4. Rhinorrhea
5. Forehead and facial sweating
6. Miosis
7. Ptosis
8. Eyelid edema

D. Frequency of attacks: from 1 every other day to 8 per day.
E. At least one of the following:
1. History and physical and neurological examinations do not suggest one of the disorders listed in groups 5–11
2. History and/or physical and/or neurological examinations do suggest such disorder, but it is ruled out by appropriate investigations
3. Such disorder is present, but cluster headache does not occur for the first time in close temporal relation to the disorder

3.1.1 Cluster Headache Periodicity Undetermined

Diagnostic criteria:

A. Criteria for 3.1 fulfilled
B. Too early to classify as 3.1.2 or 3.1.3

3.1.2 Episodic Cluster Headache

Description: Occurs in periods lasting 7 days to one year separated by pain-free periods lasting 14 days or more
Diagnostic criteria:

A. All the letter headings of 3.1.
B. At least 2 periods of headaches (cluster periods) lasting (untreated patients) from 7 days to one year, separated by remissions of at least 14 days.

Comment: Cluster periods usually last between 2 weeks and 3 months.

3.1.3 Chronic Cluster Headache

Description: Attacks occur for more than one year without remission or with remissions lasting less than 14 days.
Diagnostic criteria:

A. All letter headings of 3.1.
B. Absence of remission phases for one year or more or with remissions lasting less than 14 days.

3.1.3.1   *Chronic Cluster Headache Unremitting from Onset*
Previously used term: Primary chronic.
Diagnostic criteria:

A. All letter headings of 3.1.3.
B. Absence of remission periods lasting 14 days or more from onset.

3.1.3.2   *Chronic Cluster Headache Evolved from Episodic*
Previously used terms: Secondary chronic.
Diagnostic criteria:

A. All letter headings of 3.1.3.
B. At least one interim remission period lasting 14 days or more within one year after onset, followed by unremitting course for at least one year.

Comment: During a cluster period and in patients with the chronic form, attacks occur regularly and may be provoked by alcohol, histamine or nitroglycerine. Pain is maximal orbitally, supraorbitally and/or temporally, but may spread to other regions. Pain usually recurs on the same side of the head during an individual cluster period. During the worst attacks, the intensity of pain is excruciating. Patients are unable to lie down and typically pace the floor. Age at onset is typically 20–40 years. For unknown reasons men are afflicted 5–6 times more often than women. The mechanisms of the pain are incompletely known despite abnormalities demonstrated by studies of corneal indentation pulse, corneal temperature, forehead sweating, lacrimation and nasal secretion, or by pupillometry, thermovision, or extracranial and transcranial Doppler.

3.2   Chronic Paroxysmal Hemicrania

Previously used terms: Sjaastad's syndrome.
Description: Attacks with largely the same characteristics of pain and associated symptoms and signs as cluster headache, but they are shorter-lasting, more frequent, occur mostly in females, and there is absolute effectiveness of indomethacin.
Diagnostic criteria:

A. At least 50 attacks fulfilling B–E.
B. Attacks of severe unilateral orbital, supraorbital and/or temporal pain, always on the same side, lasting 2 to 45 minutes.
C. Attack frequency above 5 a day for more than half of the time (periods with lower frequency may occur).
D. Pain is associated with at least some of the following signs/symptoms on the pain side:
    1. Conjunctival injection

2. Lacrimation
3. Nasal congestion
4. Rhinorrhea
5. Ptosis
6. Eyelid edema

E. Absolute effectiveness of indomethacin (150 mg/day or less).
F. At least one of the following:
  1. History and physical and neurological examinations do not suggest one of the disorders listed in groups 5–11
  2. History and/or physical and/or neurological examinations do suggest such disorder, but it is ruled out by appropriate investigations
  3. Such disorder is present, but chronic paroxysmal hemicrania does not occur for the first time in close temporal relation to the disorder

Comment: Most attacks last 5–20 minutes and frequency may be as high as 30 per 24 hours. Although longer-lasting remissions are not seen in chronic paroxysmal hemicrania, frequency, duration and severity of the attacks may vary. Nausea and vomiting rarely accompany the attacks. There is great female predominance. Onset is usually in adulthood. The chronic stage may probably be preceded by an episodic stage similar to the pattern seen in cluster headache, but this has not yet been sufficiently validated.

3.3 Cluster Headache-Like Disorder Not Fulfilling Above Criteria

Description: Headache attacks which are believed to be a form of cluster headache or chronic paroxysmal hemicrania, but which do not quite meet the operational diagnostic criteria for any of the forms of cluster headache or chronic paroxysmal hemicrania.
Diagnostic criteria:

A. Fulfilling all but one of the criteria for 3.1 or 3.2.

Comment: Coded to this number are patients who do not have sufficient numbers of otherwise typical attacks as well as patients who do have enough attacks which, however, fail to fulfil one of the other criteria.

  Cluster migraine and cluster tic syndromes are not sufficiently validated.

4. MISCELLANEOUS HEADACHES UNASSOCIATED WITH STRUCTURAL LESION

4.1 Idiopathic Stabbing Headache

Previously used term: Ice-pick pains.

Description: Transient stabs of pain in the head that occur spontaneously in the absence of organic disease of underlying structures or of the cranial nerves.
Diagnostic criteria:

A. Pain confined to the head and exclusively or predominantly felt in the distribution of the first division of the trigeminal nerve (orbit, temple and parietal area).
B. Pain is stabbing in nature and lasts for a fraction of a second. Occurs as single stabs or series of stabs.
C. It recurs at irregular intervals (hours to days).
D. Diagnosis depends upon the exclusion of structural changes at the site of pain and in the distribution of the affected cranial nerve.

Comments: Stabbing pains are more commonly experienced by people subject to migraine headache, in which case they are felt in the site habitually affected by headache in about 40 per cent of patients and tend to be more frequent at the time of headache. They commonly subside with the administration of indomethacin 25 mg orally three times daily.

4.2   External Compression Headache

Previously used term: Swim-goggle headache.
Description: Headache resulting from continued stimulation of cutaneous nerves by the application of pressure, for example by a band around the head, a tight hat or goggles worn for the protection of eyes during swim-ming training.
Diagnostic criteria:

A. Results from the application of external pressure in the forehead or the scalp.
B. Is felt in the area subjected to pressure.
C. Is a constant pain.
D. Is prevented by avoiding the precipitating cause.
E. Is not associated with organic cranial or intracranial disease.

Comment: External compression may lead to a more severe migrainous headache if the stimulus is prolonged.

4.3   Cold Stimulus Headache

Description: Headache resulting from the exposure of the head to low temperatures.

4.3.1   External Application of a Cold Stimulus

Description: Generalized headache following exposure of the unprotected head to a low environmental temperature as in sub-zero weather or in diving into cold water.
Diagnostic criteria:

A.   Develops during external exposure to cold.
B.   Is bilateral.
C.   Varies in intensity with the severity and duration of the cold stimulus.
D.   Is prevented by avoiding exposure to cold.
E.   Is not associated with organic cranial or intracranial disease.

4.3.2   Ingestion of a Cold Stimulus

Previously used term: Ice-cream headache.
Description: Ice-cream headache is a pain produced in susceptible individuals by the passage of cold material, solid or liquid, over the palate and posterior pharyngeal wall.
Diagnostic criteria:

A.   Develops during ingestion of a cold food or drink.
B.   Lasts for less than five minutes.
C.   Is felt in the middle of the forehead, except in people subject to migraine, in which case the pain may be referred to the area habitually affected by migraine headache (code migraine first).
D.   Is prevented by avoiding the rapid swallowing of cold food or drinks.
E.   Is not associated with organic disease.

4.4   Benign Cough Headache

Description: Headache precipitated by coughing in the absence of any intracranial disorder.
Diagnostic criteria:

A.   Is a bilateral headache of sudden onset, lasting less than one minute, precipitated by coughing.
B.   May be prevented by avoiding coughing.
C.   May be diagnosed only after structural lesions such as posterior fossa tumour have been excluded by neuroimaging.

4.5   Benign Exertional Headache

Description: Headache precipitated by any form of exercise. Subvarieties, such as "weight-lifters headache," are recognised.

Diagnostic criteria:

A. Is specifically brought on by physical exercise.
B. Is bilateral, throbbing in nature at onset and may develop migrainous features in those patients susceptible to migraine (code for migraine first).
C. Lasts from 5 minutes to 24 hours.
D. Is prevented by avoiding excessive exertion, particularly in hot weather or at high altitude.
E. Is not associated with any systemic or intracranial disorder.

Comment: Exertional headache is prevented in some patients by the ingestion of ergotamine tartrate, methysergide, propranolol or indomethacin before exercise.

4.6 Headache Associated with Sexual Activity

Previously used terms: Benign sex headache, coital cephalalgia.
Description: Headache precipitated by masturbation or coitus, usually starting as a dull bilateral ache while sexual excitement increases and suddenly becoming intense at orgasm, in the absence of any intracranial disorder.
Diagnostic criteria:

A. Is precipitated by sexual excitement.
B. Is bilateral at onset.
C. Is prevented or eased by ceasing sexual activity before orgasm.
D. Is not associated with any intracranial disorder such as aneurysm.

4.6.1 Dull Type

Diagnostic criteria: A dull ache in the head and neck that intensifies as sexual excitement increases.

4.6.2 Explosive Type

Diagnostic criteria: A sudden severe ("explosive") headache occurring at orgasm.

4.6.3 Postural Type

Diagnostic criteria: Postural headache resembling that of low CSF pressure developing after coitus.

FOURTH DIGIT CODE NUMBER FOR GROUPS 5–11:
TYPES OF HEADACHE

Comment: Included are as many forms of headache as can be distinguished using only headache characteristics and operational criteria. Most forms are also found elsewhere in this classification.

0. Headache is as described in the diagnostic criteria for the particular disorder.

   Comment: For some disorders in groups 5–11, headache characteristics are not part of the diagnostic criteria, for some they are. Fourth digit 0 applies only to the latter.

1. Migraine—fulfilling criteria for 1.1 or 1.2 with the exception that migraine occurs for the first time in close temporal relation to one of the disorders listed in groups 5–11.

2. Tension-type headache—fulfilling criteria for 2.1 or 2.2 with the exception that tension-type headache occurs for the first time in close temporal relation to one of the disorders listed in groups 5–11.

3. Cluster headache—fulfilling criteria for 3.1 or 3.2 with the exception that cluster headache or chronic paroxysmal hemicrania occur for the first time in close temporal relation to one of the disorders listed in groups 5–11.

4. Increased intracranial pressure type (prototype: brain tumour headache).
   A. Crescendo time profile over 3 months or less
   B. Moderate or severe intensity of pain
   C. Occurs in the morning or after napping and remits or improves spontaneously after getting up
   D. Is present at least 50 per cent of all mornings

5. Decreased intracranial pressure type (prototype: post-lumbar puncture headache)
   A. Bilateral
   B. Absent or mild in the recumbent position, occurs or worsens markedly in the upright position

6. Local lesion type (prototype: pain from bone metastasis)
   A. Headache is non-pulsating and constantly present
   B. Pain has a distinct maximum in a circumscribed area of 5 cm or less, but may irradiate to surroundings or refer to more distant areas

7. Vasodilator type (prototype: nitroglycerin-, histamine- and prostacyclin-induced headache)
   A. Bifronto-temporal pulsating pain

    B. No aura, nausea or vomiting
- 8. Stabbing type (ice-pick type)
  - A. Stabbing head pains lasting less than a second
  - B. Occur as single stabs or series of stabs
  - C. Each stab or series of stabs occur in a small, sharply localized area.
- 9. Other type (specify)
- 10. Two or more types (specify)

5. HEADACHE ASSOCIATED WITH HEAD TRAUMA

Comment: Worsening of preexisting headache is coded according to preexisting headache form. Patients who develop a new form of headache (including migraine, tension-type headache or cluster headache) in close temporal relation (specified below) to a head trauma are coded to group 5. Type of headache may be specified with the fourth digit [see "Fourth Digit Code Number for Groups 5–11" above]. Traumatic intracranial hematoma is coded to group 6, posttraumatic hydrocephalus to group 7.

    A causal relation between head trauma and headache is frequent with 5.1.1, 5.1.2 and 5.2.1 and infrequent with 5.2.2. There remains, however, a group of patients especially with acceleration/deceleration injury who do not meet criterion 5.2.1 A, but who display an abrupt decline in work performance and/or social functioning or change in personality following head trauma which indicates a possible causal relationship between headache, these symptoms and trauma. Chronic post-traumatic headache (5.2.1 and 5.2.2) is often part of the post-traumatic syndrome. The complex inter-relationship between organic and psychosocial factors in these syndromes is difficult to assess.

5.1 Acute Post-Traumatic Headache

5.1.1 With Significant Head Trauma and/or Confirmatory Signs

Diagnostic criteria:

- A. Significance of head trauma documented by at least one of the following:
  1. Loss of consciousness
  2. Post-traumatic amnesia lasting more than 10 minutes
  3. At least two of the following exhibit relevant abnormality: clinical neurological examination, X-ray of skull, neuroimaging, evoked potentials, spinal fluid examination, vestibular function test, neuropsychological testing

B. Headache occurs less than 14 days after regaining consciousness (or after trauma, if there has been no loss of consciousness)
C. Headache disappears within 8 weeks after regaining consciousness (or after trauma, if there has been no loss of consciousness)

5.1.2 With Minor Head Trauma and No Confirmatory Signs

Diagnostic criteria:

A. Head trauma that does not satisfy 5.1.1 A.
B. Headache occurs less than 14 days after injury.
C. Headache disappears within 8 weeks after injury.

5.2 Chronic Post-Traumatic Headache

5.2.1 With Significant Head Trauma and/or Confirmatory Signs

Diagnostic criteria:

A. Significance of head trauma documented by at least one of the following:
   1. Loss of consciousness
   2. Post-traumatic amnesia lasting more than 10 minutes
   3. At least two of the following exhibit relevant abnormality: clinical neurological examination, X-ray of skull, neuroimaging, evoked potentials, spinal fluid examination, vestibular function test, neuro-psychological testing
B. Headache occurs less than 14 days after regaining consciousness (or after trauma, if there has been no loss of consciousness).
C. Headache continues more than 8 weeks after regaining consciousness (or after trauma, if there has been no loss of consciousness).

5.2.2 With Minor Head Trauma and No Confirmatory Signs

Diagnostic criteria:

A. Head trauma that does not satisfy 5.2.1 A
B. Headache occurs less than 14 days after injury.
C. Headache continues more than 8 weeks after injury.

Index

About the Editors

ROGER K. CADY is Medical Director of the Shealy Institute for Comprehensive Health Care, Springfield, Missouri. The author or coauthor of numerous professional papers, Dr. Cady is a member of the American Medical Association, the American Association for the Study of Headache, the American Academy of Family Physicians, the American Academy of Pain Medicine, the National Headache Foundation, and the American Academy of Pain Management, among others. He received the B.A. degree (1972) in biology from Drake University, Des Moines, Iowa, and the M.D. degree (1977) from the Mayo Medical School, Rochester, Minnesota.

ANTHONY W. FOX is Vice-President of Drug Development at Cypros Pharmaceutical Corporation, Carlsbad, California. Dr. Fox is the author or coauthor of numerous papers on topics such as drug-receptor theory, vascular smooth-muscle receptors and corresponding second messengers, and malignant hyperthermia. A member of the Faculty of Pharmaceutical Medicine of the Royal College of Physicians, he received the B.Sc. degree (1977) in pharmacology, the M.B.B.S. degree (1980) and the M.D. degree (1988) from the University of London, and the Diploma in Pharmaceutical Medicine (1989) from the Royal College of Physicians, United Kingdom.